ENVIRONMENTAL HEALTH – EMERGING ISSUES AND PRACTICE

Edited by **Jacques Oosthuizen**

Environmental Health – Emerging Issues and Practice
Edited by Jacques Oosthuizen

Published by InTech
Janeza Trdine 9, 51000 Rijeka, Croatia

Publishing Process Manager Adriana Pecar

Technical Editor Teodora Smiljanic

Cover Designer InTech Design Team

Additional hard copies can be obtained from orders@intechopen.com

Environmental Health – Emerging Issues and Practice, Edited by Jacques Oosthuizen
p. cm.
978-953-307-854-0

For EU product safety concerns:
IN TECH d.o.o., Prolaz Marije Krucifikse Kozulić 3, 51000 Rijeka, Croatia,
info@intechopen.com or visit our website at intechopen.com.

Meet the editor

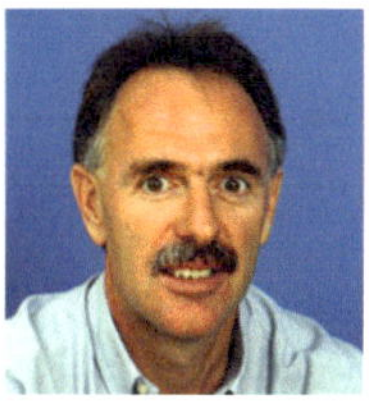

Associate Professor Jacques Oosthuizen received his Bachelor's degree, MMed Sci and PhD in Environmental Health. Dr Oosthuizen is the Director of the Occupational Health Research Group at Edith Cowan University, Perth, Australia. He coordinates the undergraduate Environmental Health and the Post Graduate Occupational Hygiene Program. Dr Oosthuizen is a certified occupational hygienist, registered with the Australian Institute of Occupational Hygienists and he is a member of Environmental Health Australia and the Safety Institute of Australia. He is responsible for the development of a number of successful courses, consulting with the industry. He has also worked closely with the industry providing consultancy and performing contract research in various areas of health, safety and occupational hygiene (exposure assessment). Dr Oosthuizen has supervised numerous Master and PhD students and has a strong track record in applied occupational health research as evidenced by his conference proceedings, journal publications, book chapters and prior as well as current industry collaborative research grants.

Contents

Preface

This book contains chapters that cover a diverse range of topics in contemporary environmental health practice. What makes this book unique is the emphasis on emerging research and translation of research into practice. Furthermore, the chapters cover issues from a range of different countries and contexts in both the developed and the developing world, thus providing an insight into the complexity of issues that face environmental health researchers and practitioners globally.

The chapters have been arranged according to topic into six broad sections that cover the state-of-the-art in current literature and introduce new and emerging methods. Some topics in the book include water, air, food, new technologies, health impacts and environmental justice.

Dr. Jacques Oosthuizen
School of Exercise, Biomedical & Health Sciences,
Edith Cowan University,
Australia

Part 1

Water Quality

1

When is Short Sea Shipping Environmentally Competitive?

Harald M. Hjelle[1] and Erik Fridell[2]
[1]*Molde University College – Specialized University in Logistics and Northern Maritime University,*
[2]*IVL Swedish Environmental Research Institute and Northern Maritime University,*
[1]*Norway*
[2]*Sweden*

1. Introduction

Maritime transport is broadly accepted as an environmentally friendly mode of transport in terms of CO_2 emissions, and is also receiving government support for promotion and development, often based on presumed performance along environmental dimensions.

There is really no debate about the superior comparative efficiency of ships with respect to fuel consumption when calculated per deadweight tonne along routes of similar length. However, the emission figures calculated per deadweight tonne is only relevant for bulk transports, and fuel consumption per cargo tonne is quite different for typical short sea shipping services based on container or RoRo technologies. Further, other emissions to air, like sulphur dioxide, nitrogen oxides and particles, are typically very high for shipping - especially when no abatement technologies are applied.

The case for short sea shipping as an environmentally-friendly mode of transport is no longer self-evident under realistic assumptions, and needs deeper analysis.

The main competitors of such shipping services are rail and road transport. Considering realistic load factors - could the environmental friendly case for maritime transport still be made? This paper is based on the latest data for comparative environmental performance and presents a set of realistic European multimodal transport chains, and their environmental outputs, focusing on fuel consumption and CO_2 emissions. Through this comparative analysis we differentiate the common comprehension of shipping being the indisputable green mode of cargo transport, and analyze necessary actions that need to be taken for short sea shipping to maintain its green label. Finally, perspectives on both regulatory regime and technology are analysed.

2. When is short sea shipping environmentally competitive?

2.1 The competition between short sea shipping and land-based modes

Short sea shipping (SSS) plays an important role in the market for regional freight transport in many areas of the world. It's relative importance compared to alternative land-based modes is, however, quite different in different regions. Whereas SSS along with inland waterways represents 40% of the intra EU27 transports and more than 60% of the total tonnekilometres in China, the equivalent market-share in the US and Russia is much smaller (Figure 1). To some extent such differences in market shares could be explained by geographical characteristics like the length of the coast-line compared to land area and population, or by the characteristics of natural inland waterways and coastal waters. Such factors may be a natural explanation for the low market share of SSS in Russia - and the equivalently high market-shares in Japan and China. However, it is harder to see how such factors could explain the very different market-shares of EU27 versus the USA. Both have a long coastline and some natural inland waterways. Differences in policy-regimes and the quality of alternative land-based infrastructure are factors that might explain the higher market-share of SSS in Europe compared to the USA.

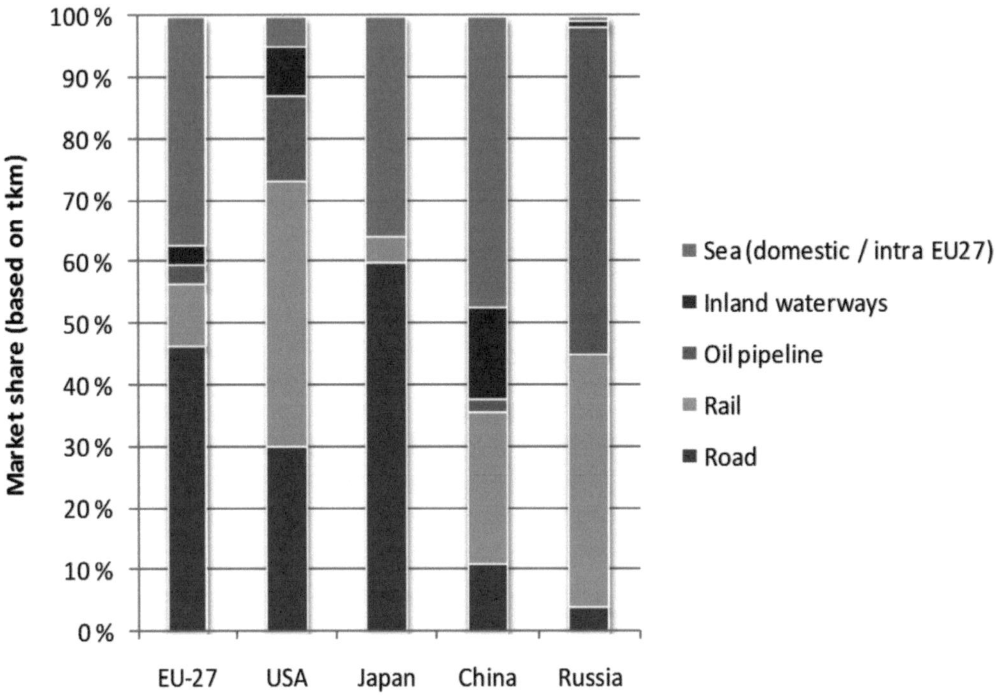

Fig. 1. Short sea shipping market-shares in 2006
Compilation: Eurostat 2009

From the mid 1990s to 2003 short sea shipping in Europe largely kept up with the growth rates of road transport (Figure 3), but in the years from 2003 to 2006 there has been a significantly lower growth in SSS relative to road transport (Figure 2). The average annual growth rates for road transport in EU27 from 1995 to 2006 was 3.5%, whereas the equivalent figure for SSS was 2.7%.

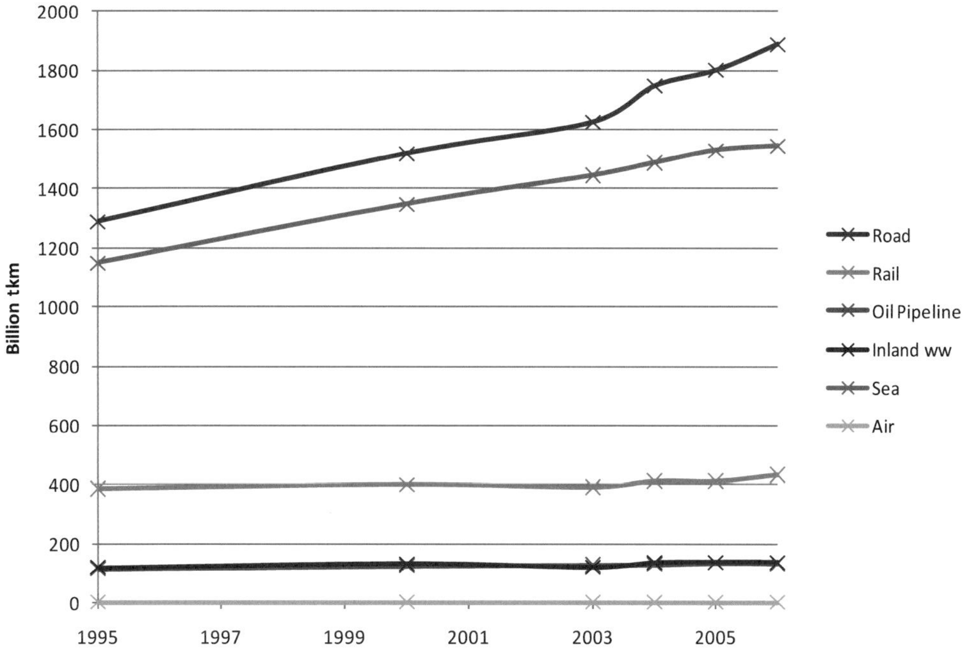

Fig. 2. Freight transport activity in EU27, billion tonne-kilometres
Source: DG Energy and Transport

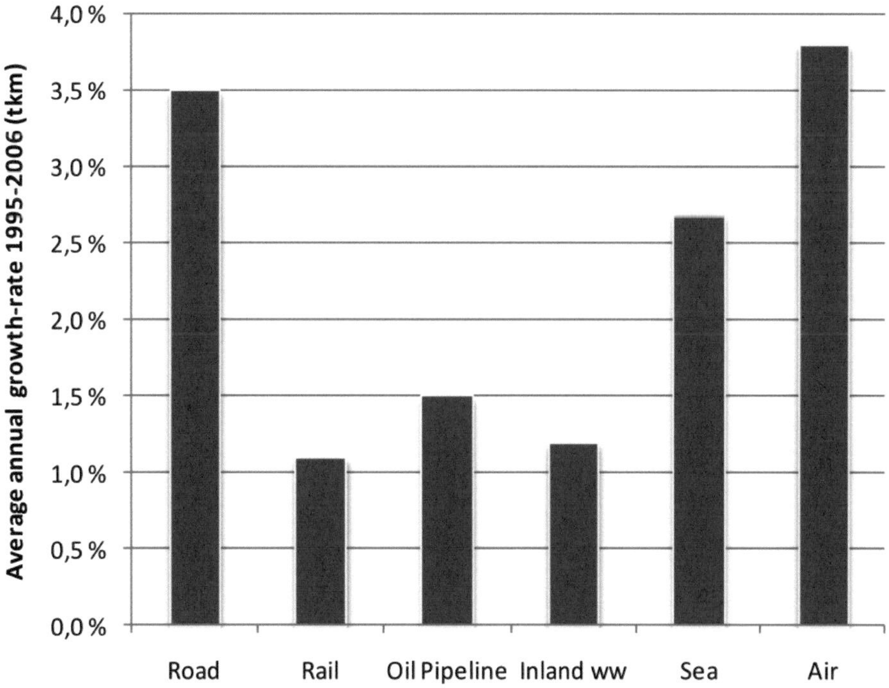

Fig. 3. Average annual growth rates of transport modes in EU27
Figures from Eurostat 2009

2.2 Short sea shipping as an instrument for greening freight transport

Since the 1970s European national and EU transport policy papers have had a relatively high focus on moving cargo from road to sea, inland waterways and rail. Partly the rationale for such a policy has been based on the environmental performance of SSS compared to road transport. In general shipping has been regarded "the green mode" of freight transport - often substantiated by empirical data on average energy use per tonne-kilometre and corresponding emission figures. Sometimes such figures have been based on energy use per deadweight tonne, calculated for big wet or dry bulk vessels. Such figures would typically show that shipping is 10-20 times more energy efficient than relevant road transport alternatives (IMO 2009) calculated per tonne-kilometre. This is why land-based modes like road and rail transport normally would not be competitive to maritime transport when it comes to the transport of commodities like iron ore or oil and chemicals, unless the sea leg is significantly longer than the land leg.

The relevant competition for the SSS industry is therefore not so much in the bulk markets, but in the markets for loose and unitized cargo (containers, trailers, pallets). The relevant vessels for such transports are general cargo vessels, container or RoRo vessels, partly in the business of feeding cargo to and from the deep sea, intercontinental, routes and partly transporting cargo within the continent. The environmental performance of these vessels is very different from the bulk vessels, mainly for three reasons. *Firstly,* the payload capacity relative to the size of the vessel is significantly lower than that of bulk vessels. *Secondly,* these vessels are typically designed for, and operated at, significantly higher operating speeds compared to the bulk vessels, and *thirdly* these vessels are operating in liner operations where average shipment sizes are much smaller than in the bulk market, necessitating a demanding consolidation activity in order to fill the available cargo capacity of the vessels. The latter factor normally means that the average load factor of such vessels may be lower than that of the bulk vessels. However, the scope for attracting back-haul cargoes - thus avoiding return trips in ballast - is definitely better for the general cargo, container and RoRo vessels than that of the bulk ships. This may mean that the average roundtrip cargo utilization does not have to be lower compared to bulk operations - which very often are operated with empty back-hauls.

For the RoRo and container industry there is an additional fourth factor - which may be called "the double load factor problem" of these modes (Hjelle 2010). The fact that containers and trailers transported are not always carrying cargo - and may be only partly filled - effectively means that the relevant load factor of such vessels is a multiple of two load factors. The number of containers / trailers compared to the container / trailer capacity - *and* the typical cargo load factor of containers and trailers. Statistics showing a 70% load factor of RoRo vessels often mean that on average 7 out of 10 available lanemetres are occupied by trucks and trailers. If these trailers have a load factor of 60%, then the relevant load factor of the RoRo vessel is not 70%, but 42%.

All of these factors (with the potential exclusion of the third one) contribute to a significantly lower fuel efficiency for relevant SSS vessels than for bulk vessels.

The level of CO_2 emissions will follow the fuel efficiency, but emissions of particles, SO_2 and NO_X are very different for trucks and ships. Under current regulations the shipping industry is allowed to use fuels with much higher sulphur content than the trucking industry in Europe. The legal emissions of NO_X and particles are also much higher for shipping than for trucks. This could be attributed to the very different policy regimes for these alternative modes of transport.

2.3 The regulatory regime of shipping vs. land-based transport modes

The global nature of the shipping industry makes it harder to regulate than the trucking business. Regulation must be imposed on a supranational scale to be efficient. This is also true to some extent for road transport, but the degree of national control is much higher on the road networks than for international waters. In Europe this means that the environmental performance of trucks has been improved significantly over the past decades through a series of emission standards gradually reducing emissions of CO, NO, HC and particles (Figure 4). From 2013 the Euro 6 limits will apply with further cuts in NO_X, HC and PM emissions. Sulphur emission levels have also been significantly reduced through stricter regulations of the sulphur content of diesel oil. The reductions in fuel use and CO_2 emissions have not been as substantial.

Trains can use either diesel or electricity. In the former case the situation is similar to that of trucks, although the specific emissions of NO_X and PM (per work of the engine) are somewhat higher for a modern train engine compared to a truck. From 2012 the emission limits in the EU will be similar to that of a Euro 5 truck. There are no direct emissions from an electric engine. However, for a fair comparison with other modes of transport one should consider the emissions that arise from electricity production. For CO_2 this means that the emissions vary significantly with the actual source of the electricity - from negligible for hydropower to relatively large for coal-power.

International shipping has not been subjected to similar regulations over the same period of time, but emissions to air was introduced to the global regulatory regime through the Annex VI of the IMO Marpol convention in 2007. Emissions of CO_2 from international shipping were exempted from the Kyoto protocol due to the complexity of allocating emission to the individual partner states. Lately, the Marpol Annex VI regulations have become stricter, especially in the so-called Environmental Control Areas (ECAs). These areas can be for either SO_2 (SECAs), NO_X (NO_X-ECAs) or both. Currently The Baltic Sea, The North Sea and The English Channel are SECAs and the North American coasts will be both SECAs and NO_X-ECAs in 2012. The sulphur content in the fuel is currently (2011) limited to 3.5% worldwide and to 1.0% in SECAs. The sulphur restrictions will be further tightened to 0.5% worldwide from 2020 and in SECAs to 0.1% from 2015. The regulation for NO_X is also gradually tightened, although through another regulatory instrument, - the NO_X-code, applying to marine engines. Engines delivered at present must comply with Tier 1 regulations. From 2012 Tier 2 regulations, giving a cut of about 20%, will apply. In NO_X-ECAs Tier 3 regulations apply from 2016, representing a cut in NO_X emissions of about 80% compared with Tier 1. The allowed emission for a slow-speed engine will then be 3.4 g/kWh. No specific regulations for particle emissions are implemented for marine engines.

Vessels have become more fuel efficient over the past decades, but the most significant advances were made in the late 1970s and the 1980s, triggered by significant increases in bunker prices. Some national regulations have been imposed, e.g. an environmentally differentiated fairway due system in Sweden and a NO_X tax in Norway. The European

Commission currently considers implementing emissions from the shipping industry into its cap and trade system of CO_2 emissions.

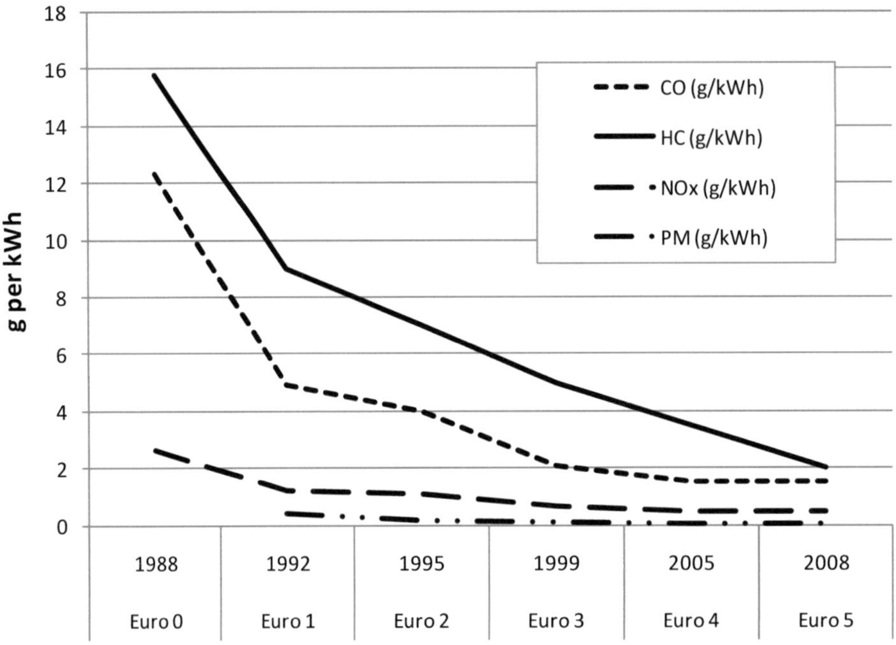

Fig. 4. Truck engine emission standards in Europe
Source: EC DG Energy & Transport

The international regulatory regime of maritime transport is moving quite slowly due to the demanding process of reaching the necessary consensus among nations. Adding to this sluggishness of new regulations is the fact that the penetration lead time of technological advances is much longer for ships than for trucks. The average age of a typical short sea vessel trading in European waters is probably around 15 years (Hjelle 2010), whereas a typical long distance truck in Western Europe has an average age of 4 years. This means that the Euro 5 standard, and in a few years Euro 6, will shortly be representative of the fleet of long distance trucks.

3. The environmental performance of vessels, trucks and trains

In order to compare different alternatives for transporting goods one needs to obtain emission factors expressed as mass of emitted substance per transported amount of goods and distance (functional unit), i.e. an emission factor with units like g/tonne-km. This requires knowledge of emissions per km for the specific vehicle/vessel and the mass of the cargo transported. The latter is often expressed as the maximum possible load multiplied with a load factor.

In this paper we compare the emissions of carbon dioxide (CO_2), sulphur dioxide (SO_2), nitrogen oxide (NO_X) and particulate matter (PM) for different transport alternatives. CO_2 emissions are directly obtained from the fuel consumption. The emitted SO_2 is formed from sulphur present in the fuel and can easily be obtained if the sulphur content in the fuel and the fuel consumption is known. Nitrogen oxides are formed in the engine and the emissions will depend on the type of engine and on the presence of NO_X after-treatment systems. PM comprises a number of different types of particles and the emissions will depend on engine type, fuel quality and after-treatment system.

3.1 Empirical evidence on fuel consumption and emissions for short sea vessels

For shipping the tabulated emission factors are usually in the form of mass of emission per energy for propulsion from a specific engine. These are normally divided into slow speed, medium speed and high speed engines. Further, the emission factors depend on the type of fuel used; residual oil or gasoil and sulphur content (Cooper and Gustafsson 2004). The emission from a specific vessel thus depends on the engine power and fuel type. In reality the emissions per transported amount of goods and distance will vary significantly depending on the type of ship (tanker, container, general cargo, RoRo etc) and the ships' size. The emissions factor for CO_2, for a ship that carries cargo up to its payload, can vary from 1.2 g/tonne-km for a large tanker, to 250 g/tonne-km for a small RoRo ship. Once the emission factor for CO_2 is established, emission factors for other substances can be obtained through the relationship with fuel consumption. However, the emissions of NO_X, PM and HC may vary significantly from engine to engine depending on model and maintenance level.

Within the Greenhouse gas working groupof the IMO, a design index for CO_2 emissions are being developed for different types of ships (IMO 2009). These are expressed as functions of the deadweight tonnage (dwt) for emissions in g/tonne-nm, and are based on data from a large number of ships. In order to get emission factors for the transported cargo, the relationship between dwt and payload needs to be known as well as typical load factors. The former relationship has been presented in the Clean Ship index (The Clean Shipping Project).

In the calculations presented below we have used the specific emission factors presented by Cooper and Gustafsson (2004) as implemented in the model documented in NTM Working Group Goods and Logistics (2008) and NTM (2009). These are obtained from a large number of measurements and correspond well with other reports (see, e.g Whall et al.(2002)). The emission factors for SO_2 and PM are adjusted for the sulphur content in the fuel both inside and outside the SECA regions. However, to get the emissions from a specific ship the power used needs to be known. Here we have used the CO_2 indexes from IMO and then calculated the corresponding emissions for NO_X, PM and SO_2. The relationship between dwt and payload used (The Clean Shipping Project) are 0.95 for tanker, 0.8 for container ship and 0.5 for RoRo ships.

3.2 Empirical evidence on fuel consumption and emissions for road transport

The emissions from trucks for the transport of a specific cargo will depend on the size of the truck, the emission classification, the fuel used, driving conditions and the load factor. The emissions of NO_X and PM decrease significantly the newer the truck is (see Figure 4). The emission of SO_2 will depend on the sulphur content in the diesel which is now at a maximum of 10 wt-ppm in Europe. The CO_2 emissions are lower the larger the truck is, when considering emissions per mass of transported goods. The fuel consumption and thus the CO_2 emissions will also depend on the type of driving. Within the European Artemis project (Andre 2005) emission factors are available for a large number of trucks and driving conditions. For example, the CO_2 emission per km for a typical Euro 4 truck of around 19 m length and capable of loading 26 tonnes of goods vary from 700 g/km (urban driving) to 580 g/km (rural) for an empty truck and from 1380 g/km to 1080 g/km for a fully loaded truck. In the calculations made here a load factor of 60% is used and the calculations are made for rural driving.

3.3 Empirical evidence on fuel consumption and emissions for rail freight

For diesel rail engines the data on fuel consumption is very limited and in this review the procedure of EcoTransIT was used to calculate emissions. In the case of electrical engines the CO_2 emissions depend on the source of electricity. For calculations an electricity mix for EU 25 obtained from EcoTransIT was utilized (Knörr 2008).

3.4 Realistic load factors and realistic speed are crucial elements in the comparative analysis

In Figure 5 the emissions per tonne-kilometre are presented for the alternative modes of transport included in this paper. These are estimated based on realistic load factors for the various modes as presented above. For the RoRo vessel a load factor of 44% is used, for the container feeder 48%, for the tanker 55%, for trains 50% and for the truck/trailer 60%. The load factor for the RoRo and container vessel represents the relation with the transported goods and the payload and takes into account both the weight of the trucks themselves and that containers are assumed to have a fill factor of 60%.

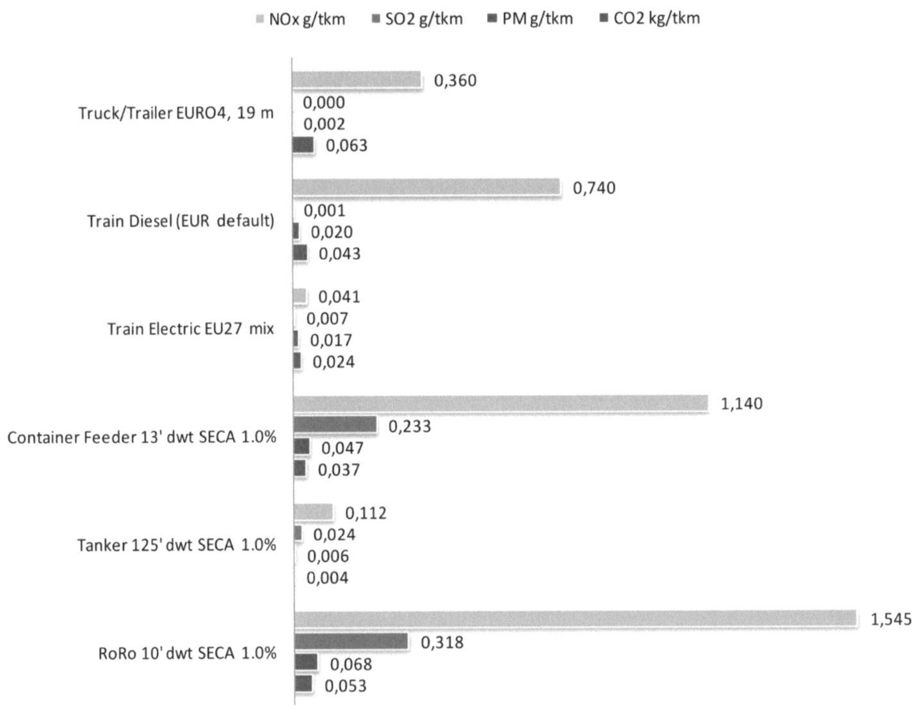

Fig. 5. Emissions per tonnekilometre for the alternative freight transport modes. CO_2 emissions in kg/tkm. NO_X, PM, and SO_2 emissions in g/tonne-km.

CO_2 emissions are directly correlated with use of fossil fuels. The most fuel efficient among the cases in Fig. 5 is the big tanker vessel, with a CO_2 emission of 4 grams per tonne-km. At the other end of the scale is the truck/trailer combination with a CO_2 emission of 63 grams per tonne-km. The RoRo vessel is marginally better with an equivalent figure of 53 grams. The CO_2 emissions from the electric train with the EU25 energy mix is 24 grams per tonne-km. The container feeder vessel performs much better than the RoRo-vessel at 37 grams per tonne-km[1].

The comparatively very high SO_2 emissions from the vessels range from 0.024 grams for the large tanker to 0.32 grams for the RoRo-vessel while it is only 80 µg/tonne-km for the truck. This is despite the fact that we have assumed that the fuel quality is according to the SECA-regulations of 1.0% sulphur content. Future stricter limits for sulphur content will to some extent make short sea shipping SO_2 emissions come closer to those of the alternative modes, but not beat them.

European trucks (Euro 4 and Euro 5 standard) have relatively low particle emissions[2]. No other mode has lower PM emissions. NO_X emissions are also low for truck transport, only beaten by the large tanker and the electric train. Further, a Euro 6 truck would have an additional cut in NO_X emissions by around 90% compared with the Euro 4 truck.

Comparative figures like these are often presented in policy papers as a rationale for promoting short sea shipping as an alternative to land based modes of transport. Sometimes the figures presented are quite different from one setting to another. One late example is the figures presented in Chapter 9 in the IMO MEPC (IMO 2009) report. Here the CO_2 emissions of a wide range of vessels are presented along with figures for road and rail. As a benchmark for the figures presented in Figure 5, we present a subset of figures representing CO_2 emissions per tonne-km from this paper in Table 1.

Vessel / Vehicle	**Total CO_2-efficiency (g/tonne-km)**
Crude oil tanker 120'-200' dwt	4.4
Container 1000-1999 TEU	32.1
Container 0-999 TEU	36.3
RoRo 2000+ lm	49.5
Road freight	150 (80-180)
Rail	10-119

Table 1. CO_2 emissions per tonne-km for alternative freight transport modes according to IMO MEPC (2009). Compiled from the text and various tables.

The data for the oil tanker used here is 3.7 g/tonne-km, as compared to 4.4 g/tonne-km in the IMO MEPC-report. The latter is an average for tankers between 120 000 and 200 000 dwt, whereas the tanker considered in this paper is a 125 000 tonner. This discrepancy may be partly explained by the fact that the model used yields a load factor of 55% for crude tankers, whereas the IMO MEPC-report applies 48%.

[1] The container feeder vessel performs better than the RoRo vessel, but it should be noted that the weight of the container itself is included when the calculations have been made.

[2] This applies to exhaust PM. Trucks will also generate resuspended particles from road dust and wear.

The two container vessels from the IMO MEPC-report yields a CO_2 emission level of 32.1-36.3 g/tonne-km. The 13 000 dwt container vessel included in our analysis would typically carry 1000 TEUs, and emits 37.3 g/tonne-km - which is somewhat higher than the IMO MEPC figures. According to the text in the IMO MEPC-report the cargo capacity of the container vessels is based on an assumed 7 tonnes per container. The 70% load factor applied in the IMO MEPC-report is probably calculated as a percentage of this figure, meaning that the assumed net cargo on a 1000 TEU vessel would be 4 900 tonnes. This is similar to our assumption which is based on a cargo capacity of 10 400 tonnes for the 13 000 dwt container feeder vessel, and a load factor of 48%, yielding 4 992 tonnes of cargo.

In our case study we have included a RoRo vessel of 10 000 dwt, emitting 52.7 g/tonne-km. This is slightly higher than the 2000+ lm RoRo-vessel in the IMO MEPC-figures above - which yields 49.5 g/tonne-km. We have applied a load-factor of 44%. This is a combination of the truck load factor and the "lanemeter loadfactor" - see Hjelle (2010) on the double load-factor problem of RoRo shipping. We have also corrected the net cargo carrying capacity of the vessel for the difference between the gross and payload weight of the truck/trailer (40 tonnes vs 26 tonnes).

The IMO MEPC figures are based on an assumption of a cargo capacity of 2 tonnes per lanemeter for the RoRo vessels. The IMO report does not state weather the term "cargo" means net cargo, or a gross term in the form of the combination of truck/trailer and cargo. A plausible interpretation would be that one has assumed only unaccompanied trailers with a payload of 26 tonnes and a lanemeter footprint of 13 meters, which yields 2 tonnes per lanemeter as the maximum net cargo capacity. In most operations one would have a mix of accompanied and unaccompanied trailers. One will also have to allow some extra space for stowage, which means that a more plausible figure probably would be in the area of 1.6 tonnes per lanemeter as a maximum capacity limit. The 2 tonnes applied in the IMO MEPC figures implies that the average lanementer capacity of the 2000+ lm category is 2577 lanemeters. According to the calculations above this corresponds to a cargo carrying capacity of 4123 tonnes. If 70% of the lanemeters are utilized on average, and the truck has an average load factor of 60%, the combined loadfactor of 42% means that this vessel category on average carries 1732 tonnes of cargo.

In our calculations we have applied the IMO GHG group's CO_2 index for a 10 000 dwt RoRo ship which is 15.1 g/tonne-km when it is full. Such a vessel is assumed by us to have a payload of 5000 tonnes (including the own weight of the trucks and trailers, 3250 tonnes without). As indicated above, we have applied a combined load factor (representing both lanemeter utilization and truck payload utilization) of 44%. Based on this we end up with a CO2 emission factor that is close to the one reported in the IMO MEPC-report.

For road freight the IMO MEPC (IMO 2009) report refers to seven different sources/studies, and concludes with an average figure of 150 g/tkm and a range from 80 to 180 g/tkm. Based on the Artemis model we end up with 63.1 g/tkm for our 19m truck/trailer combination with a load factor of 0.6. Since the IMO publication only briefly refers to external sources, it is not quite clear which settings all of these figures stem from, neither the implied load factors. It is clear though, that some of the referred sources include figures representative for smaller trucks and trucks operating in more urban environments. In a setting where truck transport is compared to short sea shipping such settings are not very relevant as the maritime transport alternatives would compete against long haul truck/trailer combinations rather than distribution vehicles in urban settings. This might explain the fact that our figure lies below the lower bound of the IMO MEPC figures.

Our rail alternatives yield CO_2 emission figures between 24.3 (electric) and 42.6 (diesel) g/tonne-km. The IMO MEPC (2009) study refers to six different studies, yielding a range between 10 to 119 g/tonne-km. The lower figure stems from the long and slow moving bulk trains in the USA, and the upper limit stems from a top-down calculation based on data for the EU region provided by Eurostat. Our data based on the EcoTransIT (Knörr 2008) model lie within these limits, but are significantly lower than the top-down calculations based on Eurostat data. Among the sources cited by the IMO MEPC-report, our figures are quite close to the ones based on US container trains (35-50 g/tonne-km). Further, it can be pointed out that an electric train using exclusively hydro electricity would in our calculations have a CO_2 emission of 0.004 g/tonne-km with a load factor of 0.5.

4. Comparing alternative modes on typical short sea legs

4.1 Four cases and seven modal alternatives

We have chosen four typical intra-European trade links which are quite different with respect to the comparative distances for alternative modes of freight transport (Figure 6). The first case is Gothenburg (Sweden) to Rotterdam (The Netherlands), which is a relatively short distance by sea, and somewhat longer by road and rail. The second case, Helsinki (Finland) to Genoa (Italy) is the longest one, and a case where the sea-link is significantly longer than the road and rail alternatives. Rotterdam to LeHavre (France) is a link where the sea-leg is almost parallel to the road and rail alternatives, which means that this third case will mainly be affected by differences in emissions per tonne-km for the alternative modes. Finally, the last case is Gothenburg to Aberdeen (Scotland). This case represents an alternative where short sea shipping has a very significant comparative advantage distance-wise. Road and rail alternatives for this case are three times as long as the maritime transport alternative.

These four geographical cases are then combined with alternative modes, also with some different varieties within the broad modal categories of sea, road and rail transport. The sea transport alternatives included in this analysis are a 10 000 dwt RoRo-vessel, a 6000 dwt container feeder vessel and a 125 000 dwt tanker. The latter one would typically be used for shuttle transports from offshore oil production sites to refineries, and thus road and rail transport is no realistic alternative to the tanker. We have included this vessel here more as a reference to illustrate how typical calculations of emissions per dwt for large bulk vessels will be very different to such figures for typical short sea cargo vessels. For rail transport, we have included one diesel train alternative, and one electric train with a typical mix of electricity production for the EU. Finally, we have included one typical long distance truck/trailer combination (19 meter) with a Euro 4 engine. As the average age of such trucks in Western Europe will in the area of 4-5 years (Sandvik 2005), this will be a representative engine type.

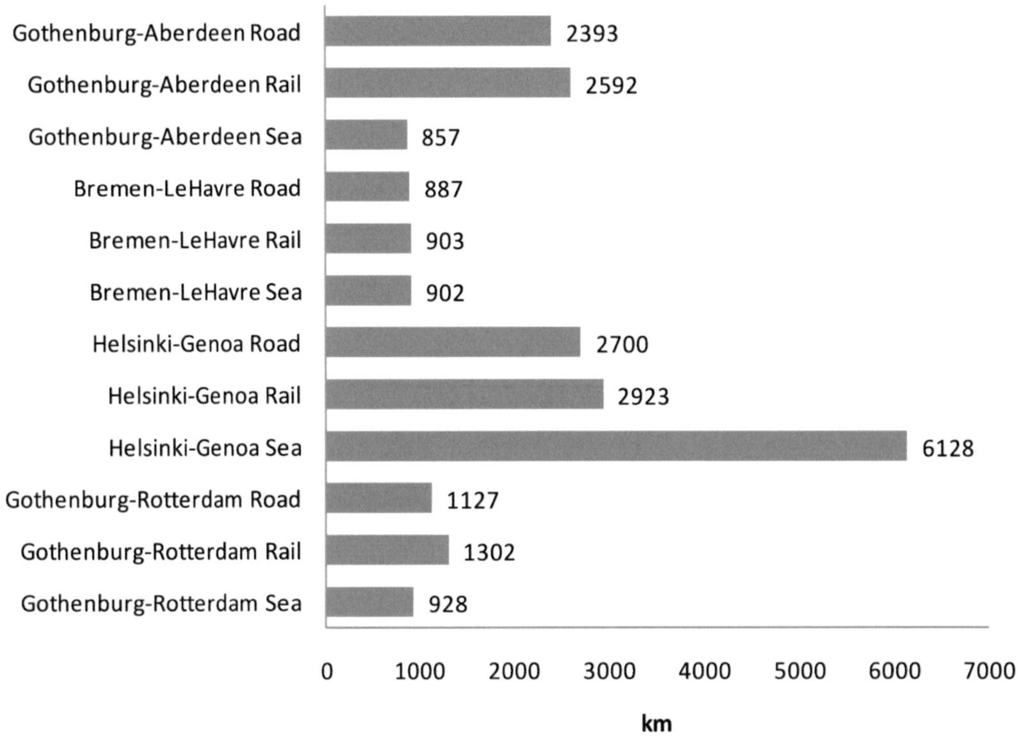

Fig. 6. Distances for alternative OD-pairs and modes (kilometres)

4.2 Emissions to air for the alternative cases

Putting these alternative modes into realistic settings, differences in relative distances also comes into play. In Figure 7 the environmental performance of the alternative modes are presented for the Gothenburg-Rotterdam link. This is a link where the sea-leg is somewhat shorter than the road and rail alternatives. This makes the RoRo and container liner alternatives the winners along with the electric train, regarding CO_2 emissions. The truck/trailer combination yields CO_2 emissions that are more than twice as high as those of the RoRo-vessel, and 4-5 times that of the container vessel.

Even with the distance advantage for the shipping alternative - the emissions of SO_2 are significantly higher from the SSS alternatives than for road and rail. The picture is more mixed for NO_x and PM emissions. The container feeder performs much better than the diesel-train regarding NO_x, whereas the RoRo alternative is comparable to the diesel train. Regarding PM-emissions both train alternatives are of the same order of magnitude as the container vessel, but yield a lower emission level compared to RoRo transport. As we have pointed out earlier, European trucks have very low particle emissions compared to alternative modes.

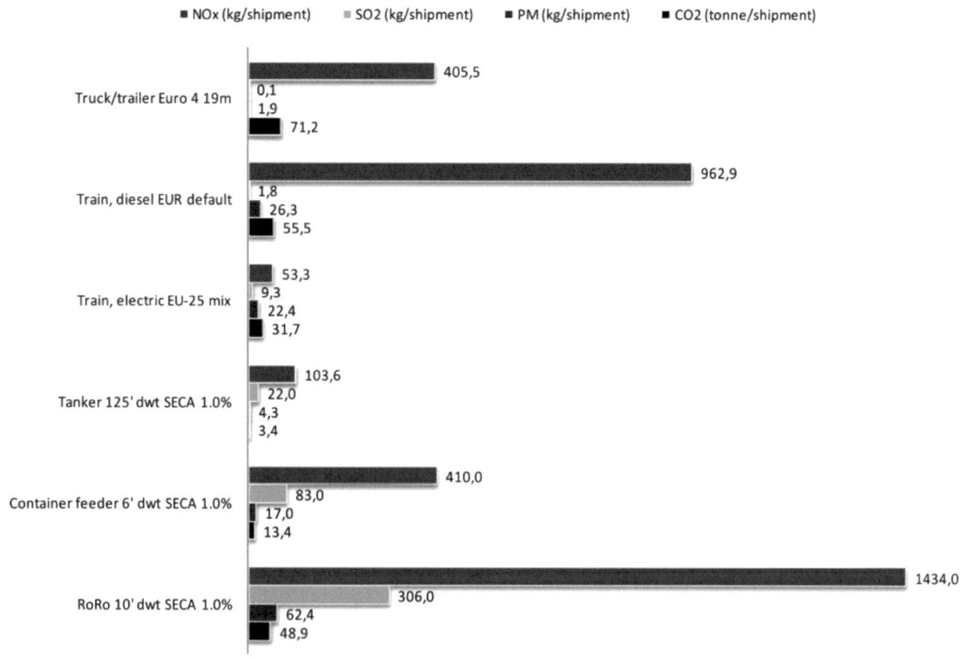

Fig. 7. Emissions of alternative freight transport modes.
One shipment of 1000 tonnes from Gothenburg to Rotterdam

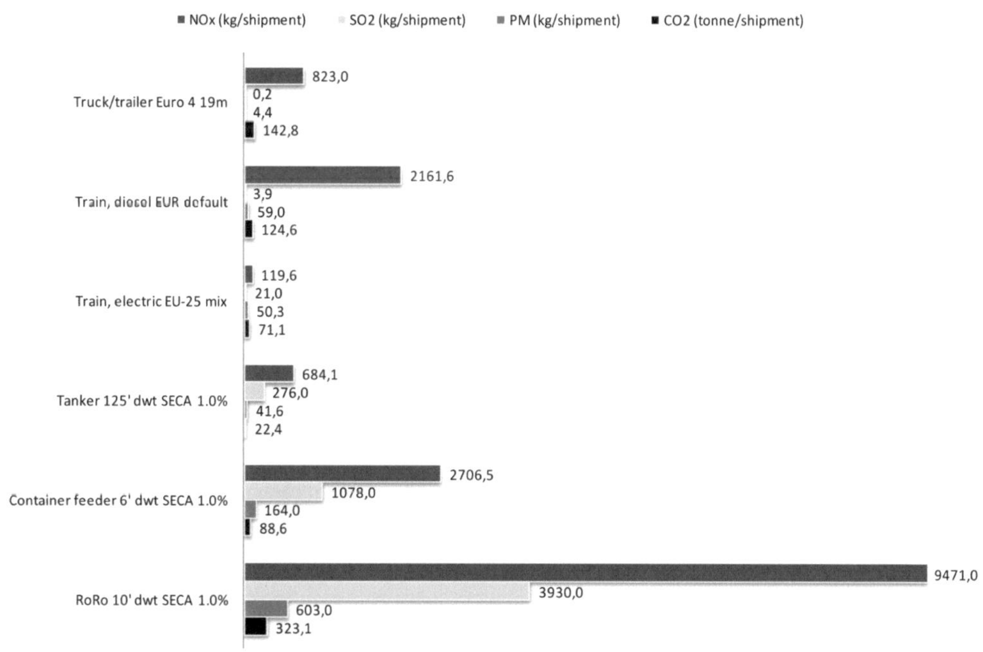

Fig. 8. Emissions of alternative freight transport modes.
One shipment of 1000 tonnes from Helsinki to Genoa

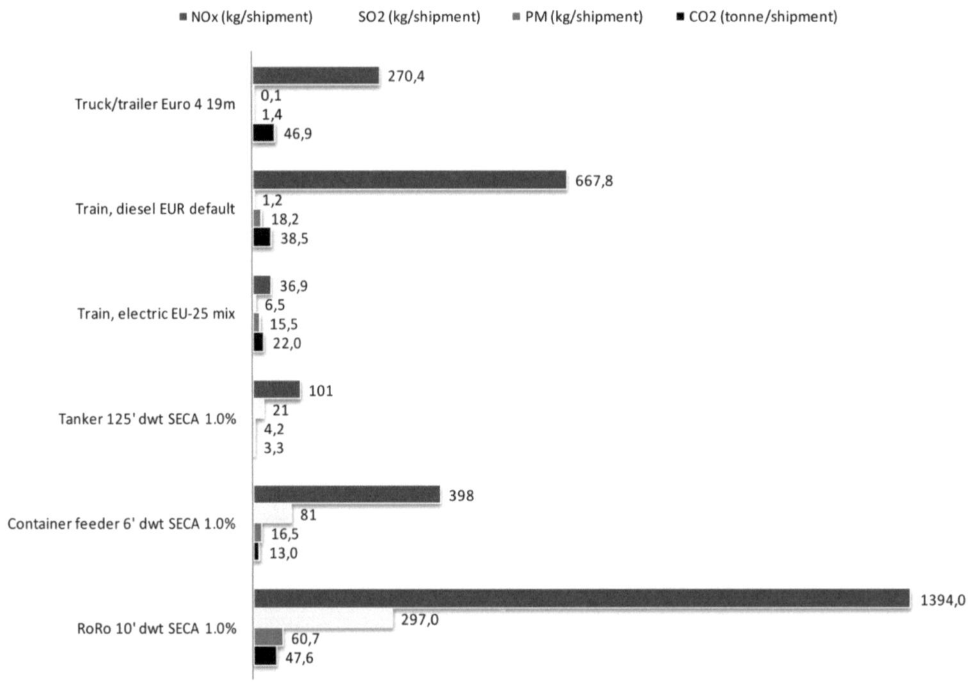

Fig. 9. Emissions of alternative freight transport modes.
One shipment of 1000 tonnes from Bremen to Le Havre

The Helsinki-Genoa case illustrates the effects of cases where the sea leg is significantly longer than the land-based alternatives. With such a big distance-disadvantage the SSS modes will lose along all environmental dimensions. Still, it may be interesting to note that our "reference" tanker vessel is more energy efficient than the land based modes even with such a huge difference in distances. The train alternatives are preferable to the truck alternative with respect to CO_2 emissions, but the picture is more mixed for other emission types.

The Bremen-Le Havre case (Figure 9) would be a typical project for the Motorways of the Seas programme of the EU, since this would be a service that might relieve traffic congestion on parallel road (and rail) networks. Would it also be good case along pure emissions-to-air dimensions? As always the maritime transport alternatives performs poorly with respect to SO_2 emissions - and also with respect to NO_X and PM when compared to truck transport. The container feeder emits much less CO_2 than the two rail alternatives, whereas the RoRo vessel emits more CO_2 than the electric rail alternative and somewhat less than the diesel train. Both SSS services perform better with respect to CO_2 than the truck/trailer combination.

Finally, our Gothenburg-Aberdeen case represents the other extreme, compared to the third case. Here the SSS-alternatives have a very large distance advantage compared to road and rail. Even with this advantage SO_2 emissions are high for the container and RoRo-alternatives. This is also true for the NO_X emissions for RoRo relative to the road transport alternative. The energy use is of course much lower for the vessels than for the road and rail alternatives.

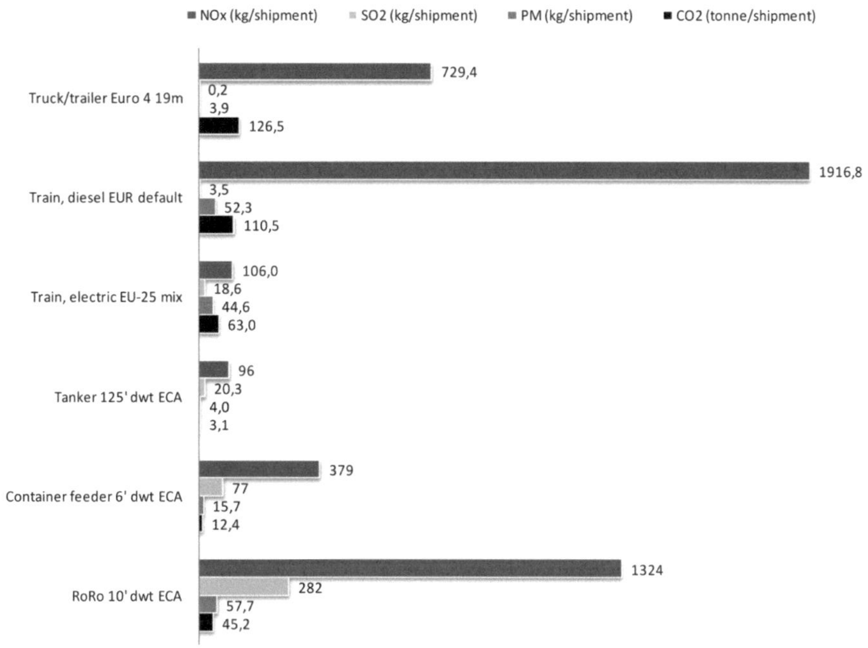

Fig. 10. Emissions of alternative freight transport modes.
One shipment of 1000 tonnes from Gothenburg to Aberdeen

5. Technological and political perspectives on green shipping

5.1 The scope for technology-based reductions of emissions from short sea shipping

The picture presented here will be altered in the future as new engine and exhaust conversion technologies are introduced. If we look at regulations already in place we can note that a Euro 6 truck would reduce the emissions of NO_X by 90% and by PM with 50% compared with the truck used in our calculations. For the ships most of the routes we studied are already within SECAs. Here the emissions of SO_2 will be reduced by 67% by 2015 compared with today. Also the PM emissions are then probably reduced by about 80% by 2015 in SECAs. If the ship were to have Tier 3 engines the NO_X emissions would be reduced by about 80%. The use of natural gas as fuel would give even further reductions in all three substances. The train with diesel engines will show better performance as the new emission regulations are put in place.

When it comes to CO_2 emissions all three transport modes have the potential for reductions through increasing the load factors. For the ships, significant improvements can be obtained through reducing the ships' speed, since the fuel consumption is strongly dependent on speed. All three modes also have the possibility to use alternative fuels. Natural gas should give a 25% reduction in CO_2 emissions but may increase the emissions of methane which is a powerful green-house gas.

The Second IMO Greenhouse Gas Study (IMO 2009) points to a number of technology-based options for improving the energy efficiency of vessels. Partly these are related to improved design (concepts, hull and superstructure, power and propulsion systems) and improved operations (fleet management, logistics, incentives, voyage optimization, energy management). The combined potential for reductions of CO_2 emission from these technologies is estimated to be between 25 and 75%. To reach the upper bound of this range, reductions in operating speed would be necessary.

5.2 The potential impact of future regulatory actions

Some of the technological options mentioned above will be financially attractive to the ship-owners, and theoretically there should be no need for regulatory actions to put them to work. Other technologies need regulatory support in the form of regulations or incentives. Such policies could be categorized into market-based instruments, command-and-control instruments and voluntary measures (Table 2). Within these categories one could think of different concrete instruments and ways of benchmarking environmental performance. Currently benchmarks like the Energy Efficiency Operational index (EEOI) and the Eneregy Efficiency Design Index (EEDI) are candidates for benchmarking the CO_2 emissions of vessels within the IMO discussions.

	Market-based instruments	**Command-and-control instruments**	**Voluntary measures**
Maritime GHG emissions	Emissions trading, e.g., METS.* Emissions levy, e.g., ICF.†		
Operational efficiency	EEOI levy. EEOI levy/benefit scheme.	Mandatory EEOI limit. Mandatory EEOI reporting. Mandatory SEMP.	Voluntary agreement to improve EEOI. Voluntary agreement to implement SEMP.
Design efficiency	EEDI levy. EEDI levy/benefit scheme.	Mandatory EEDI limit for new ships.	Voluntary agreement to improve EEDI, meet voluntary standards.
Fuel life-cycle carbon emissions	Differentiated fuel levy.	Fuel life-cycle carbon emissions standard. Biofuel standard.	

* METS - Maritime emissions trading scheme.
† ICF - International Compensation Funf

Table 2. Overview of policies to limit or reduce emissions of greenhouse gases from ships Source: IMO (IMO 2009)

As noted above, such global regulatory regimes are to a large extent dependent on achieving consensus among many nations which makes the international regulatory regime related to shipping more sluggish than the equivalent regimes applied to land based modes. This is one of the reasons why the EU "threatens" to take unilateral action by including CO_2 emissions from international shipping into the EU trading regime for CO_2-quotas.

6. Conclusions

Our case studies illustrate that short sea shipping operations, represented by RoRo and container services may very well deserve their "green label" when compared to alternative modes with respect to CO_2 emissions. This conclusion is valid under what we consider realistic operating environments with respect to vessel operation speeds and achieved load factors, and when the shipping leg is not much longer than the distances of the land based modes. This conclusion holds at least for the container vessels, but the advantage of RoRo operations versus truck transport may be marginal - and is highly dependent on the prevailing market situation and the resulting load factors achieved.

The short sea shipping alternative does generally *not* deserve a "green label" when SO_2, NO_X and PM emissions are considered. Although some improvements are in the pipeline through the stricter Marpol Annex VI regulations, the maritime transport alternatives will still not be able to compete with road transport along these dimensions unless new fuels (LNG) are introduced or abatement technologies are installed.

We have applied quite large feeder vessels, a 10 000 dwt RoRo vessel and a 13 000 dwt container vessel, in our case studies. Smaller vessels will generally yield higher emissions per tonne-km and may therefore be less competitive.

We have illustrated that the use of realistic load factors is crucial in a comparative analysis like this. Applying load factors related to the cargo *capacity* of the vessel measured in tonnes will not yield a realistic setting, especially for RoRo vessels. All emissions should be attributed to the net cargo transported - as is the intention of IMOs proposed Energy Efficiency Operational Index (EEOL).

The recent work of the IMO MEPC points out that there is a very significant potential for reductions of CO_2 emissions from ships - but that many of the possible technological and organizational measures are dependent on efficient policy regimes to come into play.

7. Acknowledgements

This paper is partly financed through the Northern Maritime University (NMU) project. The NMU project is partly funded by the EC Interreg IVB programme.

An earlier version of this paper was presented at IAME 2010 in Lisbon, Portugal.

8. References

Andre, J.-M. (2005). "Vehicle emission measurement collection of the ARTEMIS datatbase." Retrieved Feb 23, 2010, from http://www.inrets.fr/ur/lte/publications/publications-pdf/Joumard/A3312reportJMALTE0504.pdf

Cooper, D. and T. Gustafsson (2004). Methodology for calculatin emissions from ships: 1. Update of emission factors. IVL Reports. Gothenburg, IVL Svenska Miljöinstitutet.

Hjelle, H. M. (2010). The double load-factor problem of Ro-Ro shipping. 12th World Conference on Transport Research. Lisbon.

Hjelle, H. M. (2010). "Short Sea Shipping's green label at risk." Transport Reviews 30(5): 617-640.

IMO (2009). Second IMO GHG Study 2009. London, IMO.
Knörr, W. (2008). EcoTransIT: Ecological Transport Information Tool. Environmental Methodology and Date. Update 2008. Heidelberg, Germany, Institut für Energie und Umweltforschung Heidelberg GmbH.
NTM (2009). "The NTM methodology in brief." Retrieved February 23, 2010, from http://www.ntm.a.se/english/eng-index.asp.
NTM Working Group Goods and Logistics (2008). Environmental data for international cargo sea transport. Calculation methods, emission factors, mode-specific issues. Stockholm.
Sandvik, E. T. (2005). Environmental impacts of intermodal freight transport. MFM Report. Molde, Møreforsking Molde: 40 s.
Whall, C., D. Cooper, et al. (2002). Quantification of emissions from ships associated with ship movements between ports in the European Community. Northwich, UK, Entec UK Limited.

2

Speciation Methods for the Determination of Organotins (OTs) and Heavy Metals (MHs) in the Freshwater and Marine Environments

Peter P. Ndibewu, Rob I. McCrindle and Ntebogeng S. Mokgalaka
Tshwane University of Technology, South Africa

1. Introduction

Our primary goal for the development of analytical methods is their application in environmental monitoring to achieve good assessment of the contamination situation in freshwater and marine environments. As clearly stated in the endocrine disrupting contaminant (EDCs) program strategic plan for health related water issues (HRWI) of the Republic of South Africa (Version 1.2B, 7/02/2001), one of the objectives in the water research field is to protect aquatic ecosystems and human health based on sound science and defensible data through developing and validation of appropriate methods and by investigating the sources, persistence and effects of potential EDCs in water to support the risk assessment process and contribute towards a trustworthy environmental policy for endocrine disrupting contaminants.

Research goals around the globe in this area have focused on the development of speciation methods for the determination of organotins and heavy metal pollutants in both freshwater and marine environments. Research and development over the years has provided reliable and sensitive analytical techniques that can be used for water research analysis, monitoring and health risks assessment including sampling, testing and validation, although some challenges still exist in regard to the availability of efficient and cost-effective sampling techniques.

The procedures for method modification and development vary depending on the properties of the chemical, possible interferences, the desired sampling medium, the desired analytical technique, sensitivity required, and similar factors (Ombaba and Barry, 1992). The following are questions, which have to be considered and answered by any method modification or development:

- Can the analyte be collected by and removed from the sampling media?
- What are the collection and recovery factors and are they acceptable?
- Is the detection limit sufficiently low to provide meaningful data, especially when adjusted for collection and recovery factors?
- Will expected interferences produce false positive, false negative or biased results?
- If possible, can the results be verified by comparison with an accepted procedure?

This work is partitioned into two sub-sections covering the organotins (OTs) and the heavy metals which are toxic, (TMs) and in most cases are carcinogens. In the heavy metals group, only a few of them, known to cause serious health hazards are fully discussed. These are mercury (Hg), cadmium (Cd), arsenic (As), lead (Pb) and zinc (Zn), all known as endocrine disrupting contaminants (EDCs) (Fatoki and Ngassoum, 2000; HRWI, 2001; Ndibewu *et al.*, 2002). Other toxic metals including chromium (Cr) and vanadium (V) will be briefly mentioned in our discussion.

The first part of this chapter discusses speciation analysis of organotins by liquid-liquid (Espadaler et *al.*, 1997; Jiang et *al.*, 2000; Mueller, 1984) and microsolid phase extraction methods (Mueller, 1987) followed by sodium tetrahydroborate (Jiang et *al.*, 2000), sodium tetraethylborate (Cai and Bayona, 1995; Thomaidis et *al.*, 2001; Ceulemans and Adams, 1995; Pereira et *al.*, 1999) and the Grignard`s reagents (Chau et *al.*, 1996; Ceulemans and Adams, 1995; Krull et *al.*, 1985; Lucinda, 1983) derivatization. Separation and detection is usually accomplished using the GC-FPD/GC-AAS techniques (Fatoki et *al.*, 2000). In the liquid-liquid extraction phase, solvents such as tropolone, hexane-soxhlet and/or diethyl ether have been used for water (Fatoki and Ngassoum, 2000; Mueller, 1987; Leal et *al.*, 1995; Abalos et *al.*, 1997), sediment samples (Fatoki et *al.*, 2000; Abalos et *al.*, 1997; Krull et *al.*, 1985) and the biota (Kan-atireklap et *al.*, 1998). In the derivatization step, two techniques have been used. Firstly, hybridization reactions using sodium tetrahydroborate as the reagent (Abalos et *al.*, 1997) was used. Alternatively, derivatization technique based on alkylation reactions employ two reagents namely: the Grignard`s reagents (methylation or ethylation) and sodium tetraethylborate (Fatoki and Ngassoum, 2000; Cai and Bayona, 1995). While the GC-FPD (Fatoki *et al.*, 2000; Richardson and Gangolli, 1994) and GC-AAS techniques (Fatoki *et al.*, 2000) can be used for the speciation of various organotins compounds, elemental Tin (Sn) is analyzed using flame AAS (Quevauviller *et al.*, 1989) in water and sediment samples and the biota.

For the determination of cadmium (Cd), mercury (Hg), arsenic (As), and zinc (Zn), while an ion chromatography-hydride generation-atomic absorption (HG-AAS) procedure (Wade *et al.*, 1988) has been used for speciation of As, Cd and Zn are usually determined using flame AAS spectrometry (Lucinda *et al.*, 1983; Maenpa *et al.*, 2002), and Hg analyzed using the cold vapor technique (CVAAS) (Shrader *et al.*, 1983; Willis, 1965). More recently, Fatoki *et al.* (2000) has used GC-FPD for the determination of tributyltin concentrations in the coastal water and freshwater sediments from both the Port Elizabeth and East London harbors in South Africa, which contributed to resources for building regulatory data in that part of the world.

2. Background

Aquatic pollution is a major cause in the decline of resources from water. It is, thus, important to monitor the condition of water. A major concern is the need to develop accurate, reliable and efficient speciation methods for the determination of the polluting compounds within ultra-low detectable ranges. Those known so far to be particularly toxic to the aquatic ecosystems are the organotins (Fent, 1996; Mueller, 1987) and the heavy metals (Cai and Bayona, 1995; Lucinda *et al.*, 1983). The term "speciation" in analytical chemistry refers to the separation and quantification of the different oxidation states or chemical forms of a particular element (http://www.frontiergeosciences.com/ebru/).

Although the total concentration of an element is still useful to know, and sometimes essential, the determination of species is necessary to fully understand the biogeochemical and toxicological behavior of the metals. Pollution can influence aquatic life, either directly or indirectly in several ways. By pH changes (increase in acidity); decreasing dissolved oxygen (most common index for pollution); toxicity; mechanical injury to gills (for example from silt); thermal change of medium; killing food organisms through pH change or thermal changes; destruction of spawning grounds (FAO, 1978); shell malformation in oysters (Bayona and Cai, 1994), imposex in gastropods (Kuballa *et al.*, 1995); mortality of the larvae of mussels (Jiang *et al.*, 2000) and fish poisoning (Cai and Bayona, 1995; Stab *et al.*, 1992; Shrader *et al.*, 1983; Leal *et al.*, 1995).

More specifically, maritime and coastal areas, as well as freshwater are definitely amongst today`s prominent endangered ecosystems. Industrialization and other human activities have caused major changes in these reservoirs` water quality, both inland and marine (Leal *et al.*, 1995). Dumping at sea and maritime-based transport activities are mostly responsible for this problem. Polluting loads emptied into the aquatic environments are of various nature and types depending on the point or non-point source though some, like the heavy metals, occur naturally (Lucinda *et al.*, 1983; Fatoki *et al.*, 2000; Ndibewu *et al.*, 2002). The point sources are essentially discharges of sewages and industrial effluents, and are easily identifiable and controllable (Maenpa *et al.*, 2002; Lucinda *et al.*, 1983). The non-point sources arise in part from natural phenomena, for example, soil erosion; irrigation return flows; outflow from fish farms, and are often diffuse, and so difficult to identify and to control (Leal *et al.*, 1995).

3. Occurrence and ecotoxicity of heavy metals, TBT and other organotins

Unlike methyltin, which may be formed naturally in the environment, TBT is exclusively of anthropogenic origin (MCkie, 1987; Fent, 1996). This is why its occurrence in the aquatic environment has been directly attributed to its application as an antifouling agent. TBT residues in the sediments of harbors, marinas and shipping channels has been found to be considerably higher typically in the range of about 200 - 1000 $\mu g\ kg^{-1}$ (Balls, 1987). Progressive introduction of organic groups at the tin atom produces increasing biological activity (Bayona and Cai, 1994). Organotin compounds with three alkyl groups attached to the tin atom, such as tributyltin (TBT), triphenyltin and tricyclohexyltin, have found wide applications as antifouling agents in marine paints formulations, bactericides in cooling water (MCkie, 1987; Fatoki, 2000), agricultural fungicides and acaricides (Leal *et al.*, 1995). The most import of these is TBT, which is used in marine paints as an effective means of the growth of fouling organisms such as tubeworms, barnacles and mussels on seafaring vessels and marine structures (Brian, 1991).

Meech *et al.* (1998) has shown that TBT is acutely toxic to a variety of fresh water species at concentrations down to 0.1 μL^{-1}. TBT is particularly toxic (Fent, 1996; Reisch, 1996; Meech *et al.*, 1998) to mollusks (oysters) and gastropods. The decline of dog whelk populations on various coasts of France and UK has been attributed to the occurrence of TBT in these waters (Fent, 1996). Chronic toxic effects on oysters in the form of shell deformation (Fent, 1996) and marine gastropods in the form of sterilization of females have been reported occurring at concentrations of a few ng L^{-1} (Fent, 1996; Fatoki *et al.*, 2000).

Unlike TBT and organotins, metals are unique environmental and industrial pollutants in that they are found naturally distributed in all phases of the environment. The term "heavy metals" is generally interpreted to include those metals from periodic table groups IIA through VIA. The semi-metallic elements boron, arsenic, selenium, and tellurium are often included in this classification. At trace levels, many of these elements are necessary to support life. Heavy metals are elements having atomic weights between 63.546 and 200.590g (Kennish, 1992), and a specific gravity greater than 4.0 (Connell *et al.*, 1984). Living organisms require trace amounts of some heavy metals, including cobalt, copper, iron, manganese, molybdenum, vanadium, strontium, and zinc (Nriagu, 1996). Excessive levels of essential metals, however, become toxic and may build up in biological systems, and become a significant health hazard (Brickman, 1978). Non-essential heavy metals of particular concern to surface water systems are cadmium (Cd), chromium (Cr), mercury (Hg), lead (Pb), arsenic (As) and antimony (Sb) (Kennish, 1992).

During the last two decades, considerable attention has been given to problems concerning negative effects of heavy metals (HMs) on various ecosystems in different environmental media (Lucinda, 1983; Nriagu, 1996). The heavy metals rated among most of the environmental risk pollutants (Cai and Bayona, 1995) requires that, fast, accurate and reliable analytical techniques suitable for their assessment and for their determination in environmental samples at trace levels be developed. In the class of the heavy metal ecotoxicants, Hg, Cd, As and Zn are considered fairly hazardous because of their high toxicity (Schrader *et al.*, 1983; Nriagu, 1996; Fent, 1996). These metal species actually occur in the environment at sub ultra-low trace concentrations level (Cai and Bayona, 1995; Lucinda *et al.*, 1983). Therefore, accurate and sensitive determination techniques are of fundamental interest for the assessment of the effectiveness of regulatory control measures.

Heavy metals are stable and persistent environmental contaminants since they cannot be degraded or destroyed. Therefore, they tend to accumulate in soils, seawater, freshwater, and sediments (Schrader *et al.*, 1983; http://www.osha.gov/SLTC/cadmium/index.html). Excessive levels of metals in the marine environment can affect marine biota and pose risk to human consumers of seafood (http://www.msceast.org/hms/). Heavy metals are also known to have adverse effects on the environment and human health (Schrader *et al.*, 1983). Numerous field observations also indicate a significant increase of HM concentrations in agricultural and forest soils as well as in marine and inland water sediments. This increase is frequently observed in remote areas thousands of kilometers away from major anthropogenic sources and can be explained by transboundary atmospheric long-range transport only (http://www.msceast.org/hms/). An assessment of the potential ecological and health risks associated with atmospheric fluxes of heavy metals requires an understanding of the relationships between sources of emission to the atmosphere and the levels of concentrations measured in ambient air and precipitation (Ikeda *et al.*, 1996).

Since the industrial revolution, the production of heavy metals such as Pb, Cu, and Zn has increased exponentially (Lucinda, 1983; Maguire *et al.*, 1982). Between 1850 and 1990, production of these three metals increased nearly 10-fold, with emissions rising in tandem (Maguire *et al.*, 1982). The heavy metals have been used in a variety of ways for at least 2 millennia (Lu *et al.*, 1996; Lucinda, 1983; Meech *et al.*, 1998). For example, lead has been used in plumbing, and lead arsenate has been used to control insects in apple orchards. The Romans added lead to wine to improve its taste, and mercury was used as a salve to alleviate teething pain in infants (Nriagu, 1996). Once emitted, metals can reside in the environment for hundreds of years or more (Nriagu, 1996), while causing immediate or long term damage depending on the concentration released. Evidence of human exploitation of heavy metals has been found in the ice cores in Greenland and seawater in the Antarctic (Nriagu, 1996). The lead contents of ice layers deposited annually in Greenland show a steady rise that parallels the mining renaissance in Europe, reaching values 100 times the natural background level in the mid-1990s (http://h2osparc.wq.ncsu.edu/info/hmetals.html). Mining itself, not only of heavy metals but also of coal and other minerals, is another major route of exposure. Despite some noted improvements in worker safety and cleaner production, mining remains one of the most hazardous and environmentally damaging industries (Nriagu, 1996; Maenpa *et al.*, 2002). In Bolivia, toxic sludge from a zinc mine in the Andes had killed aquatic life along a 300-kilometer stretch of river systems as of 1996 (http://h2osparc.wq.ncsu.edu/info/hmetals.html). It also threatened the livelihood and health of 50,000 of the region's subsistence farmers (Nriagu, 1996; Fent, 1996). Uncontrolled smelters have produced some of the world's only environmental "dead zones" where little or no vegetation survives. For instance, toxic emissions from the Sudbury, Ontario, and nickel smelter have devastated 10,400 hectares of forests downwind of the smelter (Nriagu, 1996). All heavy metals exist in surface waters in colloidal, particulate, and dissolved phases, although dissolved concentrations are generally low (Kennish, 1992). The colloidal and particulate metal may be found in (1) hydroxides, oxides, silicates, or sulfides; or (2) adsorbed to clay, silica, or organic matter. The soluble forms are generally ions or unionized organometallic chelates or complexes. The solubility of trace metals in surface waters is predominately controlled by the water pH, the type and concentration of ligands on which the metal could adsorb, and the oxidation state of the mineral components and the redox environment of the system (Connell *et al.*, 1984).

Heavy metals in surface water systems can be from natural or anthropogenic sources. Currently, anthropogenic inputs of metals exceed natural inputs. Excess metal levels in surface water may pose a health risk to humans and to the environment (Nriagu, 1996). Considering that heavy metals are natural constituents of the Earth's crust, they are present in varying concentrations in all ecosystems and human activities have drastically changedthe biogeochemical cycles and balance of some of these heavy metals. The main anthropogenic sources of heavy metals are various industrial sources (Shrader *et al.*, 1983; Fatoki, 2000) including present and former mining activities (http://www.msceast.org/hms/), foundries and smelters (http://www.osha.gov/SLTC/cadmium/index.html), and diffuse sources such as piping (http://www.msceast.org/hms/), constituents of products, combustion by-products, traffic (Shrader *et al.*, 1983), etc. Relatively, volatile heavy metals and those that become attached to airborne particles can be widely dispersed on very large scales. Heavy metals conveyed in aqueous and sedimentary transport enter the normal coastal biogeochemical cycle and are largely retained within near-shore and shelf regions (http://www.msceast.org/hms/). The toxicity of these metals has also been documented throughout history: Greek and Roman physicians diagnosed symptoms of acute lead poisoning long before toxicology became a science (Nriagu, (1996). Today, much more is known about the health effects of heavy metals. Exposure to heavy metals has been linked with developmental retardation, various cancers, kidney damage, and even death in some instances of exposure to very high concentrations. Exposure to high levels of mercury, gold, and lead has also been associated with the development of autoimmunity, in which the immune system starts to attack its own cells, mistaking them for foreign invaders (Nriagu, 1996; http://www.mercurypolicy.org/). Autoimmunity can lead to the development of diseases of the joints and kidneys, such as rheumatoid arthritis, or diseases of the circulatory or central nervous systems. Despite abundant evidence of these deleterious health effects, exposure to heavy metals continues and may increase in the absence of concerted policy actions. Mercury is still extensively used in gold mining in many parts of Latin America. Arsenic, along with copper and chromium compounds, is a common ingredient in wood preservatives. Lead is still widely used as an additive in gasoline. Increased use of coal in the future will increase metal exposures because coal ash contains many toxic metals and can be breathed deeply into the lungs. For countries such as China, India and South Africa, which continue to rely on high-ash coal as a primary energy source, the health implications are ominous.

Mercury is a toxic metal that is liquid at room temperature (http://h2osparc.wq.ncsu.edu/info/hmetals.htm). Exposure to mercury is known to cause permanent damage to the brain, nervous system, and kidneys (http://www.mercurypolicy.org). Pregnant women are particularly vulnerable as mercury may damage the developing fetus. While mercury is released naturally from rocks, soil, and volcanoes, human activities have boosted atmospheric levels to some three times above pre-industrial levels, the experts say. Estimates vary, but the UNEP group of experts says some 5,000 to 10,000 metric tons of mercury are thought to enter the atmosphere every year and 50 to 75 percent of it from human activities (http://h2osparc.wq.ncsu.edu/info/hmetals.htm). The main human source of mercury emissions is coal combustion from electrical power plants and industrial, commercial and residential burners. Other sources include municipal solid waste incineration, mining of non-ferrous metals, and artisanal gold mining (http://www.mercurypolicy.org).

Interest in the biogeochemical cycle (Shrader *et al.*, 1983) of mercury in the environment has dramatically increased in recent years due to the observation that mercury accumulates in aquatic organisms. Moreover, methylmercury becomes magnified in the upper tropic levels as a result of bioaccumulation, from dietary intake of organisms containing methylmercury (http://www.frontiergeosciences.com/ebru/). It has been demonstrated that mercury can be methylated in the environment and bioconcentrated in the biota (Cai and Bayona, 1995). Ingestion of fish muscle is an important exposure pathway of mercury to humans (Cai and Bayona, 1995). Studying mercury in environmental systems requires a very sensitive method as typical mercury levels in aquatic environments range from 0.5 to 5.0 ng L^{-1} (http://www.frontiergeosciences.com/ebru/). Total mercury permissible in the environment is 0.005 mg L^{-1} (FAO, 1978). The high toxicity of methylmercury has been well recognized in fish (Cai and Bayona, 1995; Lucinda *et al.*, 1983; Wade *et al.*, 1988) and ingestion of fish muscle is an important exposure pathway of mercury for humans (Cai and Bayona, 1995).

Cadmium may interfere with the metallothionein's ability to regulate zinc and copper concentrations in the body. Metallothionein is a protein that binds to excess essential metals to render them unavailable when cadmium induces metallothionein's activity binding it to copper and zinc, disrupting the homeostasis levels (Kennish, 1992). Cadmium is used in industrial manufacturing processes and is a byproduct of the metallurgy of zinc. Acute cadmium toxicity may result in brain damage. Metal fume fever may result from acute exposure with flu-like symptoms of weakness, fever, headache, chills, sweating and muscular pain. Acute pulmonary edema usually develops within 24 hours and reaches a maximum by three days. If death from asphyxia does not occur, symptoms may resolve within a week. Chronic cadmium poisoning can cause eventual death. The most serious consequence of chronic cadmium poisoning is cancer (lung and prostate). The first observed chronic effect is generally kidney damage, manifested by excretion of excessive (low molecular weight) protein in the urine. Cadmium also is believed to cause pulmonary emphysema and bone disease (osteomalcia and osteoporosis). The latter has been observed in Japan ("itai-itai" disease) where residents were exposed to cadmium in rice crops irrigated with cadmium-contaminated water. Cadmium may also cause anemia, teeth discoloration (Cd forms CdS) and loss of smell (anosmia) (http://www.osha.gov/SLTC/cadmium/index.html). Arsenic ingestion can cause severe toxicity through ingestion of contaminated food and water. Ingestion causes vomiting, diarrhea, and cardiac abnormalities (Viessman and Hammer, 1985).

The behavior of metals in natural waters is a function of the substrate sediment composition, the suspended sediment composition, and the water chemistry (Nriagu, 1996). Sediment composed of fine sand and silt will generally have higher levels of adsorbed metal than will quartz, feldspar and carbonate-rich sediment. Metals also have a high affinity for humic acids, organo-clays, and oxides coated with organic matter (Connell *et al.*, 1984). The water chemistry of the system controls the rate of adsorption and desorption of metals to and from sediment. Adsorption removes the metal from the water column and stores the metal in the substrate. Desorption returns the metal to the water column, where recirculation and bio-assimilation may take place. Metals may be desorbed from the sediment if the water experiences increase in salinity, decreases in redox potential, or decreases in pH controlled by the following mechanisms:

- Salinity increase: Elevated salt concentrations create increased competition between cations and metals for binding sites. Often, metals will be driven off into the overlying water. (Estuaries are prone to this phenomenon because of fluctuating river flow inputs).
- Redox potential decrease: A decreased redox potential, as is often seen under oxygen deficient conditions, will change the composition of metal complexes and release the metal ions into the overlying water.
- pH decrease: A lower pH increases the competition between metal and hydrogen ions for binding sites. A decrease in pH may also dissolve metal-carbonate complexes, releasing free metal ions into the water column (Connell *et al.*, 1984).

3.1 Environmental effects

Aquatic organisms may be adversely affected by heavy metals in the environment. The toxicity is largely a function of the water chemistry and sediment composition in the surface water system, as clearly detailed under the section "Environmental fate/Mode of transport". Slightly elevated metal levels in natural waters may cause the following sublethal effects in aquatic organisms: (1) histological or morphological change in tissues; (2) changes in physiology, such as suppression of growth and development, poor swimming performance, changes in circulation; (3) change in biochemistry, such as enzyme activity and blood chemistry; (4) change in behaviour; (5) and changes in reproduction (Connell *et al.*, 1984). Many organisms are able to regulate the metal concentrations in their tissues. Fish and the crustacea can excrete essential metals, such as copper, zinc, and iron that are present in excess. Some can also excrete non-essential metals, such as mercury and cadmium, although this is usually met with less success (Connell *et al.*, 1984).

Research has shown that aquatic plants and bivalves are not able to successfully regulate metal uptake (Connell *et al.*, 1984). Thus, bivalves tend to suffer from metal accumulation in polluted environments. In estuarine systems, bivalves often serve as biomonitor organisms in areas of suspected pollution (Kennish, 1992). Shell fishing waters are closed if metal levels make shellfish unfit for human consumption. In comparison to freshwater fish and invertebrates, aquatic plants are equally or less sensitive to cadmium, copper, lead, mercury, nickel, and zinc. Thus, the water resource should be managed for the protection of fish and invertebrates, in order to ensure aquatic plant survival (USEPA, 1987). Metal uptake rates will vary according to the organism and the metal in question. Phytoplankton and zooplankton often assimilate available metals quickly because of their high surface area to volume ratio. The ability of fish and invertebrates to adsorb metals is largely dependent on the physical and chemical characteristics of the metal (Kennish, 1992). With the exception of mercury, little metal bioaccumulation has been observed in aquatic organisms (Kennish, 1992). Metals may enter the systems of aquatic organisms via three main pathways: (1) Free metal ions that are absorbed through respiratory surface (e.g. gills) are readily diffused into the blood stream, (2) Free metal ions that are adsorbed onto body surfaces are passively diffused into the blood stream, and (3) Metals that are sorbed onto food and particulates may be ingested, as well as free ions ingested with water (Connell *et al.*, 1984).

3.2 Irrigation effects

Irrigation water may transport dissolved heavy metals to agricultural fields. Although most heavy metals do not pose a threat to humans through crop consumption, cadmium may be incorporated into plant tissue. Accumulation usually occurs in plant roots, but may also occur throughout the plant (De Voogt *et al.*, 1980). Most irrigation systems are designed to allow for up to 30 percent of the water applied to not be absorbed and to leave the field as return flow. Return flow either joins the groundwater or runs off the field surface (tail water). Sometimes tail water must be rerouted into streams because of downstream water rights or a necessity to maintain stream flow. However, usually the tail water is collected and stored until it can be reused or delivered to another field (USEPA, 1993a). Tail water is often stored in small lakes or reservoirs, where heavy metals can accumulate as return flow is pumped in and out. These metals can adversely impact aquatic communities. An extreme example of this is the Kesterson reservoir in the San Joaquin Valley, California, which received subsurface agricultural drain water containing high levels of selenium and salts that, had been leached from the soil during irrigation. Studies in the Kesterson reservoir revealed elevated levels of selenium in water, sediments, terrestrial and aquatic vegetation, and aquatic insects. The elevated levels of selenium were cited as relating to the low reproductive success, high mortality, and developmental abnormalities in embryos and chicks of nesting aquatic birds (Schuler *et al.*, 1990).

3.3 Health effects

Ingestion of metals such as lead (Pb), cadmium (Cd), mercury (Hg), arsenic (As), barium (Ba), and chromium (Cr), may pose great risks to human health. Trace metals such as lead and cadmium will interfere with essential nutrients of similar appearance, such as calcium (Ca^{2+}) and zinc (Zn^{2+}). Amongst the heavy metals pollution, mercury pollution has become a global problem (Schrader *et al.*, 1983) because of its occurrence from natural anthropogenic sources, and its biogeochemical processes (Cai and Bayona, 1995; Coello *et al.*, 1996). As public awareness regarding the toxicity and the environmental impact of mercury contamination increases, speciation analytical methods developed, are required to distinguish between organic and inorganic forms of mercury. The determination and monitoring of mercury and arsenic is a special concern in the field of mine works and food engineering respectfully (Leal *et al.*, 1995; Nriagu, 1996). It has been reported (Leal *et al.*, 1995; Fatoki, 2000) that mercury can be methylated in the environment and bioconcentrated in the biota. Mercury poses a great risk to humans, especially in the form of methylmercury. When mercury enters water, it is often transformed by microorganisms into the toxic methyl mercury form. Symptoms of acute poisoning are pharyngitis, gasteroenteritis, vomiting, nephritis, hepatitis, and circulatory collapse. Chronic poisoning is usually a result of industrial exposure or a diet consisting of contaminated fish (mercury is the only metal that will bioaccumulate). Chronic poisoning may cause liver damage, neural damage, and teratogenesis (USEPA, 1987).

The Global mercury assessment working group of the United Nations Environment Programme (UNEP) had in the past concluded a week long meeting in Geneva (2002) with the recommendation that governments negotiate a treaty to limit the amount of mercury traded worldwide. In the meantime, countries should reduce mercury risks by cutting or eliminating the production and consumption of the chemical by substituting other products and processes. Mercury has been widely used in consumer products because it is an excellent conductor of electricity and is highly malleable. Products containing mercury include thermometers, dental fillings, fluorescent lamps and other electrical equipment, and some batteries. Mercury is used in several types of instruments common to electric utilities, municipalities and households, such as switches, barometers, meters, temperature gauges, pressure gauges and sprinkler system contacts. It has been used as an ingredient in some pesticides and biocides, certain pharmaceuticals, and cosmetics such as skin lightening creams. In some countries, mercury has ritual religious uses. People are most likely to be exposed to mercury by eating fish or shellfish contaminated with methylmercury, and many jurisdictions have issued fish consumption warnings based on the presence of mercury in fish (Cai and Bayona, 1995; Abalos *et al.*, 1997; Fatoki *et al.*, 2000; Ndibewu *et al.*, 2002). People can be exposed when breathing vapours in air from spills, incinerators, and industries that burn fuels containing mercury (Nriagu, 1996). Mercury can be released from dental work or medical treatments and dental or health service workers can be exposed from breathing contaminated workplace air or skin contact during use in the workplace. When placed in landfills, mercury can slowly seep into groundwater or evaporate into the air. It can travel over long distances and persist in the environment for lengthy periods of time. Two studies released in March (2002) (http://h2osparc.wq.ncsu.edu/info/hmetals.html) show that mercury generated by fossil fuel burning power plants is falling from the sky in Antarctica and in the Arctic, and is entering the food chain.

Cadmium is an extremely toxic metal commonly found in industrial workplaces, particularly where any ore is being processed or smelted. Due to its low permissible exposure limit (PEL), over exposures may occur even in situations where cadmium is only in trace quantities in the parent ore or smelter dust. Cadmium is used extensively in electroplating, although the nature of the operation does not generally lead to overexposures. Several deaths from acute exposure have occurred among welders who have unsuspectingly welded on cadmium-containing alloys and among silver solders. Cadmium is also found in industrial paints and may represent a hazard when spray applied. Operations involving removal of cadmium paints by scraping or blasting may similarly pose a significant hazard. Cadmium emits a characteristic brown fume (CdO) upon heating, which is relatively non-irritating, and thus, does not alarm the exposed individual (Maenpa *et al.*, 2002; Meech *et al.*, 1998).

4. Pollution source - Points of TBT and organotins

Organotin compounds have found many important industrial and agricultural applications for more than three decades (Prudente *et al.*, 1999; Leal *et al.*, 1995). These include the use of mono-methyl tins, mono-butyltins and di-butyltins as stabilizers in polyvinyl chloride (PVC) and as catalysts in industrial processes. Organotin compounds with three alkyl groups attached to the tin atom, such as tributyltin (TBT), tri-phenyltin and tri-cyclohexyltin, have found wide applications as antifouling agents in marine paints formulations, bactericides in cooling water, agricultural fungicides and acaricides (Leal *et al.*, 1995), as previously mentioned. Most import of TBT is used in marine paints as an effective means of the growth of fouling organisms such as tubeworms, barnacles and mussels on seafaring vessels and marine structures (Abalos *et al.*, 1997; Fatoki, 2000).

5. Pollution source - Points of heavy metals (HMs)

Nonpoint sources of heavy metals pollution are mostly natural. Chemical and physical weathering of igneous and metamorphic rocks and soils often releases heavy metals into the sediment and into the air. Other contributions include the decomposition of plant and animal detritus, precipitation or atmospheric deposition of airborne particles from volcanic activity, wind erosion, forest fire smoke, plant exudates, and oceanic spray (Kennish, 1992). Anthropogenic sources are contributed by surface runoffs from mining operations usually has a low pH and contains high levels of metals such as iron, manganese, zinc, copper, nickel and cobalt. The combustion of fossil fuels pollutes the atmosphere with metal particulates that eventually settle to the land surface. Urban stormwater runoffs often contain metals from roadways and atmospheric fallout (Connell *et al.*, 1984). Currently, anthropogenic inputs of metals exceed natural inputs. Point sources include domestic wastewater effluents which contains metals from metabolic wastes, corrosion of water pipes, and consumer products. Industrial effluents and waste sludges may substantially contribute to metal loading (Connell *et al.*, 1984).

6. Mode of transport and environmental fate of HMs

Transport occurs mostly in water and air. Water can transport metals that are bound to sediment particles. The primary route for sediment-metal transport is overland flow. Water also transports dissolved metals. Although dissolved metals are primarily transported in overland flow, some underground transport is possible (Nriagu, 1996). Metals that are introduced to the unsaturated zone and the saturated zone will most likely not be transported a long distance. Dissolved metals that are carried below the land surface will readily sorb to soil particles or lithic material in the unsaturated zone and the saturated zone (Nriagu, 1996). Metals introduced into the atmosphere may be carried to the land surface by precipitation and dry fallout. Additionally, because metals readily sorb to many sediment types, wind-borne sediment is a potential route for metal transport (Nriagu, 1996).

7. Regulatory measures applied to TBT and organotins

Zehra Aydin (2002) reported that by the early 1970s, there was clearly a need to promote better use and management of the seas and their resources which imposed a call on the international community to begin negotiating a comprehensive treaty on the law of the sea. What is remarkable is that, these laws had diversified in time to fit specific country`s standards and regulatory needs. For continual assessment, there had then been a growing need to develop suitable analytical tools to assess organotins and heavy metals. In response to this trend, countries with advanced economy began research in this area long ago. Today, a substantial body of knowledge on OTs and heavy metals in waters of the developed countries of Europe, America, Asia and Oceania has evolved. However, data are very scanty for developing nations' water environments (Bryan, 1991; ATRP Corp-U.S-EPA, 2000, 2001 and 2002).

Particularly, the ecotoxicological effects of TBT and other tri-organotin (Leal *et al.*, 1995) compounds in the aquatic environment have caused much concern in recent years leading to the control or banning of their use in a few developed countries (Jiang *et al.*, 2000). At present, it is doubtful if specific legislation exists controlling the use of TBT in many, if not all developing countries (Samson and Shenker, 2000). This is primarily due to the lack of supporting data on the occurrence and impact of TBT in these countries. Tributyltin has been described as "the most toxic substance ever deliberately introduced into the natural waters" (Jiang *et al.*, 2000; Leal *et al.*, 1995; Thomaidis *et al.*, 2001). Owing to its extremely toxic effects to aquatic life at low concentrations, TBT and other forms of organotin such as triphenyltin are legislatively banned to be used as antifouling paints from since the late 1980s in most European and North American countries (Jiang and Yang, 2000). The first regulatory and legislative control on the use of TBT was only adopted in France in 1982 followed by UK in 1985 (Meech *et al.*, 1998). Most of the control measures introduced since then involved banning the use of TBT in marine boats of less than 25 m length (Ceulemans and Adam, 1995). For marine water, the UK adopted an environmental quality target of 20 ng L^{-1} TBT in 1985 and environmental quality standard of 2 ng L^{-1} TBT was proposed in 1989 (Cai *et al.*, 1994). The US Environmental Protection Agency's proposed limits for TBT in fresh and marine waters were 26 ng L^{-1} (4-day average) and 10 ng L^{-1} (4-day average), respectively, (Dirkx *et al.*, 1994). The Canadian Council of the Ministers of Environment derived an Interim Water Quality Guideline of 8 ng L^{-1} TBT in estuarine or seawaters for the protection of aquatic life (Cai and Bayona, 1995).

Levels of TBT of the order of a few hundred ng L^{-1} have been reported in coastal waters with heavy marine traffic, such as ports, marinas and dockyards, as compared to open water where TBT is found to be near or below 10 ng L^{-1} or less for Europe and North America and Hong Kong (Evans *et al.*, 2000; Forstner, 1983; Maguire *et al.*, 1982).

Fatoki, (2000) have reported a preliminary study of TBT in waters and sediments from some major ports in South Africa (Port Elizabeth and East London). This study indicates significant contamination of the East London and Port Elizabeth Harbors' aquatic environment with TBT (Fatoki *et al.*, 2000). This study also indicates contamination levels of 5.5 ng L^{-1} - 22.7 ng L l^{-1} (water samples) and 1.8 ng g^{-1} - 26.2 ng g^{-1} (sediments) for Port Elizabeth. The figures for East London are 3.3 – 49.9 ng L^{-1} and 3.5 – 1103.1 ng g^{-1} for water and sediments, respectively. As such, this should be viewed as danger to the biota in the aquatic system.

8. Regulatory measures applied to heavy metals in marine environments

In 1998, in Aarhus (Denmark), 36 Parties to the Convention on Long-Range Transboundary Air Pollution signed the Protocol on HMs. The Protocol was aimed at the elimination, restriction on use, and reduction of HM emissions to the environment. An integrated program for the inter-comparison study of mercury models was developed (http://www.msceast.org/hms/).

The US Food and Drug Administration (FDA) has set an action level of 1µg g^{-1} (wet mass) for fresh fish (Cai and Bayona, 1995; Lucinda *et al.*, 1983), Canada and several US states have set consumption limits for fish at 0.5µg g^{-1}. The European Union (UE) has set environmental quality objectives of 0.3µg g^{-1} (wet mass), 1µg L^{-1} for continental water, 0.5µg L^{-1} for estuarine water, and 0.3µg L^{-1} for coastal water as total mercury (Cai and Bayona, 1995). In addition to a legally binding mercury treaty, the Global Mercury Assessment Working Group (http://www.mercurypolicy.org) urges governments to establish a non-binding global program of action, and strengthen cooperation among countries on information sharing, risk communication, assessment and related activities. The Working Group recommended immediate action to enhance outreach to vulnerable groups, such as pregnant women and provide technical and financial support to developing countries and to countries with economies in transition. Increased research, monitoring, data collection on the health, environmental aspects of mercury and development of environmentally friendly alternative chemicals to this one are among the group's recommendations. Some countries have seriously taken action to deal with mercury pollution while others still take it slightly, especially the developing countries. The European Union had faced a bill of up to 330 million Euros (US$324 million) to dispose safely of excess mercury stocks from an obsolete method of chlorine production (http://www.mercurypolicy.org/). The U.S. Senate passed legislation in early 2002 (http://h2osparc.wq.ncsu.edu/info/hmetals.html) banning the sale of mercury fever thermometers anywhere in the United States. Similarly, in the same year, the U.S. Environmental Protection Agency proposed changing waste regulations for computers, televisions and mercury containing equipment to discourage the flow of these materials to municipal landfills and incinerators (http://www.mercurypolicy.org).

9. An overview of speciation methods and determination techniques of heavy metals, TBT and other organotins in seawaters

Organotins or butyl compounds (BCs) which are generally of interest for speciation include the tributyltins (TBTs), dibutyltins (DBTs) and monobutyltins (MBTs), as well as the triphenyltins (TPTs), diphenyltins (DPTs) and monophenyltins (MPTs). Amongst them, TBT is acutely toxic to a variety of freshwater species at concentrations down to 0.1 μg L^{-1} (Prudente *et al.*, 1999; Chau *et al.*, 1996). Indeed, this toxicity limits level has been checked for only some marinas in South Africa (Fatoki *et al.*, 2000). Although, the lack of research in this area cannot be over stressed as an underlining factor in setting regulatory limits in developing countries, BT contamination should be regarded as a global pollution problem (Maguire *et al.*, 1982) particularly in countries where no regulation has been implemented such as South Africa.

We have mentioned that TBT and organotins once were the preferred universally available biocides for marine coatings (Mueller, 1987) and large amounts were used (Leal *et al.*, 1995; Kuballa *et al.*, 1995) for pleasure boats, large ship or vessels, docks and fish-nets, lumber preservatives and slimicides in cooling systems, as an effective antifouling agent in paints. Also, that dibutyltins (DBTs) and monobutyltins (MBTs) were mostly used as stabilizers in polyvinyl chlorides and as catalysts in the production of polyurethane foams, silicones, and in other industrial processes (Cai and Bayona, 1995; Fent, 1996). Finally, it suffices to recall that another well-known source (Leal *et al.*, 199) is their use in the manufacture of fungicides, acaricides and insecticides for use in agriculture. And after years of use, their effects on marine environments have brought about actions to limit the use of TBTs through laws and regulations (Kan-atireklap *et al.*, 1997; Jiang *et al.*, 2000; Fatoki *et al.*, 2000), especially in developed countries. With the growing concern regarding the impact on the environment with threats to aquatic life (Kuballa *et al.*, 1995; Kumar *et al.*, 1993) and human health (Fatoki, 2000), an international stakeholders' process (Murmansk-2000) considered a draft treaty to ban the use of TBTs on all hulls worldwide.

Actually, considerable work has been done in the area of techniques development for organotins speciation analysis elsewhere (Mueller, 1987; Prudente *et al.*, 1999; Cai and Bayona, 1995; Ikeda *et al.*, 1996; Jiang *et al.*, 2000; Meech *et al.*, 1998; Abalos *et al.*, 1997) while research efforts in most developing countries, including South Africa are still at their first endeavors at the moment (Fatoki *et al.*, 2000; Ndibewu *et al.*, 2002). Thus, lack of continual consistent research work in this field and lack of monitoring really present potential danger both to the aquatic biota and man. As reported for the case of man-generated heavy metals discharge into the environment (Lucinda *et al.*, 1983; http://www.mercurypolicy.org/), OTs, disperse on a global scale by long-range atmospheric transport and deposit into colder regions could cause an environmental disaster. If the lack of research interest in this area on a global scale stays as such, this will lead to no regular monitoring of water environments in order to avoid potential danger that can be caused by these endocrine-disrupting compounds to human and marine lives including the aquatic ecosystems.

Generally, any procedure for speciation analysis consists of five successive steps (Fatoki, 2000): (i) extraction of the analytes from the sample matrix, (ii) derivatization to form the volatile derivatives, (iii) pre-concentration (iv) clean-up and, (v) determination.

In the first step, extraction is critical, meaning that the choice of a particular extraction technique is also critical. Two extraction methods are popularly used (Abalos *et al.*, 1997), namely: the liquid-liquid (LLE) and the solid phase extraction (SPE) extraction techniques. Liquid-liquid extraction methods often require a large amount of hazardous solvents and tend to be replaced by the solid phase extraction (SPE) procedures (Fent, 1996). The advantage of SPE include a higher pre-concentration factor and ease of application in the field and in on- line systems, while a drawback has been observed in that only filtered samples can be analyzed. More recently, the solid phase microextraction (SPME) technique has been applied to organotin speciation (Attar, 1996; Abalos *et al.*, 1997). SPME offers an attractive alternative method, which minimizes some problems associated with other methods (Fatoki *et al.*, 2000).

Using Liquid-liquid extraction methods, many non-polar and polar solvents have been used for extraction in water, sediment and biological samples. During early techniques applications for organotins determination in water samples, speciation analysis were based on acidification (hydrochloric acid-HCL, hydrobromic acid-HBr or acetic acid-HOAc), to release alkyl tin compounds from the sample matrix, then converting them to the halides or acetate forms (Forstner, 1983). Relatively high polarity solvents are now being used for extraction. These methods (Abalos *et al.*, 1997) succeeded for TBT, TPT and tricyclohexyl (TCyT) and failed for other species due to their high polarity.

For sediment analysis with regard to organotins speciation, acid leaching (Kan-atireklap *et al.*, 1997; Chau *et al.*, 1995; Tanabe *et al.*, 1998) to release organotin compounds from sediment was the basic approach in early use. Hydrochloric acids (HCl), Hdrobromic acid (HBr) and acetic acids (HOAc) are used. This is done in an aqueous or methanolic medium by sonification, stirring, shaking or Soxhlet extraction with an organic solvent (Dirkx *et al.*, 1994). As mentioned above, organotin compounds are not involved in biogeochemical process. They rather bind onto the surface of the sediment, hence, the complete dissolution of the later prior to the analysis is, therefore, not considered necessary. Extraction yield is increased by the addition of complexing agents such as tropolone or DDTC (Fatoki *et al.*, 2000). While the tri- and di-substituted compounds can be extracted quantitatively, only about 60 % or less of the mono-substituted compounds are recovered. Two approaches have been evaluated to improve the extraction efficiency of mono- and di-organotin species: (i) the addition of complexing agents (e.g. diethylammonium-diethylthiocarbamate, DEA-DDC or (DDC), and (ii) alkylation in a reaction cell with Grignard reagent prior to the extraction (Fatoki *et al.*, 2000; Abalos *et al.*, 1997). On one hand, recoveries obtained by the first approach are satisfactory for di- and tri-organotin species but a clean-up step is usually needed. On the other hand, the second method yields satisfactory recoveries only for TBT and TPT. Further developments are needed to bring these methods to routine analysis. Apparently, no reliable and efficient method for extracting all organotins from sediment has yet been developed (Abalos *et al.*, 1997).

Hexane, benzene, toluene or dichloromethane (DCM) are non-polar solvents used for the extraction of organotins with complexing agent (Cai and Bayona, 1995; Jiang *et al.*, 2000; Abalos *et al.*, 1997). The efficiency with which butyltins are extracted from spiked sediment with non-polar solvents in the presence of complexing agents is satisfactory. In contrast, very poor recovery is obtained with monobutyl tin and dibutyltin with DCM without a complexing agent (Abalos *et al.*, 1997). With volatile solvents such as hexane, hexane-acetone, dichloromethane (Abalos *et al.*, 1997; Tanabe *et al.*, 1998; Dirkx *et al.*, 1992), Soxhlet extraction is applied without complexing agent (Willis, 1965), since the more polar solvents are incompatible with the Grignard reagents used later for derivatization and favor co-extraction of organic interference compounds (Fatoki *et al.*, 2000). Therefore, the current recommended procedures (Wade *et al.*, 1988; Abalos *et al.*, 1997) are based on the extraction of low polar organotin complexes with tropolone or diethyldithiocarbanate (DDTC). Tropolone is preferred to DDTC (Dirkx *et al.*, 1994), as under acidic condition, this undergoes decomposition, giving rise to extractable interference (http://h2osparc.wq.ncsu.edu/info/hmetals.html). Sample preparation procedures before analyses, such as liquid-liquid extraction of organotin chelates with fresh tropolone or diethyl dithiocarbamate (DDTC) (Fatoki et al, 2000) are also convenient.

Non-polar solvent plus acids are used in complex matrices' extraction (Tanabe *et al.*, 1998). For example, sediment sample is treated with hydrochloric acid with shaking or sonification, followed by sequential solvent extraction (Wade *et al.*, 1988). Hydrobromic acid or acetic acid or a mixture is also used (Tolosa *et al.*, 1992; Martin *et al.*, 1994). Sonification has become the most widely used stirring method for sediment matrix, whereas, energy-mixing methods are used for biotic materials. Mixtures of solvents have been used to increase the polarity of the medium, hexane-ethyl acetate, hexane -diethyl ether, and chloroform-ethyl acetate (Fatoki, 2000). The salting out effect or ion-pairing effect is used to increase the efficiency of extraction of organotins (OTs) from aqueous phase to the organic phase, when HCl is used (Dirk *et al.*, 1992; Tao *et al.*, 1999). Polar solvents have also been used to achieve extraction. The polar solvents which have been used are aqueous (i) HCl (Ceulemans and Adams, 1995); (ii) HCl or HOAc in polar organic solvents (MeOH, acetone) (Kuballa *et al.*, 1995; Cai *et al.*, 1993); (iii) acetic acid (Quevauviller, 1996); (iv) net polar organic solvents (MeOH, DCM-MeOH, butanol, MeOH-EtOAc (Han and Weber, 1988; Apte and Gardner, 1998); (v) polar organic solvents in basic conditions (Pawliszyn, 1997). In this case, sonification is used in most procedures. Very recently, a focused microwave field has been introduced to reduce extraction time from hours to several munites (Donard *et al.*, 1995). In some cases, after the acid or polar solvent extraction, a liquid-liquid extraction (LLE) with a non-miscible solvent (benzene, CH_3Cl-DCM, ETOAc-MeOH, DCM, hexane, cyclohexane, toluene, hexane-ETOAc) is used to recover OTs from the extract. Several authors (Abalos *et al.*, 1997) have used tropolone and salting out effect to increase the solubility of OTs in the organic solvent. Quite recently, as already mentioned, a more environmentally-friendly extraction technique developed is the supercritical fluid extraction (SFE). Advantages of these methods are shortened extraction time and limited amount of toxic solvents and acids used.

For biological samples analysis, tetramethyl ammonium (TMAH) hydrolysis is currently applied (Fatoki *et al.*, 2000), above room temperature (60°C) for several hours, for example 1-2 h. (Leal *et al.*, 1995). The TMAH hydrolysis can be reduced from hours to minutes when the digestion is carried out under focused microwave irradiation. OTs are isolated from the hydrolyzed tissue by hexane (LLE) in the presence of tropolone. Alternatively, after a pH adjustment, simultaneous extraction derivatization with $NaBEt_4$ is used to reduce the numbers of LLE, compared to Grignard reagents. Also, ethanolic- KOH at 60°C for 90 min or NaOH at 40°C for 20 min followed by pH adjustment and LLE has also been applied to the determination of OTs from biotic matrices (Nagase *et al.*, 1998). The digestion time in basic extraction conditions is critical due to the lack of stability of mono- and di-organotin compounds. Basic and enzymatic hydrolysis methods, which are restricted to biotic samples, lead to tissue solubilization. This makes the embedded organotin more available to extracting agent (Tanabe *et al.*, 1998).

In the case of heavy metals speciation, many extraction techniques have been reported with differences in methods approach depending on the aqueous, solid or gaseous nature of the species. Most of these techniques are in use today depending on individual situations and analytical goals. For the analysis of many metals in seawater or other matrices with strongly interfering elements, several different extraction techniques have been developed using co-precipitation with Co-APDC (ammonium pyrrolidine dithiocarbamate) or FeOH, or reductive precipitation using APDC, NaBH4, Fe, and Pd. These techniques allow quantitative extraction of metals from the interfering matrix. In addition, the extraction serves to pre-concentrate the metals, thus, improving detection limits.

After the above discussion, it is understood that, generally, testing and analysis of environmental pollutants demands the highest quality reagents for calibration and validation. Solvents used in the preparation of standard solutions must be validated free of interfering substances (Chemika-BioChemika Analytika-1995/96, 1905-1923). Quality parameters that need checking are: the physical characteristics and purity of the analytes, gravimetric data pertaining to solution preparation, actual concentration of analyte, chromatographic analysis of finished standard, and the expiration date or scheduled re-assay date. The second step involving derivatization is reviewed. For organotins speciation, GC methods require a derivatization reaction to produce volatile OT compounds for separation (Attar, 1996). The methods of conversion of ionic alkyl tins into gas chromatographable species include: (i) in situ hybridization using $NaBH_4$; (ii) ethylation with $NaBEt_4$; (iii) derivatization using Grignard reagents: methyl-, ethyl-, propyl-, pentyl-, hexyl-magnesium chlorides/bromides.

In in-situ process, Hydride generation with $NaBH_4$ has seldom been used in off-line methods, owing to the lack of hydride stability. However, this derivatization technique combined with CT-QFAAS allows for the determination of butyltins and highly volatile OTs (i.e methyltin), which cannot be determined by most off-line methods (Bayona, 1994). Furthermore; phenyltin cannot be analyzed by this method. The on-line HG-CT-QFAAS methodology allows for the reduction of the sample handling steps to a minimum, which makes this approach tone of the most rapid alternatives for the analysis of OTs (Quevauviller *et al.*, 1989). The amount of derivatization reagent needed to be optimized according to the matrix characteristics, since the matrix can inhibit the hybridization reaction. In this regard, the uncomplexed tropolone suppresses the hydride generation reaction. SPME technique has recently been used for speciation analysis of the hydride derivatives (Bayona and Cai, 1994). This method is also used in generating the hydride volatiles in the analysis of mercury using the cold vapor technique (CVAAS or CVAFS). Boron tetra-ethyl reagents have been developed (Schrader *et al.*, 1983; Leal *et al.*, 1995; Nagase *et al.*, 1995; Mueler, 1984) to minimize analyzing time. This allows carrying out the reaction in aqueous media under buffer conditions. In spiked river sediments, the derivatization yield of MBT using $NaBEt_4$ is lower than that given by hybridization methods, but matrix effects are reduced (Fatoki *et al.*, 2000; Cai *et al.*, 1993). The method is particularly successful for aqueous samples, but lower derivatization yields than those given by the Grignard reactions are observed in complexed matrix containing large amounts of co-extracted compounds. The $NaBEt_4$ procedure allows a simultaneous extraction-derivatization in the buffer medium. The ethylated derivatives are recovered with non-polar solvents (Tao *et al.*, 199). SPME technique has recently been used for speciation analysis of ethyl organotin derivatives (Millán and Pawliszyn, 2000). Alkylation with a variety of Grignard reagents (e.g. methylation, ethylation, propylation, pentylation and hexylation) is the most widely used derivatization technique for water, sediment and the biota (Tolosa et *al.*, 1996). However, the method is time consuming, and requires strict anhydrous conditions and non-protic solvents, which necessitate solvent exchange when polar solvents are used as extracting agents. Furthermore, the LLE step becomes necessary to isolate the derivatized OTs. Cai *et al.*, (1994; 1995) found the formation of dialkyl mono- and disulfide when the derivatization is performed in-situ on a sediment sample before the SFE, which necessitates large excess of Grignard reagents. Similar side reactions occur when the derivatization is performed on the extracts. A wide range of reaction times is reported (Ashby and Craig, 1989) but too long exposure of phenyl to Grignard reagent can lead to deproportionation reactions. Some workers have reported substantial losses of the most volatile tin species when the derivatization is performed with methyl and ethyl Grignard reagents. It is, thus, advisable to avoid evaporation to dryness of derivatized OTs. Another limitation of the methyl derivatives is that they do not allow for the determination of the naturally occurring methylbutyltins.

The next step, usually after the derivatization step is the clean-up phase. Most of the analytical procedures based on GC determination require a clean-up step or process, usually after the derivatization step as mentioned above. Silica is the adsorbent mostly used. Other adsorbent candidates in use are: florisil (Harino *et al.*, 1992), alumina (Dirkx and Adams, 1992), alumina-silica (Willis, 1965), amino and C_{18} cartridges, florisil-alumina, and florisil-silica (Harino *et al.*, 1992; Dirkx and Adams, 1992). In most of the methods applied to sediments that use GC-MS or GC-flame photometric detection (FPD), a desulfurization with activated copper following a clean-up is performed. However, alkylsulfides generated during the Grignard derivatization from elemental sulfur occurring in the sediment are not removed by this procedure. Alternatively, other desulfurization reagents such as tetrabutyl ammonium hydogensulfate and sodium sulfide have been successfully applied (Okamura *et al.*, 2000). Florisil is a preferred adsorbent for biotic matrix with a high lipid content. Hexane or hexane-Et_2O mixtures are the most widely used eluents during the clean-up step because they allow GC determination without evaporation to dryness. More volatile solvent such as pentane is used to minimize the evaporation losses of the most volatile species. Other analytical procedures perform the clean-up before derivatization. Since underivatized OTs have a strong interaction in these adsorbents; polar eluents are needed to achieve quantitative recovery, which leads to poor clean-up efficiency. Tropolone in hexane has been used as an eluent in this case. Today, the most preferred approach, gradually gaining popularity, is the extraction of the analyte earlier derivatized in situ, preferably using sodium tetraethylborate ($NaBEt_4$) (Thompson *et al.*, 1998) and sodium tetrahydroborate ($NaBH_4$) as a derivatization reagent (Balls, 1987). Hydride generation is more prone to interference and in the case of mono substituted organotin; it leads to very volatile derivatives, which can hardly be further pre-concentrated by evaporation of the extracting solvent. In addition, organotins are relatively reactive and decompose when subject to cleanup or harsh instrumentation conditions (Lespes *et al.*, 1998).

The last step, which allows for the compound under investigation to be speciated, is detection. Many techniques have been developed although most of these methods are not commonly used due to their poor sensitivity or cost. From the detection point of view, GC is highly flexible (Fatoki *et al.*, 2000; Ndibewu *et al.*, 2002]. In this respect, the following detector have been used for OTs speciation, GC (Fatoki *et al.*, 2000) coupled to flame ionization detection (FID), flame photometric (FPD) detection (Brickman, 1978); liquid chromatography (LC) (Fatoki *et al.*, 2000), or supercritical fluid chromatography (SFC)

(Martin and Donard, 1994) with spectrometric (AAS) detection (DWAF, 1992; Prudente *et al.*, 1999), atomic emission (AES) spectrometry (Fatoki *et al.*, 2000; Ombaba and Barry, 1992), flame photometric (FPD) detection (Kumar *et al.*, 1993; Fatoki and Ngassoum, 2000; Jiang *et al.*, 2000), electron capture detection (ECD), mass (MS) spectrometry (Fatoki *et al.*, 2000) or induced coupled-plasma (ICP-MS) spectrometry (Fatoki *et al.*, 2000). Most of these techniques are based on an extraction (Ndibewu *et al.*, 2002) step followed by derivatization using Grignard reagents (Fatoki *et al.*, 2000, Abalos *et al.*, 1997), sodium tetrahydroborate (Abalos *et al.*, 1997) or sodium ethylborate (Abalos *et al.*, 1997). However, some analytical techniques allow TBT determination by GFAAS after hybridization and selective extraction in water (Balls, 1987), sediments (Lespes *et al.*, 1998) and biological samples (Prudente *et al.*, 1992, Lespes *et al.*, 1998). ECD and FID were used in the earlier speciation studies but seldom used during the last decade. The lack of selectivity and/or sensitivity of those detection systems for organotins led to their replacement by more sensitive low cost detector such as MS in the electron impact mode, FPD equipped with an interference filter at 610 nm or AAS. The low molecular masses of diagnostic ions in the electron impact or chemical ionization modes impair moderate selectivity in case of complex matrices (Morabito *et al.*, 1995). Similarly, FPD suffers some interference associated with co-extracted sulfur species (Cai and Bayona, 1995). AED is one of the most sensitive and selective detection systems coupled to GC used in OT speciation. However the high cost and maintenance operation of the GC-microwave induced plasma (MIP)-AED system makes it unsuitable to monitoring studies involving a large number of samples.

Despite the more complex sample preparation procedure often required in GC because of insufficient volatility of the ionic organic compounds, GC is preferred (Sasaki *et al.*, 1988; Arakawa *et al.*, 1983) to the liquid chromatography-based technique (Fatoki *et al.*, 2000) which suffers from poor resolution and usually a lack of sensitivity (Yang *et al.*, 1995). Another advantage of GC over LC is the possibility of using several internal standards (IS) and surrogates, which allows the steps of analytical procedure to be traced. The main disadvantage of GC methods is that they usually require production of volatile OT derivatives to perform their separation. Packed columns are used exclusively in cold temperature (CT) when hydride derivatization is carried out. The hydrides are purged with a helium stream and trapped in a U-shaped packed column cooled by liquid N_2. The column is then heated rapidly until the purging step is complete. This method is only successful for the determination of methyl and butyl tins. Capillary column methods gained acceptance during the 1990's (Fatoki *et al.*, 2000) and nowadays, they are commonly used rather than packed or megabore columns. Sample is usually introduced into the column by splitless injection because non-volatile co-injected compound is retained in the liner. Its limitation is the low sample capacity (up to 2 μL) and the discrimination of low volatile OTs against the high volatile tin species. Cold on-column and temperature programmable injectors avoid some of the limitations of the splitless mode and then allow up to 5 μL to be injected. In order to prevent column contamination, GC Tenax packing in the injection port or uncoated deactivated tubing has been used.

The high efficiency achieved by capillary GC (cGC) allows satisfactory resolution of OTs according to carbon number even with non-polar, non-selective stationary phases, such as dimethylpolysiloxane or 5 % diphenyldimethylpolysiloxane (DB-1, HP-1, SE-30). OTs with equal number of carbon co-elute (Mueller, 1987). The mid-polarity stationary-phases such as 50 % diphenyldimethylsiloxane (OV-17) or 14 % cyanopropylphenyl 86 % dimethyl siloxanes (DB-1710) allow the resolution between specific OTs (phenyl and cyclohexyl) (Kuballa *et al.*, 1995).

The use of liquid chromatographic separation is not very popular in speciation procedures. Most of the published works with LC have been done on standards (Fatoki *et al.*, 2000), with few on environmental samples (Yang *et al.*, 1995; Suyani *et al.*, 1989). In spite of the advantage of avoiding derivatization step, LC has some limitation arising from the insufficient sensitivity of the most common detector for the levels found in environmental samples. Butyltin are the most species considered but in some cases phenyltin is considered.

Ion exchange chromatography is performed in the silica-based cation-exchange column and it has been the most applied (Rivaro *et al.*, 1995; Leal *et al.*, 1995). Mobile phases consist of mixtures of methanol or acetonitrile and water containing ammonium acetate or citrate. The separation of TBTs and DBTs amongst the other OTs is achieved at the same pH. In the separation of di- and triorganotin compounds based on normal phase mode, cyanopropyl have been used. The mobile phase consisted of high percentage of hexane together with polar solvent such as ethyl acetate, tetrahydrofuran (THF) and HOAc. A mobile phase consisting of tropolone in toluene has been used (Fatoki *et al.*, 2000). On one hand, reversed-phase with octadecyl silane stationary phase (C_{18}) has been used (Fatoki *et al.*, 2000) in the separation of butyltin compounds in sediments using a polar mobile phase containing complexing agent such as tropolone. On the other hand, reversed-phase ion pair approach has been used in the separation of tri-organotin compounds (Beyer *et al.*, 1997). Polymeric based column (PRP-1) or octylsilane column was used, where pentane sulfonate or hexane sulfonate is used as an ion-pair (Kumar *et al.*, 1993).

Several detectors or hyphenated techniques have been used in LC: AAS, ICP-MS (Beyer *et al.*, 1997), fluorimetry, MS, laser-enhanced ionization (LEI) and ICP-AES. Among different AAS modes, flame AAS with pulse nebulization and off -line GFAAS were the earliest (Fatoki *et al.*, 2000). When ICP-MS is coupled to LC, pneumatic nebulizers and spray chambers are the common systems for sample introduction. ICP methods suffer incompatibility of most of the mobile phases. When fluorimetric detection is used, derivatization with fluorogenic reagent such as flavone derivatives is mandatory. The reaction is performed after chromatographic separation (McKie, 1987).

In any analytical method, a few important parameters are important to assure quality and reliability of the method involved. Some of these parameters are: detection limits, calibration, accuracy and precision. Bearing this in mind during methods development, any analytical methods developed for speciation should, therefore, provide sufficient sensitivity allowing for the determination of individual organotin compounds and elemental heavy metals below set limits. Selected absolute detection limits according to analytical techniques and analytes are reviewed below. Among the non-chromatographic techniques, ion spray mass spectrometry (ISMS-MS) is ca. 4-order of magnitude more sensitive than GFAAS (Fatoki, 2000). In the group of the GC detection techniques, AED, MS in the electron impact (selected ion monitoring) and FPD have the detection limit in the sub-to-low picogram range (Fatoki *et al., 2000;* Ndibewu *et al.,* 2002). The FPD configuration can lead to a remarkable difference in sensitivity. Filterless operation and quartz surface-induced luminescence are the most sensitive detection mode in FPD (Attar, 1996). Unfortunately, the dramatic deterioration of the selectivity due to sulfur emission at 390 nm was found in these operational modes. Also, oxidant flames can lead to poor selectivity since the luminescence at 610 nm is attributed to tin hydride (Gomez *et al.*, 1994; Martin *et al.*, 1987). The sensitivity of the AES is strongly dependent on the plasma source. In this regard, alternating current plasma (ACP-AES) (Ombaba and Barry, 1992) has detection limit at least two orders of magnitude higher than MIP-AES.

The GC-QFAAS techniques have LODs ca. two orders of magnitude higher than the former detection systems (ECD, FPD, MS, AED) coupled to GC techniques. Nevertheless, the suitable design of the interface and GCs columns can improve the sensitivity of AAS by at least one order of magnitude (Kuballa *et al.*, 1995). Among the LC methods, ICP-MS detection (Yang *et al.*, 1995; Suyani *et al.*, 1989), either with ultrasonic or pneumatic nebulization is the most sensitive for all the OTs, and is comparable to the most sensitive GC methods (Kumar *et al.*, 1993). Concerning LC-MS interface, only thermospray has been applied to environmental studies; it has moderate sensitivity with a detection limit about 2- or 3-orders of magnitude higher than ICP-MS. The sensitivity attained with fluorimetric detection depend both on the species and the fluoregenic reagents used, and in some cases very low detection limits are achieved, only improved by LC-ICP-MS by one order of magnitude.

Calibration is another essential operation in the analytical method procedures. In some papers, especially in those devoted to environmental monitoring, little information, if any is provided on this aspect (Abalos *et al.*, 1997) is very limited. In methods based on GC, calibration is generally carried out with an internal standard; however, external standards are almost extensively used. In contrast, the standard addition method is seldom used (Abalos *et al.*, 1997). In those methods that involved cold trapping of volatile species, (hydride or ethyl derivatives) quantitation is usually performed by the method of standard addition or with matrix matched standards (Abalos *et al.*, 1997, Fatoki *et al., 2000)*. When the technique applied is LC, calibration is usually performed with external standards, although the standard addition method is sometimes used (Abalos *et al.*, 1997). When the external standards are used, the standard solution must be subjected to an entire extraction procedure (Tam and Wong, 1995; Sasaki *et al.*, 1988). In other cases, in order to account for the matrix effects, matrix- matched standards are proposed (Han and Weber, 1988). However, suitable analyte-free matrices to match sample matrices may not be available. When using internal standard methods, several approaches are proposed. In the most common approach, the substance used as internal standard (IS) is added to the extracts before the derivatization step, usually as trialkyltin, or just before the injection to the chromatograph as the tetraalkyltin (Fatoki *et al., 2000*, Abalos *et al.*, 1997). In the first case, the IS affords a compensation for the incompleteness of the derivatizatioin reaction, for the possible losses occurring in the operations subsequent to derivatization (extractions, evaporations, clean up) and for the instrumental variability. In the second case, it only compensates for the uncontrolled variations in the chromatographic measurements (Abalos *et al.*, 1997). A second approach consists of the addition of IS (in this case also called surrogate) at the beginning of the extraction process, providing the compensation for the losses taking place in the whole process, including the variability in the determination step (Arakawa *et al.*, 1983; Pereira *et al.*, 1999). Some authors used both the surrogate and IS. This allows for the calculation of the recovery of the substance added as surrogate and, on this basis, correction of the amount of the analytes recovered (Willis, 1965). The substances most commonly used as IS or surrogates are tripropyltin (TPT), tetrabutyltin (TBT), tetraphenyltin

(TePeT), and triphenyltin (TPT). Generally, only IS and or surrogate is used but some alternative approaches have been proposed: (i) the used of different IS's such as monophenyltriethyltin (MPTT), diphenyldiethyltin (DPDT), triphenylethyltin (TPEtT) and tributylmethyltin (TBMEtT), depending on the nature of OTs being determined. This has been shown to be the more accurate way for correcting variations of the alkylation step (Stab *et al.*, 1994), (ii) the use of several surrogates with different degrees of alkylation (Tripropyltin (TPrT), monophenyltin (MPT), diphenyltin (DPT) and triphenyltin (TPT)), in order to mach the behaviour of the different OTs in moieties in the extraction step (Fatoki *et al.*, 2000; Garcia-Romero *et al.*, 1993).

After considering both the detection limits and calibration, the accuracy of the analytical procedures is mostly evaluated through the analysis of either certified reference materials (CRMs) or spiked samples. In the field of OTs in sediments, nowadays, there are two CMRs available (Fatoki *et al.*, 2000): the harbor sediments, PACS-1 with certified value of MBT (280 ± 170, ng g^{-1} as Sn), DBT (1160 ± 180 ng g^{-1} as Sn) and TBT (1270 ± 220 ng g^{-1} as Sn), and the coastal sediment CRM-462 with certified values for DBT (63 ± 8 ng g^{-1} as Sn) and TBT (24 ± 6 ng g^{-1} as Sn) (Fatoki et al., 2000; Abalos *et al.*, 1997). There is also the reference material RM-424, with a reference value for TBT (8 ± 5 ng g^{-1} as Sn) and indicative value for DBT (27 ± 10 ng g^{-1} as Sn) and MBT (174 ± 36 ng g^{-1} as Sn) (Fatoki *et al.*, 2000). The situation now is that, the CRM only allows for the assessment of the accuracy of butyltin compounds, and thus, the need for more CRMs with certified values for other OTs of environmental relevance, such as phenyl tin species is necessary.

Although the analysis of CRMs is preferable to that of spiked samples, only a few papers have reported the use of sediments certified reference materials, and in most cases PACS-1 is the CRM analyzed (Abalos *et al.*, 1997). This is probably due to the fact that PACS-1 was the first CRM available for organotins, or because concentration levels of OTs are higher in PACS-1 than in CRM-462. In relation to the analysis of MBT in PACS-1, some problems have been reported though. None of the ten methods evaluated by Zhang *et al.* (1996) could recover MBT from PACS-1 satisfactorily. A higher scatter of results has also prevented the certification of MBT in CRM-462 (Martin *et al.*, 1994).

In the field of biological samples, only one CRM for OTs has been available since 1991. This is a fish tissue (sea bass) from the National Institute for Environmental Studies (NIES) in Japan, with a certified value for TBT (475 ± 36 ng g^{-1} as Sn), and indicative value of TPHT (1942 ng g^{-1} as Sn (Abalos *et al.*, 1997). Another method for the assessment of the accuracy of the analytical methods is based on the analyses of spiked samples, and the determination of the recoveries obtained for each analyte (Fatoki *et al.*, 2000). The analyses of spiked samples are carried out in most of the papers reviewed for quality assurance. In this case the main problem lies in how the spiking has been performed, probably because; this is one of the most critical points. In any case, experiments should be performed with several kinds of matrices, and at several concentration levels, always in the range of concentrations usually found in environmental samples (Cai *et al.*, 1994). Moreover, it should be taken into account that the availability of spiked analytes in the extraction step can be higher than that of the same substances incorporated into the matrices in the environment. So, using spiked samples can lead to an overestimation of the extraction efficiency, and, therefore, quantitative recoveries from spiked materials do not ensure that the same result will be achieved with natural samples (Abalos *et al.*, 1997).

SAMPLE	SAMPLE TREATMENT STEPS	DETERMINATION TECHNIQUES	SPECIES
Water	1) 50 ml water + 50 acetate buffer pH 3.3 2) 1 mL $NaBH_4$ (3 %) in water) 3) SPME 15 min	GC/FPD	TBT, DBT, MBT.
Water	1) 1000 mL water 70 °C + 0.6 g $NaBH_4$ 2) air purged and trapping Porapak cartridge, 3) CH_2Cl_2 elution, evaporation to 0.1 mL	GC/FPD	TBT, DBT, MBT
Water	1) 250 mL water + adjust pH = 6 tris + AcOH + 1 mL isooctane 0.1 ml $NaBEt_4$ (2 % sol.) stirred 30 min, separation	GC/FPD	TBT, DBT, MBT.
Water	1) 25 ml water + standard 2) + Pd solution	GFAAS	Total tin (Sn)
Water	1) 500 mL H_2O + 5-20 mL HBr (48 %) + standards + 25 mL benzene tropolone, shaking for 15 min., 2) 3 mL MeMgBr (2.5 M sol. In diethylether), for 30 min., 3) Cooling + 25 mL 1 N H_2SO_4, shaking, separation, evaporation to 25 mL	GC/MS (if possible)	TBT, DBT, MBT.
Sediment (Also suitable for water)	1) 200 mL H_2O + 20 mL buffer pH 5 or 3 g wet sediment + 15 g Na_2SO_4, mixing, Soxhlet extraction 9 hrs (110 mL hexane-acetone 9:1, 2) acetate buffer 4 + 10 mL hexane + 4 mL $NaBTEt_4$ (2% sol.), reaction 30 min, separation, evaporation to 1 mL 3) clean up, 0.5 g silica gel 80-100 or alumina elution 5 mL hexane	GC/FPD	TBT, DBT, MBT,
Sediment (Also suitable for water)	1) 1000 mL H_2O + 5 mL conc. HCl 2) + 3* 10 mL pentane extraction by shaking, separation and evaporation to 5 mL 3) + 2 mL MeMgBr sol. reaction 10 min 4) + 5 mL H_2O + 0.5 conc. HCl, separation + $CaCl_2$ evaporation to 1 ml 5) clean up, 0.5 g silica gel 60 elution pentane 1') 20 g wet sediment + conc. HCl to pH 2 2') + 4 - 10 ml diethyl ether extraction by shaking separation and evaporation to 5 ml 3' – 6') following the same steps as for water sample	GC/FPD GC/MS	TBT

SAMPLE	SAMPLE TREATMENT STEPS	DETERMINATION TECHNIQUES	SPECIES
Biological material (biota) (Also suitable for water and sediment)	1) 500-1000l mL water or 1-5 g sediment or 1g fish tissue in 10 ml TMAH + 10 mL hexane or 10-500 l air trapping on carbosive, eluted with hexane 2) Acetate buffer 4 + 10 mL hexane + 4 ml $NaBEt_4$ (2% sol.), reaction 30 min, separation, evaporation to 1 mL 3) Clean up, 0.5 g silica gel 80-100 or alumina elution 5mL hexane	GC/FPD	TBT, DBT, MBT.

Table 1. Recommended analytical procedures for the speciation analysis of organotins

Precision is the hardcore of all analytical operations. The precision of analytical methods reviewed in this chapter corresponds to the whole analytical procedure, that is to say: extraction, the derivatization and the determination technique (Cai *et al.*, 1994). An attempt is made to point out some trends about the precision of the reviewed methods. Two groups including the method commonly applied have been considered: those based on GC-FPD as determination technique and those based on CT-QFAAS. Independent of the analytical method used, the analysis of OTs in biological material gives more precise results than in sediments (Fatoki, 2000; Abalos *et al.*, 1997). For instance, in the case of TBTs, relative standard deviations (R.S.Ds) calculated as the mean of the different methods and concentration, are 12% and 8.5% for sediments and biological materials, respectively. The precision of GC-FPD seems to be, somewhat, better than those using CT-QFAAS: 10.5 versus 13 for sediment and 7 versus10 for biological materials (Fatoki, 2000). This trend is also noticeable in the results of the certification campaign of coastal sediments (CRM-462) of the European Commission (Quevauviller, 1996). One of the reasons for the higher precision for GC FPD may be the fact that ISs are used in the calibration step of this technique, whereas, in the case of CT-QFAAS, the standard addition method is usually applied. The MIP-AED was introduced in the '90s (nineties) in the field of GC. It has not been widely applied to the analysis of OTs. However, some trend in the precision of this technique can be pointed out. An inter-laboratory study carried out in the USA among ten laboratories (Sharron *et al.*, 1995) that analyzed fourteen OTs compounds in three pentylated extracts of soils and sediments gave inter-laboratory R.S.Ds between 2 and 4 % for most compounds. Some researchers have applied GC-MS to OTs analysis, the R.S.D given are higher than the techniques previously commented upon by Fatoki *et al.* (2000).

Various techniques (Unicam, 1992; Prudente *et al.*, 1999; Nriagu, 1996; Fatoki *et al.*, 2002),) have been developed and used for speciation analysis of heavy metals or analysis of total metals. The modification and development of these methods sometimes not only require acute analytical skills but do involve several steps. In order to reduce the number of steps and for optimization purposes], instrumentation design and set-ups nowadays use the combination of a number of the techniques. The validity of an analytical method is based, in part, on the procedures used for sample collection and analysis, and data interpretation. In many instances these procedures use approaches that have been refined over many years and are accepted by professionals as good practice. However, the multitude of variables within a specific workplace requires the professional to exercise judgment in the design of a particular assessment.

TECHNIQUES (Comparative methods and procedures)			Samples and species detected
Liquid-liquid (LLE)	Sodium tetrahydroborate ($NaBH_4$)	GC - AAS or GC - FPD	Tri-, Di- and Mo- clusters of the butyl compounds (TPh, DPhT, MPhT) can be monitored in water, sediment
Liquid-liquid (LLE)	Sodium tetraethylborate ($NaBEt_4$)	GC - AAS or GC - FPD	As above
Liquid-liquid (best solvent from above)	Best reagent out of three: $NaBH_4$, $NaBEt_4$ and EtMgBr	GC - AAS or GC - FPD	As above Water and sediment
Liquid-liquid (best solvent from above)	EtMgBr (Grignard reagent)	GC - MS (compared with GC-AAS/GC-FPD)	monitor both the butyltins and phenyltins (TPh, DPhT, MPh & TPh, DPhT, MPhT) ion species Water, sediment and biota
Liquid-liquid (best solvent)	Best reagent	Best detection technique	Monitoring of butyl and phenyl tins species in water, sediment and biota
Solid-phase Extraction (SPME)	Above protocol followed (slight modifications where necessary)	Slight modifications where necessary	Routine reason Sediment and biota

Table 2. Comparative extraction and detection techniques for speciation of organotins

For the analysis of total metals (including all metals, organically and inorganically bound, both dissolved and particulate) most samples will require digestion before analysis to reduce organic matter interference and to convert metal to a form that can be analyzed by atomic absorption spectroscopy or inductively coupled plasma spectrometry (APHA, 1992),

For speciation analysis, a few common direct determination methods have earlier been employed (Unicam, 1992). These are the dissolved metals by air/acetylene and direct determination with nitrous oxide/acetylene. In water samples analysis, elemental Cd, Zn and Sn have been determined directly by AAS after dissolving in air/acetylene (dissolved metals by air/acetylene). In another technique, Cd and Zn, if present in low levels is chelated, and aspired into the flame prior to detection by AAS (Mueler, 1984). This method consists of chelation with ammonium pyrrolidine dithiocarbamate (APDC) and extraction with methyl isobutyl ketone (MIBK), followed by aspiration into the flame (Liquid-Liquid Extraction Prior to Flame AAS) (Lucinda *et al.*, 1983). Results are achievable by adjusting the pH of the sample and the water blank, to the sample pH as the standard. While organic tin is extracted with solvent, the inorganic tin is determined by AAS after digestion with nitric acid (Unicam, 1992).

For reliability, efficiency and sensitivity, most trace metals analyses currently involve inductively coupled plasma-mass spectrometry (ICP-MS). The standard ICP-MS technique works quite well for many matrices. But for some element/matrix combinations, it gives poor detection limits or accuracy because of elemental or molecular interferences. In choosing the most appropriate methods to analyze any element/matrix combination, ICP-MS has been coupled to dynamic reaction cell (IC-DRC-MS) (Han and Weber, 1988). This combined technique can detect trace levels in complex matrices, where the standard ICP-MS would be prone to interferences; the standard has also been coupled to a micro-mass platform ICP-MS with collision cell technology (IC-ICP-MS) (Han and Weber, 1988). Extremely low detection limits (especially for the higher mass elements) even in matrices traditionally considered difficult are achievable in an ultra-clean sample preparation and analysis environment.

An analytical technique utilizing hydride generation and atomic fluorescence spectrometry (HG-AFS) (Unicam, 1992) or atomic absorption (HG-AAS) has been developed for the analysis of arsenic, antimony, and selenium at either ultra-trace levels or in complex matrices. With HG-AFS, we can accurately measure total arsenic, antimony, and selenium in nearly all matrices at single-digit parts-per-trillion levels [http://www.frontiergeosciences.com/ebru]. Speciation information could be determined using modifications of this technique, including cryogenic trapping/GC and ion chromatographic separation (Wade *et al.*, 1988).

For mercury speciation, relatively poor sensitivity is provided by transitional flame absorption. Alternate atomization techniques for the AA determination of this element have been developed (Cai and Bayona, 1995; Shrader *et al.*, 1983; Maguire *et al.*, 1982; Wade *et al.*, 1988). Amongst them, the cold vapor atomic absorption technique has received the greatest attention (Schrader *et al.*, 1983, Wade *et al.*, 1988). Other techniques employ cold vapor atomic fluorescence spectrometers (CVAFS) (http://www.frontiergeosciences.com/ebru/), which give unparalleled sensitivity for the determination of low-level total mercury. Using this detector in combination with gold amalgamation or aqueous phase ethylation plus gas chromatographic separation allows determination of Hg speciation at the parts-per-quadrillion level (Wade *et al.*, 1988). Furnace methods for mercury are not recommended due to the extreme volatility of mercury, which has a significant vapor pressure even at room temperature (Stab *et al.*, 1992; Maenpa *et al.*, 2002). Although the first cold vapor principle was proposed by Poluekov and co-workers in 1963, the most popular method credited to Hatch and Ott was published in 1968 (Shrader *et al.*, 1983). In this method, an acidified solution containing mercury is reacted with stannous chloride in a vessel external to the AA instrument. Ground state mercury atoms are produced which subsequently are transported by an air or inert gas flow to an absorption cell installed in the AA instrument. This method provides sensitivities approximately four orders of magnitude better than flame AA (Schrader *et al.*, 1983; Wade *et al.*, 1988). It is critical to note that, unlike in the case of organotins speciation where a global approach is favorable, heavy metals speciation will very much require methods choice to consider the thermodynamics of the elemental compound (solid/liquid or gaseous state at room temperature). Therefore, methods for each metal speciation will be specific although the principle underlining the different steps are similar.

9.1 Methods and techniques for the determination of heavy metals in water, sediment and biota samples

Generally, for direct atomic absorption spectroscopy or inductively coupled plasma spectrometry, the sample must be colourless, transparent, odourless, single phase, and have a turbidity of < 1 Nephelometric Turbidity Unit. Otherwise, the sample must first be digested. The following digestion methods are generally used:

- Digestion methods (open beaker).
- Nitric acid digestion: digestion is complete when solution is clear or light-colored.
- Nitric acid-hydrochloric acid digestion: complete when digestate is light in color.
- Nitric acid-sulphuric acid digestion: digestion is complete when solution is clear.
- Nitric acid-perchloric acid digestion: digestion is complete when solution is clear and white $HClO_4$ fumes appear.
- Nitric acid-perchloric acid-hydrofluoric acid digestion: digestion is complete when solution is clear and white $HClO_4$ fumes appear.

For individual metals analysis, requirements vary with the metal and the concentration range to be determined (APHA, 1992) as follows:

Dithizone Method: Mercury ions react with dithizone solution to form an orange solution that is measured in the spectrophotometer. This method is most accurate for samples with [Hg] > 2μ L^{-1}. Known interferences are: Copper, gold, palladium, divalent platinum, and silver react with dithizone in acid solution.

Mercury: Cold vapor atomic adsorption method (CVAAS): detection Limits: Choice of method for all samples with [Hg] < 2μ L^{-1}. Here, there are no known interferences.

For the analysis of solid samples such as sediments and tissues, direct determination is not possible due to the very large matrix effects that are encountered. In order to provide accurate determination in these complex matrices, specialized digestion procedures is required that not only brings the analyte of interest into solution, but also diminishes the interfering compounds present in the matrix as much as possible. The relative extreme low detection limits that are achievable with cold vapor atomic absorption spectrometry (CVAAS) offer the option of dilution or smaller aliquot sizes to overcome sample matrix issues.

Due to the volatile nature of mercury compounds, wet digestion methods are preferred over other trace metal preparation techniques such as dry ashing. Tissue samples can be prepared for total mercury analysis using a heated mixture of nitric and sulfuric acids. After the tissues have been fully solubilized, the digestate can be further oxidized by the addition of BrCl, to bring all the mercury to the Hg^{2+} oxidation state. At the time of analysis, a sub-aliquot of the digested sample can be reacted with $SnCl_2$ to reduce the mercury to its elemental form, which can then be concentrated on a trap filled with gold-plated sand and introduced into the CVAFS instrument by thermal desorption with argon as a carrier gas. Tissues can be digested for methylmercury using a heated mixture of potassium hydroxide and methanol. A small aliquot of this digestate can be reacted with sodium tetraethyl borate to produce the volatile methyl-ethyl mercury species. All forms of mercury can be collected on activated carbon traps, and can be introduced into an AAS with an argon carrier gas. The detection limit is somewhat elevated due to the small analytical aliquot required to overcome matrix interference. However, this procedure is preferred as it allows for complete digestion. This allows more accurate results than are possible for other methodologies such as distillations, and most tissues samples (especially from higher organisms) have sufficient methylmercury concentrations to allow the smaller aliquot size.

Sediment for methyl mercury analysis is prepared by extraction into methylene chloride from sulfuric acid/potassium bromide/copper sulfate slurry. After extraction, an aliquot of the methylene chloride layer is placed in reagent water and the solvent is purged completely from the solution with an N_2 gas stream, leaving the methylmercury in the relatively clean water matrix. A sub-aliquot of the water matrix is treated with sodium tetraethyl borate and is analyzed in the same manner as methylmercury in tissue (described above). This procedure is particularly useful as it isolates the methylmercury from the interfering matrix, and allows a large sample aliquot to be analyzed, which yields low detection limits. The extraction method was developed (Harino *et al.*, 1992) in order to overcome artifact formation that was present in the commonly used distillation procedure.

For water sample analysis, samples can be treated with 25 mL of 4% $KMnO_4$ to break up the organo-mercury compounds. Adding excess hydroxylamine sulphate and passing clean nitrogen through the sample removes free chlorine gas formed during the oxidation step. Reduction of mercury can be carried out in a similar manner to the other hydride forming elements. Samples can be placed in a reaction vessel (normally 20 mL). 1-2 mL of 20 % by weight $NaBH_4$ in concentrated HNO_3 can be placed in another vessel outside the cold vapor kit. The solutions can be conveyed into an enclosed system by a circulating peristaltic pump. The mercury vapor formed can then be flushed out of the system into a T piece aligned in the optical path of the AA instrument for recording.

For the analysis of cadmium (Cd) and lead (Pb) using the flame atomic absorption method, the sample is aspirated into a flame and atomized. The amount of light emitted is measured. Detection range may be extended (1) downward by scale expansion or by integrating the absorption signal over a long time and (2) upward by dilution of sample, using a less-sensitive wavelength, rotating the burner head, or by linearizing the calibration curve at high concentrations. Chemical interference occurs by a lack of absorption by atoms that are bound in molecular combination by the flame. By using electrothermal atomic absorption spectrometry, the high heat of a graphite furnace atomizes the element being determined and use of a larger sample volume or reduced flow rate of the purge gas increases sensitivity (detection limit: $0.1 \mu g\ L^{-1}$). Interferences by broadband molecular absorption and chemical (formation of refractory carbides) and matrix effects are common. The use of inductively coupled plasma (ICP) method with ionization of an argon gas stream by an oscillating radio frequency and high temperature dissociates molecules, creating ion emission spectra yielding detection limit $> 4.0\ 1 \mu g\ L^{-1}$. Spectral interference from light emissions originating elsewhere (other than the source) and other physical interference from changes in sample viscosity and surface tension can affect sensitivity. In the determination of Cd, and Zn by liquid-liquid extraction prior to flame AAS, ammonium pyrrolidine dithiocarbamate (APDC) is used to chelate the compounds. Aspiration into the flame follows after extraction with methyl isobuthyl ketone (MIBK). To achieve results in normal conditions, the pH of the sample and the water blank are adjusted to the same pH as the standards. pH range for maximum extraction is 1-6 for Cd and 2-4 for Zn.

Samples are placed in a 200 or 250 mL separatory funnel fitted with a teflon stopcock and 4 ml of acetate buffer of pH 6.2 added. The mixture is well agitated. 5 mL of 1% w/v mixed solution of ammonium pyrrolidinedithiocarbamate and diethylammonium diethyldithiocarbamate in water (chelating agent) is added. The total mixture is briefly agitated and 10 - 20 mL of methyl isobutyl ketone (MIBK) is be added. The mixture is vigorously agitated for 60 seconds. The layers are allowed to separate. The lower aqueous layer is removed while the MIBK layer is retained in the tightly capped glass bottles until sample is ready for analysis. A standard of Cd and Zn stock solution are prepared so that 200 mL of water that is extracted would contain 1-20 µg Cd or Zn L^{-1}. In this way, a direct concentration relationship would exist with samples. A reagent blank is run and the sample is analyzed (AAS) under instruments recommended conditions (Van Loon, 1985).

For the determination of arsenic (As) by continuous flow hydride generation (CF-HG-AAS), suitable for volatile metals that produce a metal hydride, the sample is treated with sodium borohydride in the presence of HCL, and then detected by AAS. If recovery is poor, interring organics could be removed by passing the acidified sample through a resin.

TECHNIQUES (Methods and Procedures)		Observations
Extraction/Separation	Detection	
Microsolid phase extraction (MSE)	Flame photometry AAS	Water, sediment, biota
Liquid-Liquid Extraction (LLE): Open beaker digestion and extractive Conc. methods	Flame photometry AAS	Cd and Zn in water and sediment samples, Detection of Hg
Hydride Generation	CF-HG-AAS	As in water, sediment and Biota
Cold Vapor Technique	CV - AAS	Hg in water, sediment and biota

Table 3. Summary of techniques for speciation and determination of selected heavy metals

9.2 Sampling and sample location

In the investigation of the freshwater and marine waters environment, water, sediment and the biota, samples should be taken within the study program-site time schedule from selected locations that reflect different sea regions (for example, Atlantic and Indian oceans) and related shipping activities of that particular location. Sampling for heavy metals analysis, apart from the marine sites, should include other sites such as from rivers (sampling sites can be fixed). Locations such as upstream, midstream and downstreams the rivers should be targeted. Lakes or municipal stream water environments can also be considered. For biological materials, biota, more logically, sourcing should be matched as much as possible to the various sites chosen for freshwater and marine sampling.

About 2.5 L subsurface water samples should be collected at each sampling site. Before sampling, sample bottles should be cleaned by washing with detergent and then soaked in 50 % HCl for 24 h. Finally, bottles should be washed with water and then rinsed with doubly distilled or deionized water. Core sediment samples should be collected at the same site used for water samples by divers. Both sample types should be kept at about 4 °C until analyzed. The biota should be fresh and bought from catchmen direct from source.

9.3 Quality assurance planning

The accuracy of the method should be demonstrated by analyzing the samples and by performing spiking experiments with water samples and reference sediment materials as outlined in the methods above. In order to carry out a successful quality assurance program, the following plan is necessary and should be strictly implemented.

- Staff organization and responsibilities.
- Sample control and documentation procedures.
- Standard operating procedure for each analytical method and
- Analyst training requirements.
- Preventive maintenance procedure for equipment.
- Calibration procedures and corrective actions.
- Internal quality control activities and performance audit.
- Data assessment procedures for bias and precision, validation, and reporting.

10. Conclusion and recommendations

Both organotins (OTs) and Heavy metals (HMs) have been implicated in endocrine disrupting activities (Mueller, 1987; Fatoki *et al*., 2000; Ndibewu *et al*., 2002). Despite their potential danger to man and the ecosystem, the manufacture and uses of these compounds are not currently controlled in many developing countries. TBT-based antifouling paints are still currently being manufactured in some developing countries and there appears to be no legislation regulating use in the environment. Thus, there is the potential for significant contamination of marine water environments by TBT and heavy metals; hence, they need to be regularly monitored to prevent potential danger to man and the ecosystem due to their endocrine disrupting activities. Also, it is observed that there is a shortage of research capacity in this field, particularly in Africa, explaining why data are very scanty on the occurrence and levels of these toxic compounds. The toxicity of OTs and heavy metals and the ulta-trace levels at which they exist in the aquatic environment make it extremely important to have sensitive and reliable analytical methods available for their determination. Such techniques are not yet commonly available. The need to develop some of these techniques is of topical importance to analytical scientists.

11. Acknowledgements

Information presented in this chapter was partly researched through the endocrine disrupting contaminants (EDCs) global initiative funded by the National Research Foundation (NRF) of South Africa. The remainder of the chapter has been written based on the authors' own scientific endeavour.

12. References

[1] Abalos, M., Bayona, J.M., Compano, R., Leal, C. and M. D. Prat. (1997). Analytical procedures for the determination of organotin compounds in sediment and biota: critical review. J. Chromatogr. A. 788, 1- 49.

[2] Advanced Technology Research Project Corporation (2000, 2001, 2002). ATRP Corp.; U.S. EPA, Region VI; Murmansk Marine Biological Institute.

[3] Apte, S. C. and M. J. Gardner. (1998). Determination of organotins in natural waters by toluene extraction and graphite-furnace AAS. Anal. Chem., 1989, 61, 2320.
[4] Arakawa, Y., Wada, O., and M. Manabe. (1983). Extraction and fluorimetric determination of organotin compounds with morin. J. Chromatogr. 207, 237.
[5] Ashby, J. R. and P. J. Craig. (1989). New method for the production of volatile organometallic species for analysis from the environment: some butyltin levels in UK sediments. Sci. Total Environ., 78, 219.
[6] ATSDR-ToxFAQs - Cadmium http://www.atsdr.cdc.gov/tfacts5.html[Accessed 2011]
[7] ATSDR-ToxFAQs - Mercury http://www.atsdr.cdc.gov/tfacts46.html[Accessed 2002]
[8] Attar, K. M. (1996). Analytical Methods for Speciation of Organotins in the Environment. Applied Organometallic Chemistry. 10(5). 317-337.
[9] Balls, P. W. (1987).Tributyltin (TBT) in the waters of a Scottish sea loch arising from the use of antifoulant treated netting by salmon farms. Aquaculture, 65, 227 - 237.
[10] Barjaktarovic, L., Elliott, J. E. and A. M. Scheuhammer. (2002). Metal and Metallothionein Concentrations in Scoter (*Melanitta* spp.) from the Pacific Northwest of Canada, 1989-1994. Arch. Environ. Contam. Toxicol. 43, 486-491.
[11] Bayona, J. M. and Y. Cai. (1994). The role of supercritical fluid extraction and chromatography in organotin speciation. Trends in Anal. Chem. 13(8), 327 - 332.
[12] Beyer, W. N., Spalding, M. and M. Morrison. (1997). Mercury Concentrations in Feathers of Wading Birds from Florida. Ambio. 26, 2.
[13] Bryan, G. W. And P. E. Gibbs. (1991). Impact of low concentrations of tributyltin (TBT) on marine organisms: A review. In Metal Ecotoxicology Concepts & Applications, ed. M. C. Newman & A. W. McIntosh. Lewis Punlishers, pp. 323–361.
[14] Cai, Y., Alzaga, R. and J. M. Bayona. (1994). In situ derivatization and supercritical-fluid extraction for the simultaneous determination of butyltin and phenyltin compounds in sediment. Anal. Chem. 66, 1161 - 1167.
[15] Cai, Y., and J. Bayona. (1995). Determination of methlmercury in fish and river water samples using in situ sodium tetraethlborate derivatization following by solid-phase microextraction and gas chromatography-mass spectrometry. J. Chromatogr. A. 696, 113-122.
[16] Cai, Y., Rapsomanikis, S. and O. A. Meinrat. (1993). Determination of butylin compounds in sediment using gas chromatography-atomic absorption spectrometry: comparison of sodium tetrahydroborate and sodium tetraethylborate derivatization methods. Analytica Chimica Acta, 274(3), 243-251.
[17] Ceulemans, M. and F. C. Adams. (1995). Evaluation of sample preparation methods for organotin speciation analysis in sediments - focus on monobutyltin extraction. Anal. Chim. Acta. 317, 161 - 170.
[18] Chau, Y. K, Yang, F. and R. J. Maguire. (1996). Improvement of extraction recovery for the mono butlyltin species from sediment. Anal. Chim. Acta 320, 165 - 169.
[19] Coello, W. F. and M. A. Q. Khan. (1996). Protection Against Heavy Metal Toxicity by Mucus and Scales in Fish. Arch. Environ. Contam. Toxicol. 30, 319-326.
[20] Corr, J. J. and E. H. Larsen. (1996). Arsenic Speciation by Liquid Chromatography Coupled with Ion spray Tandem Mass Spectrometry. J. Atom. Absorpt. Spetr., 12, 1225.

[21] Crighton, J. S., Carroll, J., Fairman, B., Haines, J. and M. Hinds. (1996). Industrial Analysis: Metals, Chemicals and Advanced Materials. J. Atom. Absorpt. Spetr., 1996, 12, 461R.

[22] Determination of tin species in environmental samples. (Technical Report). International Union of Pure and Applied Chemistry Oct 1998. .

[23] Dirkx, W. M. R. and Adams, F. C. (1992). Speciation of organotin compounds in water and sediments by gas chromatography - atomic-absorption spectrometry (GC - AAS). Mikrochim. Acta. 109, 79.

[24] Dirkx, W. M. R.; Lobinski, R.; and F. C. Adams. (1994). Speciation analysis of organotin in water and sediments by gas chromatography with optical spectrometric detection after extraction separation. Anal. Chim. Acta, 286, 309-318.

[25] Donard, O. F. X., Lalere, B., Martin, F. and R. Lobinski. (1995). Microwave-assisted leaching of organotin compounds from sediments for speciation analysis. Anal. Chem. 67, 4250.

[26] Donard, O. F. X. In: R. M. Harrison and S. Rapsomanikis (Eds.), Environmental Analysis Using Chromatography Interfaced with Atomic Spectroscopy, Horwood, Chichester, 1989, p. 188.

[27] DWAF (1992) Analytical Methods Manual, TR 151. Department of Water Affairs & Forestry, Pretoria.

[28] Espadaler, I., Caixach, J., Om, J., Ventura, F., Cortina, M., Paune, F. and J. Rivera. (1997). Identification of organic pollutants in Ter river and its system of reservoirs supplying water to Barcelona (Catalona, Spain): A study by GC/MS and FAB/MS. Wat.Res. 31(8), 1996-2004.

[29] Evans, S. M., Kerrigan, E. and N. Palmer. (2000). Causes of Imposex in the Dogwhelk Nucella lapillus (L.) and its Use as a Biological Indicator of Tributyltin Contamination. Marine Pollution Bulletin, 40, 212-219.

[30] Fatoki, O. S. and M. B. Ngassoum. (2000). Tributyltin Analysis in Water and Sediments from Port Elizabeth and East London Harbours by GC FPD.(Tech. note).

[31] Fatoki, O. S., Ngassoum, M. B and A. O. Ogunfowokan. (2000). Speciation Analysis of Organotins in Water, Sediment and Biota (Literature Review).

[32] Fent, K. (1996).Ecotoxicology of organotin compounds.Crit.Rev.Toxicol.,26(1),1-117.

[33] Forstner, Ulrich and Gottfried T. W. Wittmann "Metal Pollution in the Aquatic Environment" Springre-Verlag: Berlin, 1983. National Toxicology Program's Health and Safety Information Sheet on Cd.

[34] Garcia-Romero, B., Wade, T. L., Salata, G. G. and J. M. Brooks. (1993).Butyltin concentration in oysters from the Gulf of Mexico from 1989 to 1991. Environmental Pollution. 81, 103 - 111.

[35] Gomez Ariza, J. L., Morales, E., Beltran, R., Giraldez, I. and M. R. Benitez. (1994). Sampling and storage of sediment samples for organotin.Appl.Organomet.Chem.9, 51.

[36] Han, J. S. And J. H. Weber. (1988). Speciation of methyl- and butyl-tin compounds and inorganic tin in oysters by hydride-generation atomic-absorption spectrometry. Marine Chem., 25, 279.

[37] Harino, H, Fukushima, M. and M. Tanaka. (1992). Simultaneous determination of butyltin and phenyltin compounds in the aquatic environment by gas chromatography. Anal. Chim. Acta, 264, 91.

[38] http://h2osparc.wq.ncsu.edu/info/hmetals.html[Accessed 2002].
[39] http://www.frontiergeosciences.com/ebru/[Accessed 2011].
[40] http://www.igc.org/[Accessed[2011].
[41] http://www.mercurypolicy.org/[Accessed 2010].
[42] http://www.msceast.org/hms/[Accessed 2001].
[43] http://www.osha.gov/SLTC/cadmium/index.html[Accessed 2003].
[44] Ikeda, M., Zhang, Z.W., Moon, C. S., Imai,Y., Watanabe, T., Shimbo, S.M, W.C. Lee, C.C. and Y.L. Guo. (1996). Background Exposure of General Population to Cadmium & Lead in Tainan City, Taiwan. Arch. Environ. Contam. Toxicol., 30, 121 - 126.
[45] Inma, F. E. and J. M. Bayona. (1997). Supercritical fluid extraction of priority organotin contaminants from biological matrices. Anal. Chim. Acta 355, 269 - 276.
[46] Jiang, G. B., Ceulemans, M. and F. C. Adams. (1996). Optimization study for the speciation analysis of organotin and organogermanium compounds by on-column capillary gas chromatography with flame photometric detection using quartz surface-induced luminescence. Journal of Chromatography A, 727, 119-129.
[47] Jiang, G. B., Liu, J. Y. and K. W. Yang. (2000). Speciation analysis of butyltin compounds in Chinese seawater by capillary gas chromatography with flame photometric detection using insitu hydride derivatization followed by headspace sold-phase microextraction. Anal. Chim. Acta 421, 67 - 74.
[48] Jiang, G., Liu, J. and K. Yang. (2000). Speciation analysis of butyltin compounds in Chinese seawater by capillary gas chromatography with flame photmetric detection using in-situ hdride derivatization followed by headspace solid-phase microextraction. Anal. Chim. Acta 421, 67 - 74.
[49] Kan-atireklap, S., Tanabe, S. and J. Sanguansin. (1997). Contamination by Butyltin Compounds in Sediments from Thailand. Marine Pollution Bulletin. 34(11),894 - 899.
[50] Kan-atireklap, S., Tanabe, S. and Sanguansin, J., Tabucanon, M. S. and Hungspreugs (1997). Contamination by Butyltin Compounds and Orgamochlorine Residues in Green Mussel (*Perna viridis, L.)* from Thailand Coastal Waters. Environmental Pollution. 97(1-2), 79 - 89.
[51] Kan-atireklap, S., Yen, N. T. H., Tanabe, S. and A. N. Subramanian. (1998). Butyltins, organochlorines and Organochlorine residues in green mussels (*Perna viridis, L.)* from India. Toxicological and Environmental Chemistry. 67, 409 - 424.
[52] Krull, I. S. And K. W. Panaro. (1985). Trace analysis and speciation for methylated organotins by HPLC - hydride generation – direct-current plasma emission spectroscopy. Appl. Organomet. Chem., 3,295.
[53] Kuballa, J., Wilken, R. D., Jantzen, E., Kwan, K. K. and Y. K. Chau. (1995). Speciation and genotoxicity of butyltin compounds. Analyst 120 (3), 667 - 673.
[54] Kumar, T. U., Dorsey, G. J., Caruso, J. A. and E. H. Evans. (1993). Speciation of inorganic and organotin compounds in biological samples by liquid chromatography with ICP-MS detection. J. Chromatogr. A, 654, 261-268.
[55] Leal, C., Grandos, M., Prat, M. D. and R. Compano. (1995). Labelling of organotin compounds for fluorometric detection. Anal. Chim. Acta, 314, 175.
[56] Lespes, G., Desauziers, V, Montigny, C. and M. P. Gautier. (1998). Optimization of solid-phase microextraction for the speciation of butyl- and phenyltins using experimental designs. J. Chromatographr. A. 826(1), 67 – 76.

[57] Lespes, G., Pinasseau,C. C., Gautier, M. P. and M. Astruc. (1998). Direct Determination of Butyl- and Phenyltin Compounds as Chlorides Using Gas Chromatography and Flame Photometric Detection. Analyst. 123 (5), 1091 - 1094.

[58] Looser, P. W., Berg, M., Fent, K., Muhlemann, J., and R. P. Schwarzenbach. (2000). Phenyl- and Butyltin Analysis in Small Samples by Cold Methanolic Digestion and GC/MS. Anal. Chem. 72, 5136 - 5141.

[59] Lu, J. Y., Chakrabarti, C. L., Back, M. H. Sekaly, A. L. R., Gregoire, D. C. and W. H. Schroeder. (1996). Speciation of Some Metals in River Surface Water, Rain and Snow, and the Interactions of These Metals With Selected Soil Matrices. J. Atom. Absorpt. Spetr., 12, 203.

[60] Lucinda, M. V. (1983). Determination of the priority pollutant metals - Regulations and Methodology.Varian Instruments at Work, Varian Atomic Absorption. AA-34,(9).

[61] Lucinda, M. V. (1983). Dealing with matrix interferences in the determination of priority pollutant metals by furnace AA. Varian Instruments at Work, Varian Atomic Absorption. No. AA-35(9).

[62] Lucinda, M. V., Covick, L. A and D. E. Shrader. (1983). The Determination of the priority pollutant metals using the CRA-90 Carbon Rod Atomizer. Varian Instruments at Work, Varian Atomic Absorption. No. AA-33(9).

[63] Maenpa, K. A., Kukkonen, J. V. K. and M. J. Lydy. (2002). Remediation of Heavy Metal-Contaminated Soils Using Phosphorus: Evaluation of Bioavailability Using an Earthworm Bioassay. Arch. Environ. Contam. Toxicol. 43, 389-398.

[64] Maguire, R. J., Chau, Y. K., Bengert, G. A., Hale, E. J.,Wong, P. T. S. and O. Kramar. (1982). Occurrence of organotin compounds in Ontario lakes and rivers. Environ. Sc. Technol. 16, 698 - 702.

[65] Martin-Landa, I., De Pablos, F., and I. L. Marr. (1989). Determination of organotins in fish and sediments by gas chromatography with flame photometric detection. Appl. Organomet. Chem., 5, 399.

[66] Martin, F. M., Tseng, C. M., Belin, C., Quevauviller, P. and F. X. Donard. (1994). Interferences generated by organic and inorganic compounds during organotin speciation using hydride generation coupled with cryogenic trapping, gas chromatographic separation and detection by atomic absorption spectrometry. Analytica Chimica Acta, 286(2), 343-355.

[67] Martin, F. M. and O. F. X. Donard. (1994). Interference mechanisms and reduction during the speciation of organotin compounds by hydride generation, cryoseparation and detection by atomic absorption spectrometry. Trends in Anal. Chem., 11, 17.

[68] Martin, P. J. and P. S. Rainbow. (1998). The kinetics of zinc and cadmium in the haemolymph of the shore crab *Carcinus maenas* (L.), Aquatic Toxicology. 40, 2-3, 203-231.

[69] Matschullat, J. (1997).Trace Element Fluxes to the Baltic Sea: Problems of Input Budgets. Ambio. 26, 6.

[70] MCkie, J. C. (1987). Determination of total Tin and Tributyltin in marine biological materials by electrothermal Atomic Absorption Spectrometry. Anal. Chim. Acta 197, 303-308.

[71] Meech, J. A., Veiga, M. M. and D. Tromans. (1998). Reactivity of Mercury from Gold Mining Activities in Darkwater Ecosystems. Ambio. 26, 2.

[72] Millán, E. and J. Pawliszyn. (2000). Determination of butyltin species in water and sediment by solid-phase microextraction–gas chromatography–flame ionization detection. Journal of Chromatography A, 873, 63 -71.
[73] Morabito, R., Chiavarini, S. and C. Cremisini, in Ph. Quevauviller (ed.), Quality Assurance for Environmental Analysis, Elsevier,Amsterdam, 1995, Chapter 19, p.435.
[74] Mueler, M. D. (1984). Tributyltin Detection at Trace levels in water and sediments using GC with Flame-Photometric Detection and GC-MS. Anal. Chem. 317, 32 - 36.
[75] Mueller, M. D. (1987). Comprehensive trace level determination of organotin compounds in environmental samples using high-resolution gas chromatography with flame photometric detection. Anal. Chem. 59, 617.
[76] Muyssen, B. T. A. and C. R., Janssen. (2002). Accumulation and Regulation of Zinc in *Daphnia magna*: Links with Homeostasis and Toxicity. Arch. Environ. Contam. Toxicol. 43, 492-496.
[77] Nagase, M., Kondo, H. and K. Hasebe. (1995). Determination of tributyltin and triphenyltin compounds in hair and fish using a hydrolysis technique and gas chromatography with flame photometric detection. Analyst. 120, 1923.
[78] Nagase, M., Toba, M., Kondo, H. and K. Hasebe. (1998). Determination of dibutyltin compounds in soft polyurethane foam by gas chromatography with flame photometric detection. Analyst. 1091 - 1094.
[79] National Toxicology Program's Health and Safety Information Sheet on Cd. http://ntp-b.niehs.nih.gov/NTP_Reports/NTP_Chem_H&S/NTP_Chem7/
Radian7440.
[80] Ndibewu, P. P. And O. S. Fatoki. (2002). Development of speciation methods for the determination of organotins and heavy metals in the freshwater and marine environments. Unpublished.
[81] Nriagu, J. O. (1996). History of Global Metal Pollution. Science,Vol. 272 (4),223-224.
[82] Okamura, H., Aoyama, I., Takami, T., Maruyama, Y., Suzuki, M., Matsumoto, I., Katsuyama, J., Hamada, T., Beppu, O., Tanaka, R. J., Maguire, D., Liu, Y. L., Lau and G. J. Pacepavicius. (2000). Phytotoxicity of the New Antifouling Compound Irgarol 1051 and a Major Degradation Product. Marine Pollution Bulletin.40, 754-763.
[83] Ombaba, J. M. and E. F. Barry. (1992). Determination of organotin species by capillary gas chromatography with alternating current plasma emission detection. Journal of Chromatography A, 598(5), 97-103.
[84] Organometals and Organometalloids, ocurrence and fate in environment, ACS Symposium Series 82 (Brickman Bella J. M. (eds) (1978) Zuckermann JJ, Reisdorf PR, E11 HV, Wilkinson RR,-Washington, p 388.
[85] Pascoe, G. A., Blanchet, R. J. and G. Linder. (1996). Food Chain Analysis of Exposures and Risks to Wildlife at a Metals-Contaminated Wetland. Arch. Environ. Contam. Toxicol. 30, 306-318.
[86] Pawliszyn, J. (1997). Solid Phase Microextraction. John Wiley & sons Ltd, New York.
[87] Pereira, W. E., Wade, T. L., Hostettler, F. D. and F. Parchaso. (1999). Accumulation of Butyltins in Sediments and Lipid Tissues of the Asian Clam, Potamocorbula amurensis, Near Mare Island Naval Shipyard, San Francisco Bay. Marine Pollution Bulletin, 38 1005-1010.

[88] Prudente, M., Ichihashi, H., Kan-atireklap, S., Watanabe, I. and S. Tanabe. (1999). Butyltins, organochlorines and metals in green mussels, *perna viridis L.* from coastal waters of the Phillipines. Fisheries Science 65(3), 44 -447.

[89] Quevauviller, P., Lavigne, R., Pinel, R. and Astruc, M. (1989). Organotins in sediments and mussels from the Sado Estuarine system (Portugal). Environ. Pollut., 1989, 57, 149 - 166.

[90] Quevauviller, Ph. (1996). Atomic Spectrometry Hyphenated to Chromatography for Elemental Speciation: Performance Assessment Within the Standards, Measurements and Testing Programme (Community Bureau of Reference) of the European Union. J. Atom. Absorpt. Spetr., 12.

[91] Regoli, F.,Nigro,M. and E.Orlando.(1998).Lysosomal & antioxidant responses to metals in Antarcticscallop *Adamussium colbecki*, AquaticToxicology.40(4),375-392.

[92] Reisch, M. S. Paints and coatings. Chemical Engineering News 1996, 44049.

[93] Richardson and S. Gangolli. In: The Dictionary of Substances and Their Effects Royal Society of Chemistry, Cambridge (1994), p. 288 and 344.

[94] Rivaro, P., Zaratin, L., Frache, R. and A. Mazzucotelli. (1995). Determination of organotin compounds in marine mussel samples by using high-performance liquid chromatography - hydride-generation inductively coupled plasma atomic-emission `pectrometry. Analyst, 120, 1937.

[95] Roos, J. T. H. and W. J. Price. (1971). Mechanisms of interference and releasing action in atomic absorption spectroscopy-III, Interference of iron on chromium absorption. Spectrochimica Acta. 26B, 441 - 444.

[96] Samson, J. C. and J. Shenker. (2000). The teratogenic effects of methylmercury on early development of the zebrafish, *Danio rerio.* Aquatic Toxicology.40, 2,3,203- 231.

[97] Sasaki, K., Suzuki, T. and Y. Saito. (1988). Determination of tributyltin and dibutyltin compounds in yellowtails. Bull. Environ. Contam. Toxicol. 41, 888.

[98] Sasaki, K., Ishizaka, T., Suzuki, T. and Saito, Y. (1988). Determination of tributyltin and dibutyltin compounds in fish by gas chromatography with flame photometric detection. Assoc. of Anal. Chem. 126.

[99] Sharron, D., Swami, K. And R. L. Jansing. (1995). Rapid ultratrace analysis of tributyltin in aqueous matrixes by purge-and-trap gas chromatography with flame-photometric detection. J. AOAC Int., 78(5), 1317 - 1321.

[100] Shrader, D. E, and W. B. Hobbins. (1983). The Determination of Mercury by Cold Vapor Atomic Absorption. Varian Instruments at Work, Varian Atomic Absorption. No. AA-32, September.

[101] Shrader, D. E, Lucinda, M. V. and L. A. Covick. (1983). The Determination of toxic metals in waters and wastes by furnace Atomic Absorption. Varian Instruments at Work, Varian Atomic Absorption. No. AA-31, June.

[102] Stab, J. A., Van Hattum, B., De Voogt, P. and U. A. T. Brinkman. (1992). Preparation of pentylated organotin standards for use in trace analysis with gas chromatography. J. Chromtogr. A, 609, 1955.

[103] Stab, J. A. Cofino, W. P., Van Hattum, B. and U. A. T. Brinkman. (1994). Assessment of transport routes of triphenyltin used in potato culture in the Netherlands. Appl. Organomet. Chem. 8,577.

[104] Stewart, F. M., Furness, R. W., Monteiro, L. R. and L. R. Monteiro. (1996). Relationships Between Heavy Metal and Metallothionein Concentrations in Lesser Black-Backed Gulls, *Larus fuscus*, & Cory's. Arch. Environ. Contam. Toxicol. 30, 299-305.

[105] Strategic plan for the Health Related Water Issues (HRWI) research field. Version 1.2B (7/02/2001). p9.

[106] Suyani, H., Creed, J., Davidson, T. and J. Caruso. (1989). Inductively coupled plasma mass spectrometry and atomic-emission spectrometry coupled to high-performance liquid chromatography for speciation and detection of organotin compounds. Appl. Spectr.6, 962 - 967.

[107] Tam, N. F. Y., and Y. S. Wong. (1995). Spatial and temporal variations of heavy metal concentration in sediments of a mangrove swamp in Hong Kong. Marine Pollution Bulletin 31, 54–261.

[108] Tanabe, S., Prudente,M., Mizuno., Hasegawa, T., Iwata, H. and N. Miyazaki. (1998). Bututyltin contamination in marine mammals from north Pacific and Asian coastal waters. Environmental Science and Technology. 32, 193 -198.

[109] Tao, H., Rajendran, R. B., Quetel, C. R., Nakazato, T., Tominaga, M. and A. Miyazaki. (1999). Tin speciation in the femtogram range in open ocean seawater by gas chromatography/inductively coupled plasma spectrometry using a sheild torch at normal plasma conditions. Anal. Chem. 71, 4208 - 4215.

[110] Thomaidis, N. S., Adams, F. C., and Lekkas, T. D. (2001). A simple method for the speciation of organotin compounds in water samples using ethylation & GC-QFAAS.

[111] Thompson, J. A, J., Douglas, Y. K. S., Chau, Y. K. and R. J. Maguire. (1998). Recent studies of residual tributyltin in coastal British Columbia sediments. Applied Organometallic Chemistry. 129(8-9), 643-650.

[112] Tolosa, I., Merlini, L., de Bertrand, N., Bayona, J. and J. Albageis. (1992). Occurrence and fate of tributyl-andtriphenyltin compounds in western Mediterranean coastal enclosures. Environmental and Toxicological Chemistry. 11, 145-155.

[113] Toth, S., Becker-van Slooten, K., Spack, L., de Alencastro, L. F. and J. Tarradellas. (1996). Irgarol 1051, an antifouling compound in freshwater, sediment, and biota of Lake Geneva. Bull. Environ. Contam. Toxicol. 57, 426-433.

[114] Unicam AAS Methods Manual (1992). 1.1-27. 207.

[115] Wade, T. L., Garcia-Romero, B., Brooks, J. M. (1988). Tributyltin contamination in bivalves from United States coastal estuaries. Environ. Sci. Technol. 22,1488.

[116] Willis, J. B. `The analysis of biological materials by Atomic-absorption Spectroscopy`, from the Division of Chemical Physics, Commonwealth Scientific and Industrial Organization, Melbourne, Australia, Vol. 11, No. 2, Supp.,1965. pp251-258.

[117] Woller, A., Garraud, H., Martin, F., Donard, O. F. X. and Péter. (1996). Determination of Total Mercury in Sediments by Microwave-assisted Digestion-Flow Injection-Inductively Coupled Plasma Mass Spectrometry. J. Atom. Absorpt. Spetr., 2, 461R.

[118] Yang, H. J., Jiang, S., Yang, Y. and C. Hwang. (1995). Speciation of tin by reversed liquid gas chromatography with inductivedly coupled plasma mass spectrometric detection. Anal. Chim. Acta 312, 141 - 148.

3

Use of *Enterococcus*, BST and Sterols for Poultry Pollution Source Tracking in Surface and Groundwater

Vesna Furtula[1], Charlene R. Jackson[2], Rozita Osman[3] and Patricia A. Chambers[1]
[1]*Aquatic Ecosystem Impacts Research Division, Environment Canada, North Vancouver, British Columbia,*
[2]*Bacterial Epidemiology and Antimicrobial Resistance Research Unit, USDA-ARS, Athens, Georgia,*
[3]*Faculty of Applied Sciences, Universiti Teknologi MARA, Shah Alam, Selangor,*
[1]*Canada*
[2]*USA*
[3]*Malaysia*

1. Introduction

Maintaining and preserving the quality of surface and ground waters involves many challenges, one of the most serious being bacteriological contamination caused by discharge of human and animal waste. Water resources may become contaminated with pathogens from human or animal feces as a result of malfunctioning wastewater operations (treatment plants or septic systems), stormwater or combined sewer overflows, poor management practices for storing or land-applying livestock manure, and defecation by livestock and wildlife in or near surface waters. Pollution source identification is crucial in order to improve best management practices and eliminate consequent health risks to the general public and aquatic ecosystems. Distinguishing between human and animal sources of fecal pollution in water has been a subject of many studies (Tyagi et al., 2009a). Microbial source tracking methods have employed a wide range of micro-organisms (e.g., fecal coliforms, total coliforms, bifidobacteria, *E. coli*, enterococci) for identifying sources of water pollution, but each has certain limitations (Tyagi et al., 2009a). Moreover, many microbes are not host-specific, making them ineffective for source identification. Chemical methods for fecal source tracking include analysis of sterols, bile acids, caffeine, whitening agents etc., with sterols being the most widely used indicator compound (Bull et al., 2002; Saim et al., 2009; Tyagi et al., 2009b). Both classes of methods have been somewhat successful in identifying pollution sources but not fully evaluated and accepted as established methods in environmental studies.

Enterococci are the second most studied group of bacteria in the field of microbial source tracking (following *E. coli*) due to their connection to humans and animals as well as their recent significance as a clinical pathogen (Figueras et al., 2000; Aarestrup et al., 2002; Scott et al., 2005) and ability to persist in the environment (Harwood et al., 2000). Different strains of enterococci populate the digestive tracts of humans and animals, making them a good indicator of water contamination. A metabolic fingerprint database developed by Ahmed et al., (2005) for enterococci was able to distinguish between human and animal sources despite the fact that a number of biochemical phenotypes were found in multiple host groups. Bacterial Source Tracking (BST) uses unique genetic markers in *Bacteroides* (naturally occurring bacteria in the intestinal flora) to identify organisms responsible for fecal pollution in aquatic environments, and has been used for detection of bacteriological contamination from different sources such as humans, ruminant animals, dogs, pigs, horses, and elk (Bernhard et al., 2000a,b; Dick et al., 2005a,b). Unfortunately, primers for poultry and other birds are not available.

Sterols are organic molecules, a family of compounds that occur naturally in animals, plants and fungi. They have a steroid ring structure and varying functional groups that confer specific characteristics (such as polarity, bioactivity and lipophilicity) to the molecule. Coprostanol, the major compound in human faeces and a product of the microbial reduction of cholesterol in the higher animal guts, has been considered an indicator of faecal pollution. Other cholesterol congeners (campesterol, sitosterol and stigmasterol) are also degraded by bacteria in the intestinal tract of higher mammals to stanols. Higher concentrations of coprostanol have been found in human sewage than in animal wastewater and concentrations of stigmastanol and epicoprostanol were usually higher in animal (cows, pigs, and poultry) than in human wastewater (Blanch et al., 2004). Sterol analysis, a widely used chemical method for identifying fecal pollution sources is based on the fact that different sterol compounds are associated with human or animal waste and their presence/absence and relative concentrations and ratios can be used as an indication of the origin of water contamination (Chou & Liu, 2004; Devane et al., 2006; Gilpin et al., 2003; Bull et al., 2002; Jardé et al., 2007a, b; Saim et al., 2009).

Interpretation of findings from these and other markers can be improved by the application of chemometric techniques which are gaining ground in evaluation of environmental data (Brodnjak-Voncina et al., 2002; Mendiguchía et al., 2004; Singh et al., 2005; Terrado et al., 2011). The most common chemometric methods are cluster analysis (CA) and principal component analysis (PCA) with factor analysis (FA). The goal of CA is to identify groups of objects (such as sampling sites) that give similar, homogenous results with respect to extent or type of fecal pollution, whereas PCA enables a reduction in data and description of a given multidimensional system by a smaller number of new variables (Loska & Wiechula, 2003). Pollution sources and dischargers can also be identified using PCA (Einax et al., 1998; Loska & Wiechula, 2003).

The Fraser River valley of British Columbia is considered the poultry capital of Canada. The poultry waste generated from the industry is used as fertilizer and spread onto the fields, thus creating a non-point source run-off type of surface and ground water pollution. The objective of this study was to determine the extent and sources of fecal contamination in surface and ground water in this poultry dominated agricultural area. In particular, we tested *Enterococcus* isolates as source tracking indicators for poultry in combination with chemical indicators sterols, BST and chemometric analysis.

2. Materials and methods

2.1 Sample collection

Surface water was collected from 12 sites and ground water was sampled at 28 sites in the Abbotsford area of British Columbia, Canada, near poultry farms and berry farms that use poultry litter as fertilizer (Figure 1). Surface water was sampled for bacteriological water quality and for sterol analysis in December 2009; all samples were grab water collections. Ground water was sampled in April, August and December 2009 for microbial water quality and sterols. At each site, three full well volumes were pumped out of the piezometer (purged) using a submersive Hydrofit pump prior to sampling with low density polyethalene (LDPE) tubing (dedicated for each well) located close to the well screen. A minimum of three line volumes were purged from the sample tubing prior to sample collection.

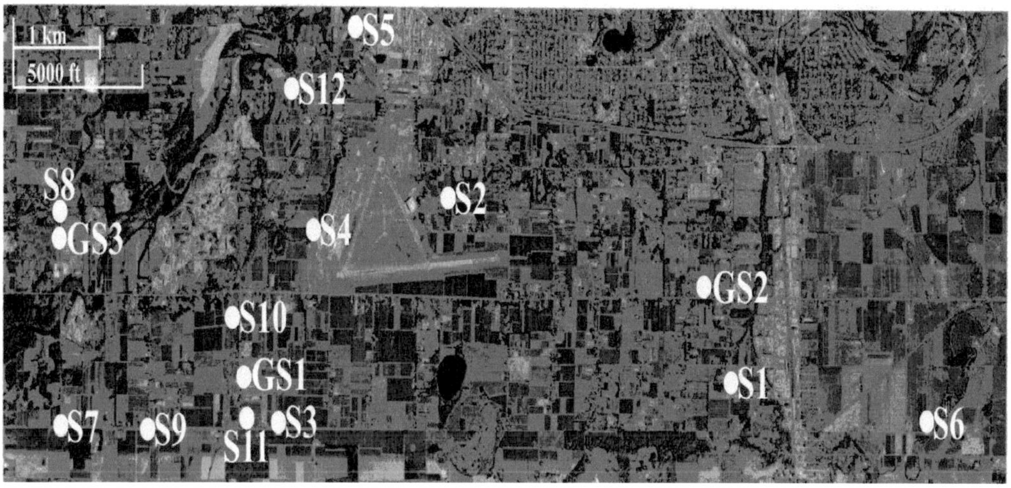

Fig. 1. Aerial map of the sampling area located in the Lower Fraser Valley region of British Columbia, Canada. "S" and "GS" indicate surface water and groundwater sampling sites, respectively. The map was generated using Google Maps

Water samples were collected in: (1) 250-mL sterile polypropylene bottles for bacteriological analyses (total and fecal coliform, *E. coli* and *Enterococcus*); (2) certified clean one liter amber glass bottles for sterol analysis and (3) one liter sterile polypropylene bottles for BST analysis. Samples were placed on ice packs in coolers (~ 4°C) and shipped to the laboratory where they were kept in a cold-room (≤4°C) until analyzed. Samples for BST analysis were filtered within 24 h of collection.

Litter samples were collected from two different poultry farms: a broiler farm and a layer farm, in at least three different locations in the poultry barn. Samples from broiler barns (total of 4) were collected at the beginning (day 3) and end of the production cycle (day 35). Samples were collected by an analyst wearing gloves and using a sterile scoop, and placed into sterile falcon tubes. The samples were kept on ice until analysis, which was performed within 24 h of collection (samples from broiler farm). Samples from layer farms were collected once, frozen after collection and analyzed at a later date.

2.2 Bacteriological analysis

Analysis of enterococci in water samples was performed using a membrane filtration technique whereby samples retained on filter paper were incubated on mE agar for 48 h at 41°C followed by incubation on Esculin Iron Agar (EIA) for 20 minutes at 41°C (USEPA, 2000). Colonies that appeared pink to red with dark precipitation on EIA were verified using Biolog Microbial ID system in combination with Biolog Gram Positive Aerobic Bacteria Database (Release 6.01, Biolog, Hayward, CA) Results are reported as colony-forming units (cfu) per unit volume.

For enterococci in poultry litter samples, 5-6 g of litter was weighed into 10-ml of 0.85% sterile saline in a sterile 50-mL falcon tube. The tube was vortexed on high for one minute and serial dilutions were plated on KF streptococcal agar (Difco, Detroit, MI). Red or pink colonies on the KF agar were verified using Biolog Microbial ID system in combination with Biolog Gram Positive Aerobic Bacteria Database (Release 6.01, Biolog). Isolated colonies of confirmed *Enterococcus* were inoculated into 5 ml of tryptic soy broth containing 6.5% NaCl and incubated for 5 - 12 hours at 35°C; one milliliter of this culture was then combined with 325 µL 80% glycerol (20% glycerol final concentration) and stored at -40°C until further analysis. Confirmed *Enterococcus* isolates were identified to species level using multiplex PCR (Jackson et al., 2004).

Total and fecal coliform and *E coli* analyses of water samples were performed using procedures based on "British Columbia Environmental Laboratory Manual for the Analysis of Water, Wastewater, Sediment and Biological Materials" (2005 Edition) (Horvath, 2009).

2.3 Sterol analysis

Analytical grade standards were purchased from Sigma-Aldrich (Oakville, ON) for 17 compounds (mestranol, norethindrone, equol, estrone, equilin, norgestrel, 17 α-ethinylestradiol, 17 α-estradiol, 17 β-estradiol, estriol, coprostanol, epicoprostanol (cholestanol), cholesterol, desmosterol, campesterol, stigmasterol and β-sitosterol); equol was purchased from Fluka (Oakville, ON). Primary standards were made in acetone at a concentration of 1 mg/ml and stored at -20°C. Acetylated mixture calibration standards of 0.02 to 0.5 µg/L were made every two months and stored at -20°C. Surrogate 17 β-estradiol-d3 and internal standard p-terphenyl-d14 were added to every sample. Solvents, sodium chloride and potassium carbonate were purchased from VWR (Edmonton, AL) and all chemical reagents were of analytical grade.

Sterol extraction and detection were conducted according to the sterol method used at the Pacific Environmental Science Centre, North Vancouver BC, Canada (Environment Canada, 2005). Briefly, 800 mL of unfiltered sample was acidified with sulfuric acid to pH ~ 3 and surrogate β-estradiol-d_3 was added. After stirring samples with 100 ml of dichloromethane for two hours, they were transferred into separatory funnels and the organic layers separated. Samples were then concentrated and derivatized with pyridine/acetic acid and re-extracted with petroleum ether in the presence of 10% potassium carbonate solution. The organic layers were concentrated to near dryness and reconstituted in 200 µl of internal standard (p-terphenyl-d_{14}).

Extracted samples for sterol analysis were injected into Agilent 5973 MS system (injector 280°C), carried by helium flow of 1.2 mL/min, separated on Rtx-5ms column (30 m x 0.25

mm x 0.25 µm film thickness) by the following temperature gradient: initial temperature 70°C hold for 1 min, 30°C/min to 180°C, 5°C/min to 310°C and hold on 310°C for 4 min. Eluting compounds were analyzed by mass spectrometer and ChemStation software (revision A.01.01, Palo Alto, CA) and sterols quantitated using internal standard method. List of sterols and their limits of quantification are presented in Table 1. Quality control blanks and spikes were run with each batch of samples. Various sterol ratios were calculated to determine the presence of fecal contamination and its likely source (Table 2).

2.4 Bacterial Source Tracking (BST)

BST analysis was conducted according to the BST method used at the Pacific Environmental Science Centre, North Vancouver BC, Canada (Environment Canada, 2006). One liter water samples were filtered through AP15 prefilters (Millipore Corporation, Billerica, MA) to remove large pieces of material. Prefiltrate was split into two aliquots (500 ml each), which were then filtered through 0.22 µm filters (Supor-200, PALL Corporation, Ann Arbour, MI). The filters were stored individually in 15 mL tubes containing 0.5 mL of GITC lysis buffer (5M guanidine isothiocyanate, 100 mM EDTA and 0.5% sarkosyl) at -20°C.

Sterol	Common names	Formula	LOQ (µg/L)
24*α*-Methyl-5-cholesten-3*β*-ol	Campesterol	$C_{28}H_{48}O$	0.005
Cholest-5-en-3 *β*-ol	Cholesterol	$C_{27}H_{46}O$	0.009
5*β*-Cholestan-3*β*-ol	Coprostanol	$C_{27}H_{48}O$	0.005
3*β*-cholesta-5,24-dien-3-ol	Desmosterol	$C_{27}H_{44}O$	0.008
3- *β*-5- *β* -cholestan-3-ol,	Dihydrocholesterol (cholestanol)	$C_{27}H_{48}O$	0.007
Cholest-5-en-3 *α*-ol	Epicoprostanol	$C_{27}H_{18}O$	0.005
1,3,5,7-Estratetraen-3-ol-17-one	Equilin	$C_{18}H_{20}O_2$	0.07
3,4-Dihydro-3-(4-hydroxyphenyl)-2H-1-benzopyran-7-ol	Equol	$C_{15}H_{15}O_3$	0.1
	17α-Estradiol	$C_{18}H_{24}0_2$	0.01
	17β-Estradiol	$C_{18}H_{24}0_2$	0.01
1,3,5(10)-Estratriene-3,16α,17β-triol	Estriol	$C_{18}H_{24}O_3$	0.01
3-Hydroxyestra-1,3,5(10)-trien-17-one	Estrone	$C_{18}H_{22}O_2$	0.02
19-Norpregna-1,3,5(10)-trien-20-yne-3,17-diol	17α-Ethinylestradiol	C_{20}-H_{24}-O_2	0.1
17α-Ethynyl-1,3,5(10)-estratriene-3,17β-diol 3-methyl ether	Mestranol	$C_{21}H_{26}O_2$	0.01
13β-Ethyl-17α-ethynyl-17β-hydroxygon-4-en-3-one	Norgestrel	$C_{21}H_{28}O_2$	0.07
19-nor-17alpha-ethynyl-17beta-hydroxy-4-androsten-3-one	Norethindrone	$C_{20}H_{26}O_2$	0.08
5-Stigmasten-3β-ol	β-Sitosterol	$C_{29}H_{50}O$	0.007
24-Ethylcolesta-5,22E-dien-3*β*-ol	Stigmasterol	$C_{29}H_{48}O$	0.007

Table 1. Sterols and limits of quantification (LOQ)

For each sample, DNA was extracted from one AP15 pre-filter and one 0.22 µm filter. DNA extraction was performed with the Qiagen DNeasy kit (Mississauga, ON), and the manufacturer's instructions were followed with the following exception: for the first steps,

Buffer AL (provided with the kit) and 100% ethanol (Commercial Alcohols, Langley, BC) were added to the 15 ml tubes (containing filters and GITC buffer) in 1:1:1 ratios with 1 minute of vortexing after each addition of a liquid.

Ratio #	Sterol Compound Ratio	Human Fecal Contamination (a)			Literature Reference
		Yes	Unsure	No	
1	Coprostanol / (Coprostanol + Cholestanol) 5β/(5β+5α)	> 0.7	0.3 - 0.7	< 0.3	Devane 2006; Bull 2002; Fattore 1996; Chan 1998; Grimalt 1990; Carreira 2004; Froehner 2009; Marvin 2001; Patton 1999; Reeves 2005; Zhang 2008; de Castro Martin 2007
2	(Coprostanol + Epicoprostanol) / (Coprostanol + Epicoprostanol + Cholestanol)	> 0.7	0.3 - 0.7	< 0.3	Bull 2002; Reeves 2005
3	Epicoprostanol / Coprostanol	< 0.2	0.2 - 0.8	> 0.8	Froehner 2009; de Castro Martin 2007
4	Coprostanol / Cholesterol	> 0.5	-	< 0.5	Gilpin 2003; Fattore 1996; Carreira 2004; Patton 1999; Reeves 2005; Zhang 2008
5	Coprostanol / Cholestanol	> 0.5 >0.4	0.3 - 0.5	< 0.3	Devane 2006; Roser 2006 Shah 2007
6	Coprostanol / (Cholestanol + Cholesterol)	> 0.2	0.15 - 0.2	< 0.15	Chan 1998
7	Coprostanol / Epicoprostanol	> 1.5	-	< 1.5	Fattore 1996; Marvin 2001; Patton 1999; Reeves 2005; Zhang 2008

Ratios for Differentiating Sources of Fecal Contamination (b)

#	Ratio	Value*	Source	
8	(Coprostanol + Epicoprostanol) / Cholesterol	>3.7 <0.7	pig chicken and/or cow	Jardé 2007
9	(Campesterol + Sitosterol) / Cholesterol	>1.5 <1	pig/chicken/cow human	Jardé 2007
10	Epicoprostanol / (Coprostanol + Cholestanol)	<0.01 >0.1	human cattle/horse/deer	Standley 2005

Table 2. Sterol ratios for identifying (a) human fecal contamination and (b) differentiating sources of fecal contamination

Three aliquots (600 µl each) were loaded onto the DNeasy columns and washed according to the manufacturer's protocol. The pure genomic DNA samples were stored at -20°C in sterile 1.5 ml tubes (Fisher Scientific, Ottawa, ON). Extracted DNA was amplified by Polymerase Chain Reaction (PCR) carried out with a DNA engine Tetrad 2 (Bio-Rad Laboratories Canada, Toronto, ON). The samples were tested with all *Bacteroides* primers available (Table 3), which identify feces from humans, ruminant animals, pigs, horses, dogs, elk, and general *Bacteroides*. After agarose gel electrophoresis of PCR samples, gels were visualized and scored in a bio-imaging system (Gene Genius, Fisher Scientific, Ottawa, ON) and the program GeneSnap was used to capture the image from a CCD camera. Positive matches were made by correlating the bands with the DNA ladder and the known size of the positive bands as published (Bernhard et al., 2000a,b, Dick et al., 2005a,b). All negative controls (included at every stage) were blank and all positive controls worked appropriately.

Organism	Primer Set	reference
Human	HF134F / HF654R	Bernhard et al., 2000b
	HF183F / Bac708R	Bernhard et al., 2000b
Ruminant Animal	CF128F / Bac708R	Bernhard et al., 2000b
	CF193F / Bac708R	Bernhard et al., 2000b
Pig	PF134F / Bac708R	Donation from K. Field
	PF163F / Bac708R	Dick et al., 2005b
Horse	HoF597F / Bac708R	Dick et al., 2005b
Dog	DF475F / Bac708R	Dick at al., 2005a
Elk	EF447F / EF990R	Dick at al., 2005a
General *Bacteroides*	Bac32F / Bac708R	Bernhard et al., 2000a

Table 3. Bacterial Source Tracking (BST) primers

2.5 Chemometric approach

The goal of the chemometrics approach is to display the most significant patterns in the complex data sets. The most popular statistical methods are principal component analysis (PCA) which provides information on the most meaningful parameters to describe a large data set and cluster analysis (CA) which identifies natural groupings within a data set. Sterol data were used in both PCA and CA; the statistical analyses were performed by XLStat2009 statistical program.

Principal component analysis (PCA) generated principal components (PCs). Varimax rotation was applied on the PCs with eigenvalues greater than 1 (Kim & Mueller, 1987) in order to obtain new groups of variables called varimax factors (VFs) that better interpret the data set (Juahir et al., 2009). Cluster analysis applied on surface water samples data identified similarities in the sterol composition and grouped sampling sites accordingly.

3. Results

3.1 Bacterial contamination

Total coliform, fecal coliform and *E. coli* in surface water ranged from 100-17,000 cfu/100 mL, <1-700 cfu/100 ml and <1-690 cfu/100 mL, respectively (Table 4). Several groundwater locations also tested positive for total coliform ranging from 25-17000 cfu/100 ml, although the majority of groundwater samples showed no evidence of total coliform contamination (Table 5). Only one location, BC-008, consistently tested positive for total coliform.

Enterococcus was detected in all surface water samples and at 3 groundwater sites. *Enterococcus* counts ranged from 2 to 2100 cfu/100 mL for surface water samples (Table 4) and 1 to 5 cfu/100 ml for groundwater samples (Table 5). Seven enterococci were isolated from groundwater, 85 were isolated from surface water samples and 163 were isolated from poultry litter, for a total of 255 isolates. In the August 2009 sampling, the groundwater site 94-SH-29 had one presumptive *Enterococcus* isolate but the confirmation test did not verify this result. Previous samplings of the 94-SH-26 site and 94-SH-29 site in November 2008 (data not presented) had similar issues, yielding 49 and 74 presumptive enterococci respectively, but none of the presumptive results were confirmed.

Sample location	Total Coliforms	Fecal Coliforms	E. coli	Enterococcus
S1	2700	26	7	9
S2	500	5	4	6
S3	17000	<1	<1	12
S4.	800	95	95	10
S5	560	2	1	2
S6	2500	56	22	52
S7	100	7	6	29
S8	2500	700	690	2100
S9	3200	2	2	71
S10	1300	13	6	2
S11	1200	6	6	7
S12	2800	5	5	11

Table 4. Bacterial counts for surface water sites

	Apr-09		Aug-09		Dec-09	
Field ID	Total Coliforms	*Enterococcus*	Total Coliforms	*Enterococcus*	Total Coliforms	*Enterococcus*
94Q14	<1	<1	2	<1	n/s*	n/s
94Q20	<1	<1	1	<1	n/s	n/s
94Q27	<1	<1	<1	<1	n/s	n/s
PC25	<1	<1	<1	<1	n/s	n/s
PC35	<1	<1	2	<1	n/s	n/s
PC55	<1	<1	440	<1	<1	<1
PC75	<1	<1	<1	<1	n/s	n/s
PB55	<1	<1	2	<1	n/s	n/s
PB75	<1	<1	<1	<1	n/s	n/s
91-11	<1	<1	240	1	n/s	n/s
91-12	<1	<1	30	<1	n/s	n/s
91-15	n/s	n/s	n/s	n/s	<1	<1
ABB5	<1	<1	390	<1	n/s	n/s
ABB3	60	<1	4	<1	n/s	n/s
ABB-10	n/s	n/s	n/s	n/s	8	<1
ABB-06	n/s	n/s	n/s	n/s	1500	<1
ABB-02	n/s	n/s	n/s	n/s	3	<1
91-3	7	<1	230	<1	n/s	n/s
91-1	<1	<1	<1	<1	<1	<1
94-SH-26	1400	<1	<1	<1	22	<1
94-SH-29	3100	<1	<1	1**	2200	<1
BC-008	25	<1	17000	5	4400, 4800	<1
BC349	<1	<1	5	<1	1	<1
US-04	n/s	n/s	n/s	n/s	1	<1
US-02	n/s	n/s	n/s	n/s	10	1
FT7-22	n/s	n/s	n/s	n/s	2500	<1
FT5-12	n/s	n/s	n/s	n/s	1	<1
FT1-24	n/s	n/s	n/s	n/s	14	<1

Table 5. Bacterial counts for groundwater (colony counts in cfu/100 mL).*n/s-not sampled, **not confirmed as *Enterococcus*

3.2 Identification of enterococci

From speciation analysis, *E. faecalis* accounted for the largest portion of the environmental isolates at 26.6% (n=25), but *E. faecium* was a close second at 24.5% (n=23). *E. mundtii* (n=12), *E. durans* (n=9), *E. casseliflavus* (n=8), *E. hirae* (n=4), *E. gallinarum* (n=2) and *E. raffinosus* (n=1) were also present. All 29 isolates from the litter samples from the layers farm were *E. faecium*. Broiler barns were tested for *Enterococcus* on Day 3 (close to beginning of production cycle) and Day 35 (end of the production cycle). Samples collected on Day 3 contained a fairly even mix of *E. gallinarum* (27.6%; n=29), *E. faecalis* (26.7%; n=28), *E. faecium* (16.2%; n=17) and *E. hirae* (25.7%; n=27) as well as smaller numbers of *E. cassiflavus* (n=1), *E. durans* (n=1), and two isolates that reacted positively with the *Enterococcus* genus primers but not with any of the species primers. For Day 35 samples, *E. faecium* was the dominant species at 72.4% (n=21) followed by *E. faecalis* at 20.7% (n=6), *E. durans* at 3.5% (n=1), and *E. hirae* at 3.5% (n=1).

3.3 Sterols in surface and groundwater

Surface water samples were tested for a total of 18 sterols (Table 1) but only 8 sterols were detected (Figure 2). The fecal sterols cholesterol, dihydrocholesterol (cholestanol) and desmosterol were detected in all 12 sampling sites ranging from 0.275-7.710 μg/L, 0.022-1.040 μg/L and 0.031-1.119 μg/L, respectively. Coprostanol was detected in all but two sites and ranged from 0.006-0.086 μg/L. Epicoprostanol was detected in six sampling sites ranging from 0.005-0.048 μg/L. The plant sterols campesterol, stigmasterol and β-sitosterol were detected in all 12 sampling sites ranging from 0.044~1.692 μg/L, 0.072~2.928 μg/L and 0.361-10.072 μg/L, respectively.

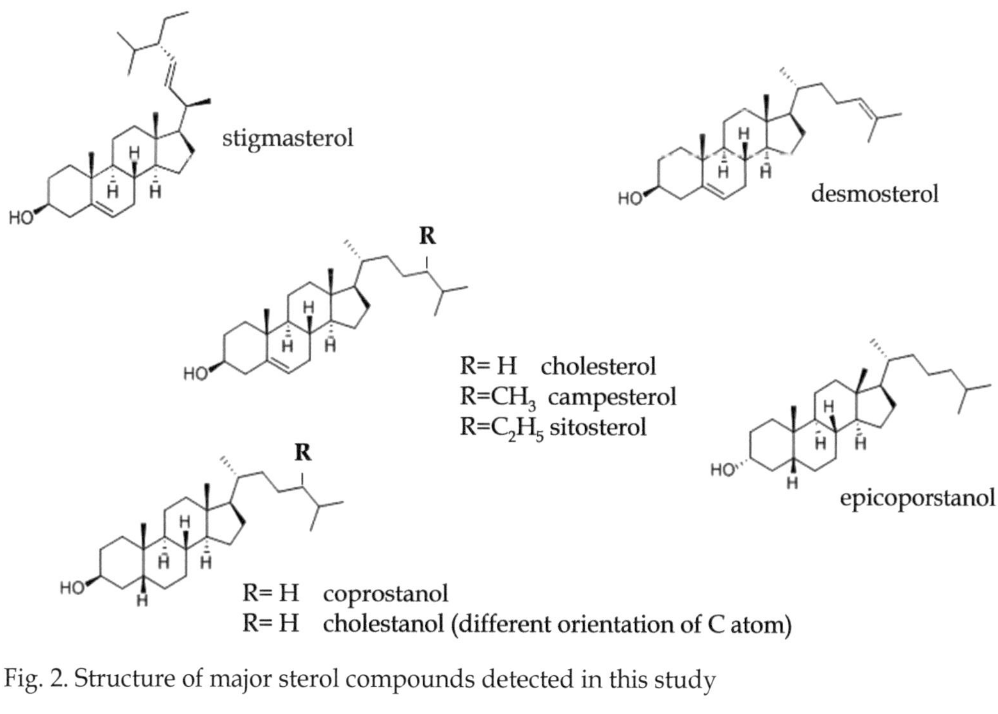

Fig. 2. Structure of major sterol compounds detected in this study

Cholesterol was present in all groundwater samples ranging from 0.022-0.480 μg/L, 0.023-0.590 μg/L and 0.009-0.155 μg/L in April 2009, August 2009 and December 2009 respectively. A few sites regularly tested positive for low concentrations of beta-sitosterol, campesterol, signmasterol, desmosterol, and dihydrochloresterol. Coprostanol was sporadically detected. In December 2009, 15 groundwater sites were sampled for sterols, and six sterols were detected. Cholesterol was detected in all 15 sampling sites ranging from 0.018~0.209 μg/L. Desmosterol was only detected in two sampling sites (FT7-22 and PC-55) ranging from 0.018~0.035 μg/L. Dihydrocholesterol was detected in four sampling sites (ABB-06, FT1-24, FT7-22 and PC-55) ranging from 0.011~0.030 μg/L. Plant sterol campesterol was detected in eight sampling sites (ABB-06, ABB-02, BC008, US-04, US-02, FT1-24, FT7-22 and PC-55) ranging from 0.005~0.032 μg/L. Stigmasterol was detected in all but five sampling sites (ABB-10, 94SH-29, BC349, 91-15 and 91-11) ranging from 0.015~0.668 μg/L. β-sitosterol was detected in all but one (91-11) sampling site ranging from 0.012~0.956 μg/L. Coprostanol was not detected in groundwater during this sampling period.

Based on sterol analyses, ten sterol ratios were calculated and presented in Table 6.

	Identifying Human Fecal Contamination							Differentiating Source of Contamination		
	sterol ratio#									
Field ID	1	2	3	4	5	6	7	8	9	10
Surface water										
S1	n/a	n/a	n/a	n/a	n/a	n/a	n/a	n/a	**1.53**[c]	n/a
S2	n/a	n/a	n/a	n/a	n/a	n/a	n/a	n/a	1.33	n/a
S3	0.046	0.089	1.000	0.002	0.049	0.002	1.00	0.003[b]	1.43	0.046
S4	0.413	0.526	0.579	0.091	0.703[a]	0.081	1.73[a]	0.144[b]	2.03[c]	0.239[d]
S5	0.415	0.529	0.588	0.092	0.708[a]	0.081	1.70[a]	0.145[b]	1.42	0.244[d]
S6	0.358	0.469	0.583	0.065	0.558[a]	0.058	1.71[a]	0.103[b]	1.49	0.209[d]
S7	0.135	n/a	n/a	0.014	0.156	0.013	n/a	n/a	2.79[c]	n/a
S8	0.077	0.114	0.556	0.016	0.083	0.014	1.80[a]	0.025[b]	0.889[a]	0.043
S9	0.047	0.083	0.833	0.001	0.049	0.001	1.20	0.002[b]	0.535[a]	0.039
S10	0.296	n/a	n/a	0.048	0.421[a]	0.043	n/a	n/a	1.64[c]	n/a
S11	0.280	n/a	n/a	0.039	0.389	0.036	n/a	n/a	1.64[c]	n/a
S11rep	0.280	n/a	n/a	0.040	0.389	0.036	n/a	n/a	1.50[c]	n/a
S12	0.250	n/a	n/a	0.038	0.333	0.034	n/a	n/a	2.31[c]	n/a
Groundwater										
91-11 (GS1)	n/a	n/a	n/a	n/a	n/a	n/a	n/a	n/a	n/a	n/a
BC-008 (GS2)	n/a	n/a	n/a	n/a	n/a	n/a	n/a	n/a	0.563[a]	n/a
BC-008 (GS2)-D	n/a	n/a	n/a	n/a	n/a	n/a	n/a	n/a	0.613[a]	n/a
US-02 (GS3)	n/a	n/a	n/a	n/a	n/a	n/a	n/a	n/a	0.527[a]	n/a

Table 6. Sterol ratios for surface and groundwater samples. Underlined values indicate contamination from (a) humans; (b) chicken and/or cow; (c) pig/chicken/cow; (d) cattle/horse/deer

3.4 Fecal pollution source identification using bacterial and chemical indicators

Sterol ratios (calculated from the sterol concentrations) showed that 6 of the 12 surface water samples coded for chicken or cow (ratio #8) contamination (Table 6). Six surface water samples coded for pig/chicken/or cow (ratio #9) contamination, five samples coded for human contamination (ratios #5 and #7), and 3 samples coded for cattle/horse/deer contamination (ratio #10). In the case of the three groundwater samples analyzed for sterol content, 2 samples showed evidence of human fecal contamination. BST analyses of surface water showed that 10 samples tested positive for markers for general fecal contamination while 5 of 12 samples tested positive for one of two markers for ruminant animals (consistently marker CF193F/Bac708R). Comparison of enteric isolates for environmental samples with isolates from poultry litter showed that 10 of 12 surface water samples and 2 of 3 groundwater samples, contained enterococci isolates that grouped with isolates from poultry litter (Table 7).

		Bacterial Source Tracking (BST)					
Field ID	Result from Sterol Ratio	human fecal contamination	pig fecal contamination	ruminant animal fecal contamination	Positive Fecal Contamination	*Enterococcus* isolates group with isolates from litter	Summary contribution to contamination
Surface Water							
S1	pig, chicken, or cow	absent	absent	absent	present	no	
S2	none	absent	absent	1 of 2 markers	present	yes	ruminant
S3	chicken or cow	absent	absent	absent	absent	yes	chicken
S4	human; human pig, chicken or cow chicken or cow cattle, horse or deer	absent	absent	absent	present	yes	chicken human
S5	human human chicken or cow chicken cattle, horse or deer	1 of 2 markers	absent	absent	present	yes	chicken human
S6	human human chicken or cow cattle, horse or deer	absent	absent	absent	present	yes	chicken human
S7	pig, chicken, or cow	absent	absent	absent	absent	yes	chicken
S8	human human chicken or cow	absent	absent	absent	present	no	human
S9	human chicken or cow	absent	absent	1 of 2 markers	present	yes	ruminant chicken
S10	pig, chicken, or cow	absent	absent	1 of 2 markers	present	yes	ruminant chicken
S11	pig, chicken, or cow	absent	absent	present	present	yes	ruminant chicken
S12	pig, chicken, or cow	absent	absent	1 of 2 markers	present	yes	ruminant chicken
Ground Water							
91-11 (GS1)	n/a	absent	absent	absent	absent	yes	
BC-008 (GS2)	human	absent	absent	absent	absent	yes	
US-02 (GS3)	human	absent	absent	absent	absent	no	human

Table 7. Summary of sterols, BST and *Enterococcus* results

Comparison amongst the indicators of fecal pollution showed that for site S5, two (#5 and #7) of seven sterol ratios indicative of human fecal contamination tested positive for human contamination and three ratios (#1, #2 and #3) were "unsure" (Table 6). For the same site, BST analysis indicated one of two markers present for human contamination. The same sterol ratios (#5 and #7) indicating human contamination were found for sites S4 and S6; however for these sites, sterols results were not confirmed by BST analysis. For site S8, two sterol ratios belonging to different groups [(coprostanol/episoprostanol) and (campesterol+sitosterol)/cholesterol)] identified a human pollution source; the epicoprostanol/coprostanol ratio gave a "unsure" result for human contamination (Table 6). Interestingly, site S8 also had the highest *Enterococcus* count but none of the environmental *Enterococcus* isolates grouped with isolates from poultry litter. Because BST analysis of S8 did not detect a ruminant contribution, all indicators point to human fecal contamination. For sites S3 and S7, sterol ratios indicated poultry contamination since BST did not detect any ruminant or pig contributions and some of the enterococci isolates from both locations grouped with the poultry litter isolates. For sites S10, S11 and S12, the sterol ratio for differentiating source of contamination indicated ruminant animals (cow) or chicken as a source. Ruminant contribution was confirmed by BST analysis (both markers present); some of the enterococci isolates for this location also grouped with isolates from poultry litter, indicating contribution from both animal sources. PCA showed that site S9 grouped with sites S3 and S7 (Figure 3): enterococci isolates grouped with the isolates from poultry litter and BST analyses showed one of two markers for ruminant fecal contamination, indicating ruminant and chicken sources contributed to pollution of these sites.

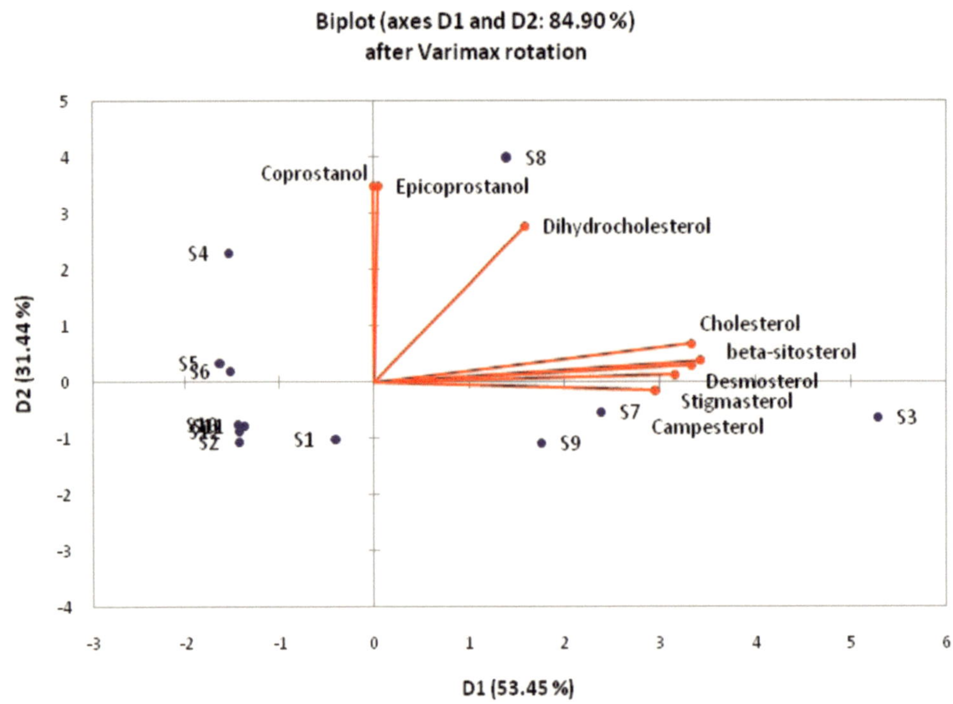

Fig. 3. Biplot (loadings and scores) on the first two principal components (sterol data)

3.5 Chemometric analysis

Most of the variation in the sterol data for surface water was explained by first two PCA factors (Table 8). The first factor (VF1) contributed 53.45% of the total variance and consisted of mostly plant sterols (cholesterol, desmosterol, campesterol, stigmasterol and β-sitosterol). The second factor, VF2 (31.44%), showed high positive loading of coprostanol, epicoprostanol and dihydrocholesterol (animal sterols). The strong loadings of coprostanol, episcoprostanols and dihydrocholesterol in VF2

(Table 8) suggested the possibility of sewage contamination since these compounds are widely used as chemical markers, especially coprostanol (Carreira et al., 2004; Isobe et al., 2004).

Parameters	VF1	VF2
Coprostanol	-0.002	**0.966**
Epicoprostanol	0.013	**0.967**
Cholesterol	**0.927**	0.188
Dihydrocholesterol	0.440	**0.769**
Desmosterol	**0.880**	0.034
Campesterol	**0.822**	-0.046
Stigmasterol	**0.929**	0.080
β-sitosterol	**0.955**	0.106
Eigenvalue	4.515	2.277
Variability (%)	53.45	31.44
Cumulative %	53.45	84.89

Table 8. Factor loadings (after varimax rotation) of sterols in surface water samples. Strong loadings (>0.75) are shown in bold

CA applied to the surface water sterol data grouped by site identified three clusters: cluster 1 consisted of samples from sites S1, S2, S4, S5, S6, S10, S11 and S12; cluster 2 consisted of samples from S3, S7 and S9; cluster 3 contained only site S8 (Figure 4). Analyses of cluster I showed that sites were grouped by sources of contamination: chicken and human (S4, S5, S6) versus ruminant and chicken (S10, S11, S12). For cluster 2 sorces of contamination were chicken whereas for cluster 3 human contamination is evident. The CA analysis on sterols generated three groups (Figure 5). Cluster 1 consisted of 3 sterols namely campesterol, β-sitosterol and stigmasterol (all plant sterols); cluster 2 consisted of cholesterol and desmosterol, while cluster 3 consisted of animal sterols (coprostanol, epicoprostanol and dihydrocholestrol). Cluster analysis supported the PCA analysis that suggested there are two potential sources of fecal contamination (human and animal) in surface water samples, which is in an agreement with the sterol ratio data.

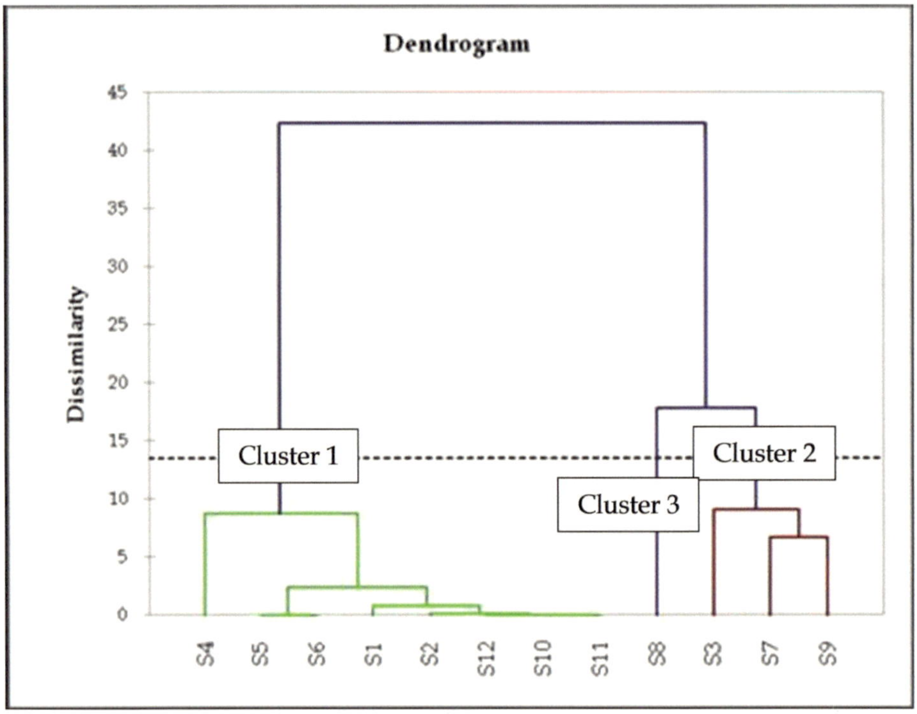

Fig. 4. Dendrogram showing the clustering of sampling sites based on sterols data

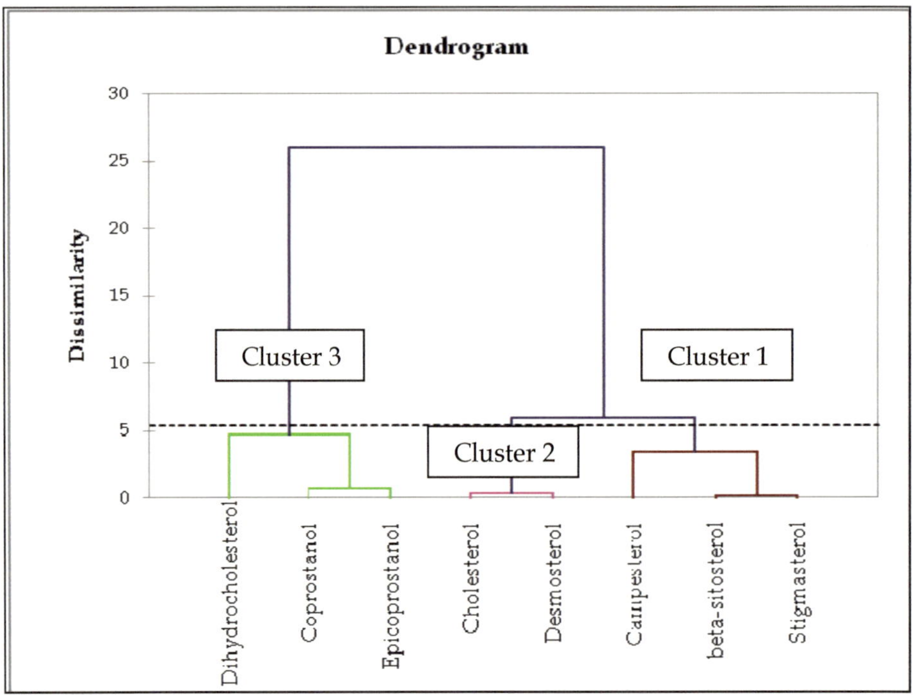

Fig. 5. Dendrogram showing clustering of sterols as variables

4. Discussion

Impacts of human and agricultural activities on surface and ground water quality are a fact of life around the globe as evidenced by studies in Australia, Europe, United States and Canada where results indicate that fecal pollution is a pervasive problem (Betcher et al., 1996; Blanch et al., 2004; O'Leary et al., 1999). Recent study in US indicated that human impacts on watershed hydrology affected 86% of assessed streams (Carlisle et al., 2010). Within the European Union, a project on tracking fecal pollution in surface water involved scientists from seven countries and a battery of microbial and chemical indicators with the objective to generate knowledge on the best methodologies for tracking sources of fecal pollution in surface water (Blanch et al., 2004). EU is committed to improve overall water quality through Integrated River Basin Management program which is a part of the European Water Framework Directive. Comparison of bacteriological water quality, sterol concentrations and ratios, and BST results for water samples collected from an agricultural (poultry-dominated) area in southern British Columbia, Canada showed that 100% (n=12) of surface water sites and 15% (n=20) groundwater sites had fecal contamination. Of the surface water sites, most (75%) showed evidence of poultry fecal contamination, 33% also showed evidence of human fecal contamination while 42% tested positive for ruminant contamination.

The broad extent of fecal pollution in surface and ground water has provided impetus for scientific studies and regulatory actions to identify fecal pollution sources and undertake corrective measures; however, such regulatory actions are only as effective as the methods employed to identify fecal pollution sources. As a result, microbiologists and organic chemists have explored the usefulness of many different markers for conclusively isolating sources of fecal pollution (Balleste et al., 2010; Blanch et al., 2004; Tyagi et al., 2009a). The over-arching conclusion of these studies was that a battery of markers is required to accurately ascribe fecal pollution source. Yet to our knowledge, few if any studies have examined a multi-metric approach for poultry pollution source tracking in surface and ground water. In our study, microbial markers, BST and enterococci were investigated for fecal source tracking.

4.1 Microbial markers for source tracking of poultry fecal pollution

Our results showed that BST was useful for detection of human and ruminant pollution in surface water; BST is the most specific of all microbial methods and can distinguish among human and animal fecal contamination, but the drawback is that primers are not available for many species, birds being one of them. A possible issue with the BST may be the method detection limit which is not easy to establish and needs to be addressed in the future.

Analysis of *Enterococcus* showed that isolates in water samples grouped with isolates from litter for 10 out of 12 surface water sites and for 2 out of three groundwater sites. *Enterococcus* has been explored as a microbial source tracking indicator for human fecal pollution specifically enterococcal surface protein (*esp*) in *Enterococcus faecium* (Scott et al., 2005). Primers developed by these authors were successful in 97% of sewage and septic samples and did not react with birds and different livestock samples. Fingerprinting or pattern matching of enterococcal isolates from poultry farms with ones found in the environment has been introduced by our group (unpublished data) and does not rely on libraries as do some MST methodologies (Balleste et al., 2010 and references within). Our method is very sensitive with only one enterococcal CFU required as opposed to 58 enterococcal CFU necessary for *esp* gene for human detection (Scott et al., 2005). In our study, nine *Enterococcus* environmental isolates and two from day 35 from layers farm reacted positively with the *Enterococcus* genus marker but did not react with any of the species markers used in the multiplex PCR. These unknown isolates could either belong to a species not tested in the multiplex PCR, or they could belong to one of the tested species but have a mutation in the *sodA* gene such that the species-specific primers do not bind.

Other bacterial total coliform, fecal coliform and *E. coli* were also measured and are useful only as general indicators of the fecal pollution. Total and fecal coliform have been regulated as indicators for rapid sanitary quality of different water bodies but they are not useful for source tracking. There is no regulation in regards to *Enterococcus* bacteria for surface water in general in Canada, but the one surface water location was above the 350 cfu/L *Enterococcus* guideline for Canadian Recreational Water Quality (Health and Welfare Canada, 1992) although the guideline values is based on a geometric mean of at least five samples taken over 30 days.

Although different bacteria and combinations of bacteria have been used in the literature for fecal source tracking (Blanch et al., 2004; Tyagi et al., 2009 and references within), the approach used in this study represents a unique integration of BST and enterococci as indicators of fecal pollution.

4.2 Chemical markers for source tracking of fecal pollution

To provide further scientific support for our microbiological findings, BST analysis and *Enterococcus* results, sterol analyses were conducted on surface and groundwater. Sterols indicative of fecal source pollution (cholesterol, coprostanol epicoprostanol desmosterol and dihydrocholesterol) were detected in all surface water samples; phytosterols (campesterol, stigmasterol and b-sitosterol), an indication of herbivores pollution sources, were detected (Leming et al., 1996; Reeves & Patton, 2005). The presence of individual sterols is generally not sufficient for tracking of fecal pollution in the environment although, for example, coprostanol is considered a marker for sewage contamination (Leeming et al., 1996, Shah et al., 2007). Sterol ratios are more reliable and widely used in the literature for source pollution tracking (References in Table 2). Sterol ratio criteria for human fecal contamination have been developed based on experimental data mainly from analysis of sterols in sediment although they have been tested and applied in water environments in the connection with discharge from waste water treatment plant discharge (Chan et al., 1998; Chou & Liu, 2004). Although there are numerous studies using sterol ratios for tracking human fecal contamination, few studies have used these ratios for differentiating sources of fecal contamination. Sterol ratio criteria for differentiating sources of fecal contamination are derived mostly from studies of agricultural environment manures and slurries matrices (Jardé et al., 2007; Standley et al., 2000), with the later study showing that ratios #8 and #9 successfully discriminated pig slurry from poultry and dairy manure. These two ratios were also successful in this study. Ratio #10 was found to be the most useful ratio for tracking agricultural activities in 19 North American watersheds (Standley et al., 2000). In our study, 5 ratios (#5, 7, 8, 9 and 10) proved useful for fecal pollution source tracking. In cases of contamination from human and animal sources, ratios for identifying human fecal contamination that contain cholesterol may be failing due to increased concentrations of cholesterol from animal sources. For sampling site 9, only one ratio for differentiating sources of contamination (namely campesterol+citosterol)/cholesterol) indicated human fecal contamination. In this case, increased concentration of cholesterol from animal sources is probably decreasing the ratio so this may be false positive, particularly as this result was not confirmed by a any other indicator. Thus, we recommend use of as many ratios as can be calculated based on the sterol analysis in suite in order to positively identify sources of contamination.

The combination of bacteriological and chemical indicators presented in this study represents a unique integration of indicators. To our knowledge, no similar study has been conducted and reported in the literature. Furthermore, this approach was able to indicate several sources of fecal contamination simultaneously.

4.3 Chemometric approach for source tracking of human and poultry fecal pollution

Although microbiological and chemical indicators were used in the combination for fecal pollution tracking, there are few studies where they were further supported by the chemometric analysis. A study of an Australian water supply system comprised of rivers, channels and drains monitored only two sterols (coprostanol and cholesterol) for a longer period of time (12 months) and used cluster analyses to detect similarities among the sampling sites (Hussain et al., 2010). In this study, clustering of sites by sterol profile suggested four clusters that differed by the source. Shah et al. (2007) showed that cluster analysis of fecal sterols of humans, herbivores, birds and carnivores could distinguish between birds and the other three categories, with humans and herbivores and also herbivores and birds being well separated whereas humans and carnivores were more closely associated. Saim et al. (2009) applied cluster analysis on their sterol data (only 5 sterols analyzed) from various point sources (sites included sewage treatment plants, chicken farms, quail farms and horse stables) and concluded that chicken and quail generated a separate cluster that can be distinguished. In this study, CA also grouped sites by sources of contamination: chicken and human, ruminant and chicken, human only and chicken only. Furthermore, CA of sterols resulted in three groups: plant sterols, human fecal sterols and animal sterols. Thus the CA results provide further corroboration of our predictions of fecal sources contamination based on BST, *Enterococcus* and sterol ratio results.

Principal Component Analysis is another chemometric technique for pattern recognition that is often used in the combination with CA. To improve interpretation of principal components, Varimax rotation is recommended. Resulting VF coefficients with values greater that 0.75 are considered to have strong correlation and in our data, all eight sterols (coprostanol, epicoprostanol, cholesterol, cholestanol-dihydrocholesterol, desmosterol, campesterol stigmasterol and β-sitosterol) were strongly correlated. Plot of discriminate functions in Saim et al. (2009) also showed clear separation of human and chicken sources. Similar PCA results presented by Leeming et al. (1996) showed human, hens and cow and sheep were clearly separated on the PCA plot. Results of PCA in this study further supported CA analyses results. Biplot on first two principal components clearly identified two groups of sterols. Moreover, sampling sites on the same biplot are grouped as per the CA clusters. For sites S3 and S7, sterol ratios indicated only poultry contamination; BST did not detect any ruminant or pig contributions and some of the enterococci isolates from both locations grouped with the poultry litter isolates. These findings were further supported by the high loading of β-sitosterol from PCA analysis. Previous studies (Leeming et al 1996; Saim et al 2009) reported β-sitosterol as major sterol in chicken and other bird species. Combination of chemometric analyses with bacteriological and chemical indicators for site 8 clearly indicated only human contamination. Surprisingly, groundwater site GS3 is located close to site S8 (Figure 1) and for both locations enterococci did not group with chicken isolates. Because the entire area is serviced by septic tanks, human fecal contamination from sewage is a possibility. Hence, for other sites where there was more that one possible source of contamination, our multi-indicator approach was able to identify sources. To our knowledge, such a comprehensive approach has not been reported in the literature for fecal source tracking.

5. Conclusion

Our study showed that application of multi-indicator approach consisting of *Enterococcus*, bacterial source tracking (BST), sterol analysis and chemometric analyses could successfully identify sources of fecal contamination in agricultural areas dominated by poultry operations and associated human activities. An ability to ascribe sources when confronted with a complex pollution situation is essential for planning management actions and implementing best management practices. Our results will assist further efforts to protect and preserve surface and ground water quality from the impacts of human and agricultural activities.

6. Acknowledgement

The authors thank Health Canada for providing the funds for this research. Many thanks to Gwyn Graham, Martin Suchey (Water Management and Indicators Section, Strategic Integration and Partnerships Division Pacific Yukon Region, Environment Canada) and Gwenn Farrell for technical assistance with this study. We also thank reviewers for inputs and review of the chapter.

7. References

Aarestrup, F.M.; Butaye, P. & Witte, W. (2002). Nonhuman Reservoirs of Enterococci, In: *The Enterococci: Pathogenesis, Molecular Biology, and Antibiotic Resistance,* M.S. Gilmore (Ed.), 55-100, ASM Press, ISBN 1-55581-234-1, Washington, DC

Ahmed, W.; Neller, R. & Katouli, M. (2005). Host Species-specific Metabolic Fingerprint Database for Enterococci and *Escherichia coli* and Its Application to Identify Sources of Fecal Contamination in Surface Waters. *Applied and Environmental Microbiology,* Vol.71, No.8, (August 2005), pp. 4461-4468, ISSN 0099-2240

Balleste E.; Bonjoch, X.; Belanche, L. A. & Blanch, A. R. (2010). Molecular Indicators Used in the Development of Predictive Models for Microbial Source Tracking. *Applied and Environmental Microbiology,* Vol.76, No.6, (March 2010), pp. 1789-1795, ISSN 0099-2240

Bernhard, A. E. & Field, K. G. (2000 a). Identification of Nonpoint Sources of Fecal Pollution in Coastal Waters by Using Host-specific 16s ribosomal DNA Genetic Markers from Fecal Anaerobes. *Applied and Environmental Microbiology,* Vol.66, No.4, (April 2000), pp. 1587-1594, ISSN 0099-2240

Bernhard, A.E. & Field, K.G. (2000 b). A PCR Assay to Discriminate Human and Ruminant Feces on the Basis of Host Difference in *Bacteroides-Prevotella* genes Encoding 16S rRNA. *Applied and Environmental Microbiology*, Vol.66, No.10, (October 2000), pp. 4571-4574, ISSN 0099-2240

Betcher, R.N.; Rudolph, D. L. & Nicholson, R. (1996). Impacts of Agricultural Activities on Groundwater Quality, *Proceedings of Manure Management Symposium*, pp. 53-62, ISBN 0-662-26811-3, Winnipeg, Manitoba, Canada, March 20-21, 1996

Blanch, A.R.; Belanche-Muñoz, L.; Bonjoch, X.; Ebdon, J.; Gantzer, C.; Lucena, F.; Ottoson, J.; Kourtis, C.; Iversen, A.; Kühn, I.; Moce L.; Muniesa, M.; Schwartzbrod, J.; Skraber, S.; Papageorgiou, G.; Huw D.; Taylor, H.D.; Wallis, J. & Jofre, J. (2004). Tracking the Origin of Faecal Pollution in Surface Water: An Ongoing Project within the European Union Research Programme. *Journal of Water and Health*, Vol.2, No.4, (June 2004), pp. 249-260, ISSN 1477-8920

Brodnjak-Vončina, D.; Dobčnik, D.; Novič, M. & Zupan, J. (2002). Chemometrics Characterisation of the Quality of River Water. *Analytica Chimica Acta*, Vol.462, No.1, (June 2002), pp. 87–100, ISSN 0003-2670

Bull, I. D.; Lockheart, M. J.; Elhmmali, M. M.; Roberts, D. J. & Evershed, R. P. (2002). The Origin of Faeces by Means of Biomarker Detection. *Environment International*, Vol.27, No.8, (March 2002), pp. 647-654, ISSN 0160-4120

Carlisle, D.M.; Wolock, D.M. & Meador, M.R. (2010). Alteration of Streamflow Magnitudes and Potential Ecological Consequences: A Multiregional Assessment. *Frontiers in Ecology and the Environment*, Vol.5, No.5, (June 2011), pp. 264-270, ISSN 1540-9295

Carreira, R. S.; Wagener, A. L. R. & Readman, J. W. (2004). Sterols as Markers of Sewage Contamination in a Tropical Urban Estuary (Guanabara Bay, Brazil): Space-time Variations. *Estuarine, Coastal and Shelf Science*, Vol.60, No.4, (April 2004), pp. 587-598, ISSN 02727714

Chan, K.H., Lam, M.H.W.; Poon, K.F.; Yeung, H.Y. & Chiu, T.K.T. (1998). Application of Sedimentary Fecal Stanols and Sterols in Tracing Sewage Pollution in Coastal Waters. *Water Research*, Vol.32, No.1, (January 1998), pp. 225-235, ISSN 0043-1354

Chou, C.C. & Liu, Y.P. (2004). Determination of Fecal Sterols in the Sediment of Different Wastewater Outputs by GC-MS. *International Journal of Environmental and Analytical Chemistry*, Vol.84, No.5 (January 2007), pp. 379-388, ISSN 0306-7319

de Castro Martins, C.; Fillmann, G. & Montone, R.C. (2007). Natural and Anthropogenic Sterols Inputs in Surface Sediments of Patos Lagoon, Brazil. *Journal of the Brazilian Chemical Society*, Vol.18, No.1, (January 2007), pp. 106-115, ISSN 01035053

Devane, M.; Saunders, D. & Gilpin, B. (2006). Faecal Sterols and Fluorescent Whiteners as Indicators of the Source of Faecal Contamination. *Chemistry in New Zealand*, Vol.70, No. 3, (October 2006), pp. 74-77, ISSN 0110-5566

Dick, L.K.; Simonich, M.T. & Field, K.G. (2005 a). Microplate Subtractive Hybridization to Enrich for *Bacteroidales* Genetic Markers for Fecal Source Identification. *Applied and Environmental Microbiology*, Vol.71, No.6, (June 2005), pp. 3179 – 3183, ISSN 0099-2240

Dick, L.K.; Bernhard, A.E.; Brodeur, T.J.; Santo Domingo, J.W.; Simpson, J.M.; Walters, S.P. & Field, K.G. (2005 b). Host Distributions of Uncultivated Fecal *Bacteroidales* Bacteria Reveal Genetic Markers for Fecal Source Identification. *Applied and Environmental Microbiology*, Vol.71, No.6, (June 2005), pp. 3184 - 3191, ISSN 0099-2240

Einax, J. W.; Truckenbrodt, D. & Kampe, O. (1998). River Pollution Data Interpreted by Means of Chemometric Methods. *Microchemical Journal*, Vol.58, No.3, (March 1998), pp. 315–324, ISSN 0026-265X

Environment Canada, Pacific Environmental Science Centre. (2005). *Sterol Method, version 1.1*, Environment Canada, Vancouver, Canada.

Environment Canada, Pacific Environmental Science Centre. (2006). *Bacterial Source Tracking Methods version 1.0*, Environment Canada, Vancouver, Canada.

USEPA. (2000). Improved Enumeration Methods for the Recreational Water Quality Indicators: Enterococci and *Escherichia coli*, Office of Science and Technology, USEPA, Document No. EPA/821/R-97/004, Washington, D.C.

Fattore, E.; Benfenati, E.; Marelli, R.; Cools, E. & Ranelli, R. (1996). Sterols in Sediment Samples from Venice Lagoon, Italy. *Chemosphere*, Vol. 33, No.12, (December 1996), pp. 2383-2393, ISSN 0045-6535

Figueras, M.J.; Borrego, J.J.; Pike, E.B.; Robertson, W. & Ashbolt, N. (2000). Sanitary Inspection and Microbiological Water Quality, In: *Monitoring Bathing Waters: Practical Guide to the Design and Implementation of Assessments and Monitoring Programmes*, J. Bartram & G. Rees (Eds.), 106-157, E & FN Spon, ISBN 0-419-24390-1, New York, New York

Froehner, S.; Martins, R.F. & Errera, M.R. (2009). Assessment of Fecal Sterols in Barigui River sediments in Curitiba, Brazil. *Environmental Monitoring and Assessment*, Vol.157, No.1, (April 2008), pp. 591-600, ISSN 0167-6369

Gilpin, B.; James, T.; Nourozi, F.; Saunders, D.; Scholes, P. & Savill, M. (2003). The Use of Chemical and Molecular Microbial Indicators for Faecal Source Identification. *Water Science and Technology*, Vol.7, No.3, (March 2003), pp. 39-43, ISSN 0273-1223

Grimalt , J.O.; Fernandez, P.; Bayona, J. M. & Albaiges, J. (1990). Assessment of Fecal Sterols and Ketones as Indicators of Urban Sewage Inputs to Coastal Waters. *Environmental Science and Technology*, Vol.24, No.3, (March 1990), pp. 357-363, ISSN 0013-936X

Harwood, V. J.; Whitlock, J. & Withington, V. (2000). Classification of Antibiotic Resistance Patterns of Indicator Bacteria by Discriminate Analysis: Use in Predicting the Source of Fecal Contamination in Tropical Waters. *Applied and Environmental Microbiology*, Vol.66, No.3, (September 2000), pp: 3698-3704, ISSN 0099-2240

Health and Welfare Canada. (1992). *Guidelines for Canadian Recreational Water Quality*, Ministry of Services and Supply, ISBN 0-660-14239-2, Ottawa, Canada

Horvath, S. (Ed.). (2009). *British Columbia Environmental Laboratory Manual*, Water and Air Monitoring and Reporting, Environmental Quality Branch, Ministry of Environment, Victoria, BC, Canada.

Hussain, M.A.; Ford, R. & Hill, J. (2010). Determination of Fecal Contamination Indicator Sterols in an Australian Water Supply System, *Environmental Monitoring and Assessment*, Vol.165, No.1, (June 2010), pp. 147-157, ISSN 0167-6369

Isobe, K. O.; Tarao, M.; Chiem, N. H. & Minh, L. Y. (2004). Effect of Environmental Factors on the Relationship between Concentrations of Coprostanol and Fecal Indicator Bacteria in Tropical (Mekong Delta) and Temperate (Tokyo) Freshwaters. *Applied and Environmental Microbiology*, Vol.70, No.2, (February 2004), pp. 814–821, ISSN 0099-2240

Jackson, C. R.; Fedorka-Cray, P.J. & Barrett, J. B. (2006). Use of a genus- and species-specific multiplex PCR for identification of enterococci. *Journal of Clinical Microbiology*, Vol.42, No.8, (August 2004), pp. 3558-3565, ISSN 0095-1137

Jardé, E. ; Gruau, G. ; Mansuy-Huault, L. ; Peu, P. & Martinez, J. (2007). Using Sterols to Detect Pig Slurry Contribution to Soil Organic Matter. *Water, Air, and Soil Pollution*, Vol.178, No.1, (January 2007), pp. 169-178, ISSN 0049-6979

Juahir, H.; Zain, S. M.; Khan, R. A.; Yusoff, M. K.; Mokhtar, M. B. & Toriman, M. E. (2009). Using Chemometrics in Assessing Langat River Water Quality and Designing a Cost-effective Water Sampling Strategy. *Maejo International Journal of Science and Technology,* Vol.3, No.1, (January 2009), pp. 26-42, ISSN 1905-7873

Kim, J.O. & Mueller, C. W. (1987). *Introduction to Factor Analysis: What it is and How to do it. Quantitative Applications in the Social Sciences Series,* Sage University Press, ISBN 0-8039-1165-3, Newbury Park, California.

Leeming, R.; Ball, A.; Ashbolt, N. & Nichols, P. (1996). Using Faecal Sterols from Humans and Animals to Distinguish Faecal Pollution in Receiving Waters. *Water Research,* Vol.30, No.12, (December 1996), pp. 2893-2900, ISSN 0043-1354

Loska, K. & Wiechuła, D. (2003). Application of Principal Component Analysis for the Estimation of Source of Heavy Metal Contamination in Surface Sediments from the Rybnik Reservoir. *Chemosphere,* Vol.51, No.8, (June 2003), pp. 723–733, ISSN 0045-6534

Marvin, C.; Coakley, J.; Mayer, T.; Brown, M. & Thiessen, L. (2001). Application of Faecal Sterol Ratios in Sediments and Effluents as Source Tracers. *Water Quality Research Journal of Canada,* Vol.36, No.4, (April 2001), pp. 781-792, ISSN 1201-3080

Mendiguchía, C.; Moreno, C.; Galindo-Raiño, D. & Garcia-Vegas, M. (2004). Using Chemometric Tools to Assess Anthropogenic Effects in River Water A Case Study: Guadalquivir River (Spain). Analytica Chimica Acta, Vol.515, No.1, (July 2004), pp. 143-149, ISSN 0003-2670

O'Leary, T.; Leeming, R.; Nicolas, P.D. & Volkman, J.K. (1999). Assessment of the Sources, Transport and Fate of Sewage-derived Organic Matter in Port Philip Bay, Australia, using the Signature Lipid Coprostanol. *Marine and Freshwater Research,* Vol.50, No.6, (June 1999), pp. 547-556, ISSN 1323-1650

Patton, D. & Reeves, A. D. (1999). Sterol Concentrations and Temporal Variations on the North Shore Mudflats of Firth of Tay, Scotland. *Marine Pollution Bulletin,* Vol.38, No.7, (July 1999), pp. 613-618, ISSN 0025-326X

Reeves, A.D. & Patton, D. (2005). Faecal Sterols as Indicators of Sewage Contamination in Estuarine Sediments of the Tay Estuary, Scotland: An Extended Baseline Survey. *Hydrology and Earth Systems Sciences,* Vol.9, No.1, (June 2005), pp. 81-94, ISSN 1027-5606

Roser, D.; Leeming, R.; Ashbolt, N.; Gardner, T. & Stewart, J. (2006). Estimating Non-point Source Contamination Loads using Faecal Sterols, Bacterial Indicators and Hydrology. *9th International Riversymposium 'Managing Rivers with Climate Change and Expanding Populations',* pp. 1-12, ISBN 9781843394525: 1843394529, Brisbane, Australia, September, 4-7, 2006

Saim, N.; Osman, R.; Spian, D.R.S.A.; Jaafar, M.Z.; Juahir, H.; Abdullah, M.P. & F.A. Ghani. (2009). Chemometric Approach to Validating Faecal Sterols as Source Tracer for Faecal Contamination in Water. *Water Research,* Vol.43, No.20, (October 2009), pp. 5023-5030, ISSN 0043-1354

Scott, T.M.; Jenkins, T.M.; Lukasik, J. & Rose, J.B. (2005). Potential of Use of a Host Associated Molecular Markers in *Enterococcus faecium* as an Index of Human Fecal Pollution. *Environmental Science and Technology,* Vol.39, No.1, (November 2004), pp. 283-287, ISSN 0013-936X

Shah, V.G.; Dunstan, R.H.; Geary, P.M.; Coombes, P.; Roberts, T.K. & Von Nagy-Felsobuki, E. (2007). Evaluationg Potential Applications of Faecal Sterols in Distinguishing Sources of Faecal Contamination from Mixed Faecal Samples. *Water Research,* Vol.41, No.16, (August 2007), pp. 3691-3700, ISSN 0043-1354

Singh, K. P.; Malik, A.; Singh, V. K.; Mohan, D. & Sinha, S. (2005). Chemometric Analysis of Groundwater Quality Data of Alluvial Aquifer of Gangetic plain, North India. *Analytica Chimica Acta*, Vol.550, No.1, (September 2005), pp. 82-91, ISSN 0003-2670

Standley, J. L.; Kaplan, A. L. & Smith, D. (2000). Molecular Tracers of Organic Matter Sources to Surface Water Resources. *Environmental Science and Technology*, Vol.34, No.15, (June 2000), pp. 3124-3130, ISSN 0013-936X

Terrado, M.; Barceló, D. & Tauler, R. Chemometric Analysis and Mapping of Environmental Pollution Sources in the Ebro River Basin. In: *The Handbook of Environmental Chemistry*, D. Barcelo & A.G. Kostianoy, (Eds.), 331-372, Springer-Verlag, ISBN 978-3-642-18031-6, Berlin, Germany

Tyagi, P.; Edwards, R. D. & Coyne, S. M. (2009a). Distinguishing Between Human and Animal Sources of Fecal Pollution in Waters: a Review. *International Journal of Water*, Vol.5, No.1, (January 2009), pp. 15-34, ISSN 1465-6620

Tyagi, P.; Edwards, R. D. & Coyne, S. M. (2009b). Fecal Sterol and Bile Acid Biomarkers: Runoff Concentrations in Animal Waste-amended Pastures. *Water, Air, and Soil Pollution*, Vol.198, No.1, (March 2009), pp. 45-54, ISSN 0049-6979

Zhang, C.; Wang, Y. & Qi, S. (2008). Identification and Significance of Sterols in MSW Landfill Leachate. *Journal of Chromatography B*, Vol.874, No.1, (August 2008), pp. 1-6, ISSN 1570-0232

Part 2

Air Quality

4

Understanding Human Illness and Death Following Exposure to Particulate Matter Air Pollution

Erin M. Tranfield and David C. Walker
The James Hogg Research Centre, Providence Heart and Lung Institute, St. Paul's Hospital, University of British Columbia, Vancouver, Canada

1. Introduction

The World Health Organization (WHO) estimates that more than two million deaths occur each year as a consequence of air pollution exposure (Mackay et al., 2004). This estimate, which some scientists consider conservative, is based on hundreds of scientific studies showing an association between exposure to air pollution and heart as well as lung related illness and death. However, scientists do not understand the sequence of events in the human body that link air pollution exposure to illness and death. Understanding these events and their order is a major focus of ongoing medical research.

The aims of this chapter are to first introduce the reader to air pollution and then to briefly present the current scientific understanding of the biological events that link particulate matter air pollution exposure to illness and death. The chapter concludes with suggestions for future actions to reduce the health consequence of air pollution exposure. This chapter does not consider the effects of indoor air pollutants such as tobacco smoke, or smoke from cooking fires because these topics are considered elsewhere in this book.

Air pollution is a complicated mixture of airborne particulates combined with gases, mist and fog. Its composition is highly variable with differences observed between rural locations and cities, between individual cities, and even between regions within cities. The gases in air pollution such as ozone, carbon monoxide, sulphur dioxide and nitrogen dioxide are considered pollutants at high levels because they have a moderate association with human illness (morbidity) and death (mortality) (Lipfert et al., 1995; Morris et al., 1995; Sheppard et al., 1999; Wichmann et al., 1989). When small enough to enter the deep regions of the body, particles in air pollution have been shown to have a strong association with human morbidity and mortality, particularly with heart (cardiovascular) and lung (pulmonary) morbidity and mortality (Dockery et al., 1993; Hong et al., 1999; Lin et al., 2005; Pope, 1989; Samet et al., 2000; Stieb et al., 2002; Wichmann et al., 1989). These small particles are called particulate matter.

1.1 Particulate matter

> **PM_{10}** - Atmospheric particles with an aerodynamic diameter smaller than 0.00001 meter or 10 micrometer

The WHO defines particulate matter (PM) as a stable atmospheric suspension of solid and liquid particles with variable composition, origin and an aerodynamic diameter ranging from ~0.000000002 to ~0.0001 meter (m). Particles with an aerodynamic diameter smaller than 0.00001 m, or 10 micrometer (μm), are strongly associated with human morbidity and mortality and are commonly referred to as PM_{10}.

1.1.1 Particle size

Particle size plays a central role in determining the biological consequences of PM exposure (Finlayson-Pitts et al., 2000; Oberdorster, 2001). Particle size has been shown to determine: 1. the location of particle deposition in the airway and lungs, 2. the amount of surface area that can contact tissues, and 3. the rate of particle clearance from the lungs (Kendall et al., 2002; Oberdorster et al., 1994; Sioutas et al., 2005; West et al., 2003).

Particles larger than 10 μm in diameter have such high inertia that they cannot turn the tight corners of the airway. As a result these particles run into the mucous covered walls of the nose and upper airway where they become trapped. The mucous holds these particles until the particles are cleared through mucociliary clearance. Due to the location of deposition in the upper airway, particles larger than 10 μm in diameter are not associated with human illness. Mucociliary clearance is a cleaning system in the airway made of small hairs called cilia. Cilia transport mucous and any debris the mucous has trapped to the upper airway for clearance through the nose or swallowing into the stomach.

Particles smaller than 10 μm in diameter have a small enough inertia that the particles can navigate the upper airway and be inhaled deep into the lungs. Particle deposition on the alveolar surface, which is where gas exchange occurs in the lungs, is linked to pulmonary and cardiovascular morbidity and mortality (Dockery et al., 1993; Seaton et al., 1995). Analysis of PM_{10} has recently revealed three fractions of PM_{10} with distinct regions of deposition in the lungs. These three fractions are the coarse fraction, the fine fraction and the ultrafine fraction. Each fraction has different formation processes, composition, atmospheric lifetimes and biological consequences (Sioutas et al., 2005).

The coarse fraction is composed of particles between 10 and 2.5 μm in aerodynamic diameter that are produced by mechanical processes such as wind erosion. These larger particulates are affected by gravitational settling and typically settle out of the lower atmosphere within hours of formation (Hinds, 1999; Sioutas et al., 2005). The coarse fraction is thought to deposit in the upper airway, and to penetrate only as deep as the pharynx and occasionally into the trachea. Similar to the greater-than-10 μm fraction, particles deposited in these areas are cleared from the body through the nose or by coughing and swallowing. The particles that enter deep into the pulmonary system are carried up the trachea by the mucociliary escalator and swallowed into the stomach.

The fine fraction is composed of particles between 2.5 and 0.1 μm in size and is called $PM_{2.5}$. These particles account for the greatest mass of airborne particulates and are generally formed through human activities. Fine particle formation typically occurs when gas molecules condense together to form particles through heterogeneous and homogeneous nucleation, as well as condensation onto already existing atmospheric particles (Finlayson-Pitts et al., 2000; Hinds, 1999; Sioutas et al., 2005). The small size of this fraction of particles makes them less susceptible to gravitational settling resulting in atmospheric lifetimes in the order of days, and the ability to be transported long distances by wind currents. The fine particles are inhaled into the conducting airways of the lungs. The mucociliary escalator also clears particles deposited in these areas. Some particles travel beyond the conducting airways into the alveoli where they become trapped in the fluid layer of the alveolar wall. In the alveoli, a population of resident white blood cells, called alveolar macrophages, patrols the alveolar surfaces immediately below the layer of fluid. Particles deposited on the alveolar wall are taken up by these alveolar macrophages. The macrophages are then transported out of the lungs by the mucociliary escalator (Dockery et al., 1994) or taken to the pulmonary lymph nodes (Harmsen et al., 1985). A small population of free particles that are not taken up by alveolar macrophages may move into the lung tissue, and then be taken into the lymphatic vessels for processing in the pulmonary lymph nodes (Dockery et al., 1994). Depending on their solubility, particles may remain in the pulmonary lymph nodes from several days to thousands of days (Brain et al., 1994).

Coarse - PM_{10}: Deposited in the upper airway; until recently associated with human illness.

Fine - $PM_{2.5}$: Deposited deep into the lungs, some deposition on the alveolar surface; associated with human illness.

Ultrafine - $PM_{0.1}$: Deposited on the alveolar surface, may enter the blood stream; associated with human illness.

The ultrafine fraction is composed of particles that are smaller than 0.1 μm in aerodynamic diameter ($PM_{0.1}$). These particles have traditionally been considered the fresh emissions in pollution that have yet to undergo condensation or modification processes. The composition of fine particles is varied, characteristically composed of ammonium, carbon, nitrate and sulphate as well as trace metals formed in the combustion processes (Sioutas et al., 2005). This fraction of the smallest particles accounts for the greatest number of atmospheric particles with the largest surface area-to-mass ratio. These particles are primarily deposited on the alveolar surface (Naga et al., 2005; Wang et al., 2002; West et al., 2003). Smaller particles are thought to move into the pulmonary circulation as evidenced by their accumulation in the lymph nodes, spleen, heart, liver and even the bladder and brain (Brain et al., 1994; Harmsen et al., 1985; Nemmar et al., 2002; Oberdorster et al., 2000; Oberdorster et al., 2004; Peters et al., 2006; Semmler et al., 2004).

The large surface-area-to-volume/mass ratios of fine and ultrafine particles may account for their negative effect on human health. Evidence suggests that the larger the surface area the greater the impact of the particle. Smaller particles are known to have the greatest surface area relative to their volume or mass (Oberdorster et al., 1994) as well as the greatest efficiency at penetrating deep into the lungs (Sioutas et al., 2005).

Collecting air pollution particles without modifying them has been a problem for scientists. Furthermore, once the particles are collected it has been difficult to separate PM into the above mentioned size fractions. Because of this, most research is done using material fractioned only by the upper size limit. As such, PM_{10} used in research is composed of PM_{10} + $PM_{2.5}$ + $PM_{0.1}$, and $PM_{2.5}$ is composed of $PM_{2.5}$ + $PM_{0.1}$. In the rest of this book chapter, the use of PM_X represents particulate matter *up to* X micrometers in aerodynamic diameter.

1.1.2 Particle formation

In general, two main processes form PM. The first process is the condensation of gases in the lower atmosphere. The second process is direct introduction of PM through mechanical means such as wind blowing over exposed soil or human activities that stir up dust particulates such as farming and construction activities (Figure 1). Industry and combustion also directly introduce particulates into the atmosphere. Source variability and formation processes affect size distribution and particle composition of PM. Particles larger than 10 μm in diameter are primarily generated by wind blowing over soil whereas human activities, particularly the combustion of fossil fuels, are by far the greatest generators of PM_{10}.

1.2 Regulation of particulate matter

In 2005, the World Health Organization updated the daily and annual mean guidelines of acceptable air pollution. These standards are still in effect and advise that within a 24-hour period, the mean level of $PM_{2.5}$ should not exceed 25 μg/m^3 and the mean level of PM_{10} should not exceed 50 μg/m^3. Furthermore, over the course of a year, the mean level of $PM_{2.5}$ should not exceed 10 μg/m^3 and the mean level of PM_{10} should not exceed 20 μg/m^3. Mean standards per 24-hours are higher than mean standards per year to allow for infrequent air pollution events caused by non-controllable factors such as wild fires or weather pattern changes. Data gathered prior to 2000 suggest that most large American cities would not have met these updated standards (Peng et al., 2005); however, PM_{10} levels are gradually decreasing with the implementation of pollution-minimization measures.

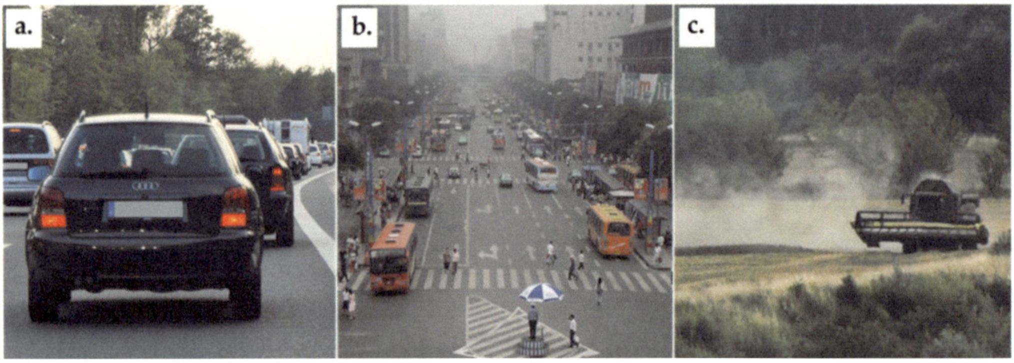

Fig. 1. Particulate matter is introduced into the atmosphere through many human activities including vehicle emissions (panel a), industrial towns in developing countries like China (panel b) and general farming practices (panel c). Image credits E Tranfield.

1.3 Worldwide air pollution standards

The guidelines set by the World Health Organization in 2005 are not followed by all countries (Table 1). Current efforts are being made by most developed countries to reduce the levels of air pollution and achieve these guidelines. Although a lot of progress has been made to reduce air pollution production in general, and PM production specifically, further reductions are required. Moreover, in rapidly developing countries like China, and India, which are currently some of the greatest sources of pollution, only minimal efforts are being made to reduce the generation of pollution.

1.4 The global nature of air pollution

Fine particulates are small enough to remain suspended in the air for long periods of time and to be transported by prevailing winds over long distances. This means that pollutant production can have a global impact and there is evidence that pollution from China has reached the west coast of North America. Efforts by individual countries will have local effects on air quality but to generate long-term global health benefits air pollution will need to be prevented, regulated and monitored on a global scale.

Country	Pollutant	Targeted limits	References
Australia	PM_{10}	24 hr maximum: 50 μg/m³	Australian Government, 2009
	$PM_{2.5}$	24 hr maximum: 25 μg/m³; Annual maximum: 8 μg/m³	
Canada	$PM_{2.5}$	24 hr maximum: 30 μg/m³	Canadian Council of Ministers of the Environment, 2000
European Union	PM_{10}	24 hr maximum: 50 μg/m³; Annual maximum: 40 μg/m³	European Commission Environment, 2011
	$PM_{2.5}$	Annual maximum: 25 μg/m³	
United States of America	PM_{10}	24 hr maximum: 150 μg/m³	United States Environmental Protection Agency, 2011
	$PM_{2.5}$	24 hr maximum: 35 μg/m³; Annual maximum: 15 μg/m³	
World Health Organization Recommendations	**PM_{10}**	**24 hr maximum: 50 μg/m³; Annual maximum: 20 μg/m³**	**World Health Organization, 2005**
	$PM_{2.5}$	**24 hr maximum: 25 μg/m³; Annual maximum: 10 μg/m³**	

Table 1. Examples of ambient particulate matter guidelines.

2. Understanding particulate matter induced human morbidity and mortality

Efforts to understand the sequence of events and the mechanisms through which air pollution affects human health have relied on two complimentary approaches.

The first approach is to use epidemiological investigations to study an illness in a large group of people and determine trends and patterns between the illness and potential causes of this illness. Epidemiological investigations are an effective public-health approach used to rapidly narrow down the potential causes of an illness but with little understanding of the underlying biochemical processes taking place.

> *Epidemiological* investigations and *medical* research are two complementary approaches that are used to understand how air pollution affects human health.

The second approach is to use medical research to understand the biochemical processes that are occurring within each person at the organ, tissue and even protein level. Medical research is more specific than epidemiological investigations in determining the cause of a medical event through a detailed understanding of the sequence of processes happening in the body. However, since medical research is very time consuming, epidemiological investigations help to rule out potential causes of illness, thus efficiently reducing the scope for medical investigations.

Scientists have been using a combination of these two approaches to understand how exposure to air pollution, particularly PM, is impacting processes within the body and leading to cardiovascular and pulmonary morbidity and mortality.

2.1 Epidemiological investigations

2.1.1 Human awareness of the impact of air quality on health

The first known environmental legislation was documented in Israel about 2000 years ago. Practitioners of the Jewish religion suspected a relationship between human illness and the foul odors of tanneries as well as the airborne waste products from threshing floors. Laws stipulated that industries should be located down-wind of cities and towns to minimize the exposure of citizens to airborne pollutants (Mamane, 1987).

Over 1600 years later, in 1661, John Evelyn wrote to the King of England regarding the soot in the air over London. He attributed chronic coughs and pulmonary mortalities to the air quality and he put forward recommendations to move industry outside the city to reduce air pollution (Evelyn, 1965). The suggestions of John Evelyn were ignored and air pollution levels continued to rise, pushed upwards by the 18th century industrial revolution.

In 1930, 63 people died during an air pollution episode in the Belgian Meuse Valley (Nemery et al., 2001). In 1948, 20 people died, several animals died and 43% of the 14,000 inhabitants became ill after a weather inversion in the highly industrialized town of Donora, Pennsylvania, trapped coal smoke, sulphur dioxide, soluble sulphates, and fluorides over the city (Schrenk et al., 1949). Yet, the event cited as the major turning point in air pollution awareness and public policy did not occur until 1952. In December of that year, London, England, suffered an absence of wind and a temperature inversion resulting in a very dense fog over the Greater London area. PM produced by the burning of coal was trapped within the fog, leading to a rapid and extreme rise in air pollution followed closely by a rapid and extreme rise in mortality rates. During the infamous four day pollution event in excess of 4000 deaths above typical levels occurred (Logan, 1953). In response to the startling number of air pollution related deaths, the British Parliament passed a Clean Air Act in 1956 to reduce emissions of airborne pollutants.

Since 1952 the search for the causative agent of air pollution related mortality has been pursued and gradually narrowed down to PM_{10}. In 1979 an epidemiological investigation suggested airborne particulates were responsible for some of the observed cardiopulmonary health effects (Holland et al., 1979). Nonetheless, it was not until a standardized definition of PM was introduced in 1987 by the United States Environmental Protection Agency, and statistical analysis was used to remove major confounding factors including smoking, socioeconomic status, and body-mass index that the first robust positive association between mortality and PM air pollution was established in 1993 (Dockery et al., 1993).

2.1.2 Epidemiological evidence

Today epidemiological studies present strong evidence that exposure to ambient PM_{10} contributes to cardiopulmonary morbidity and mortality (Dockery et al., 1993; Pope, 1989; Samet et al., 2000). Cardiovascular diseases are much more common in the world than pulmonary diseases and so there are more cardiovascular events following PM_{10} exposure than there are pulmonary events. Specifically, the number of heart attacks, strokes, aggravations of heart failure, cardiac arrhythmias and sudden deaths increase within hours of exposure to elevated levels of PM_{10} (Hong et al., 2002; Peters et al., 2000; Peters et al., 2004; Pope et al., 2004; Schwartz, 1994).

2.1.3 Limitations of epidemiological investigations

Epidemiological investigations can establish strong patterns and associations between an event and a cause, in this case between cardiovascular morbidity and mortality and ambient PM_{10} exposure. Epidemiological investigations can suggest organs, and tissues of interest that should be studied in detail by medical research but epidemiological investigations cannot explain the detailed biochemical processes that are occurring in the body as a result of air pollution exposure - for that scientists rely on medical research.

2.2 Medical research

2.2.1 Pulmonary health concerns

Air pollution predominately enters the body during breathing; therefore, investigating the effects of PM inhalation on the lungs was an initial focus of many research groups interested in air pollution. There is an extensive amount of literature in this field and the authors refer readers to the following reviews for more information on this topic (Ko et al., 2009; Laumbach, 2010; Ling et al., 2009; Liu et al., 2008).

To briefly summarize the progress made in the field, it has been found that short-term exposure to high levels of PM_{10} and ozone lead to altered pulmonary function in children and in adults (Kelly et al., 2011; Sheppard et al., 1999). The consequences of long-term exposure to high levels of PM_{10} include worsening of chronic obstructive pulmonary disease

(COPD)(Liu et al., 2008), and the development of chronic bronchitis and potentially lung cancer, although the later is still under debate (Gamble, 2010). Additionally, research has shown compromised lung development in children (Gauderman et al., 2007) and an increased risk of developing asthma and allergies (Kelly et al., 2011). Populations at risk of serious pulmonary consequences when exposed to elevated levels of pollutants are the elderly (Schwartz, 1995) or individuals with existing conditions such as pneumonia (Knox, 2008), asthma or COPD (Pope et al., 1995).

As the epidemiological evidence became stronger that exposure to PM also had an effect on the cardiovascular system, research groups began to study the underlying processes that might be responsible for cardiovascular related morbidity and mortality.

2.2.2 Cardiovascular health concerns

Introduction to cardiovascular disease and terminology

Before we look in detail at some of the medical research on this topic, it is important to understand the basic architecture of a healthy blood vessel. A blood vessel has three layers: the adventitia, the media and the endothelium. The media is the middle layer and the muscle layer of the blood vessel. It is populated with many smooth muscle cells. For arteries the media is quite thick, but for veins the media is rather thin. The innermost layer of the blood vessel is the endothelium, which is made of a single layer of endothelial cells that are anchored to a thin layer of structural proteins called the extracellular matrix (ECM). The endothelium is the barrier between the blood in the blood vessel and the cells and proteins of the blood vessel. Just like the liner of a swimming pool, if small holes appear in the endothelium it will cause problems. Blood clots, medically called a thrombosis, will form to prevent leakage of the blood vessel. A large thrombosis can block blood flow where it forms, or it can break off and travel in the blood until it gets stuck fully blocking a small blood vessel. A blocked blood vessel in the heart results in a heart attack (medically called a myocardial infarction), a blocked blood vessel in the brain results in a stroke. Events such as these are very rare when the blood vessel wall is healthy, but these events increase when the blood vessel is diseased such as when a person has atherosclerosis. Atherosclerosis is a disease of the medium and large blood vessels, typically characterized by fatty deposits under the endothelium of the vessel wall. A stable atherosclerotic plaque has lipid accumulation at the core, and a "cap" of smooth muscle cells and ECM (Virmani et al., 2002) (Figure 2a). This cap is important in keeping the lipid away from the blood and providing a stable anchoring surface for the endothelial cells. Myocardial infarctions and strokes typically occur when an area of an atherosclerotic plaque does not have a dense cap, and becomes unstable. The plaque may rip, crack or a region may break off. In all cases the contents of the plaque will come in contact with blood and a thrombosis will form blocking blood flow, either at the plaque or further downstream in the blood vessel. Individuals at risk of myocardial infarctions or strokes have large fatty atherosclerotic plaques that do not have a stable, dense cap (Virmani et al., 2002).

White blood cells play an important role in atherosclerotic plaques. There are several different kinds of white blood cells, but the most important in atherosclerotic plaque development is the monocyte / macrophage. These cells are important cells in the immune system. In their young form they circulate in the blood and are called monocytes. In response to a local immune signal indicated by signaling proteins called cytokines, monocytes can move out of the blood into the tissues and mature into immune cells called macrophages. Macrophages attempt to clear the foreign object, or infectious agent from the body. In the development of atherosclerotic plaques, monocytes easily enter the leaky blood vessel wall, become macrophages and take up the lipid that is accumulating in the wall. Fat filled macrophages are called macrophage-derived foam cells.

Research has also shown that cytokines are produced in response to particles deposited in the lungs. Monocytes move into the lungs, where they become alveolar macrophages. Alveolar macrophages take up the particles in an effort to clear the particles from the body.

The three mechanisms to explain how air pollution affects the heart

The epidemiological link between PM_{10} exposure and cardiovascular related morbidity and mortality is convincing; however, the underlying biological mechanism(s) remain(s) unclear. There are three primary mechanisms by which PM air pollution may bring about cardiovascular events. These are the inflammatory mechanism, the dysfunction of the autonomic nervous system mechanism and the cardiac malfunction mechanism.

> The three mechanisms that attempt to explain how air pollution affects the heart are the *inflammatory* mechanism, the *dysfunction of the autonomic nervous system* mechanism and the *cardiac malfunction* mechanism.

The inflammatory mechanism was originally proposed by Seaton and colleagues (Seaton et al., 1995). They hypothesized that exposure to air pollution irritates the lungs, particularly in patients with existing pulmonary conditions such as asthma and chronic obstructive pulmonary disease. This results in the release of cytokines in the lungs. The cytokines enter into the blood and begin a low level immune response (also called an inflammatory response) through the body. Seaton and colleagues proposed that the resulting low-grade systemic inflammatory response was involved in the observed cardiovascular events following air pollution exposure. In 1999, Seaton and colleagues showed a correlation between a decrease in the number of circulating red blood cells and PM_{10} exposure (Seaton et al., 1999). Subsequent medical studies have shown that PM_{10} exposure results in platelet activation, (Nemmar et al., 2003) and early release of white blood cells, specifically neutrophils (Mukae et al., 2000) and monocytes (Goto et al., 2004), into the circulation. Furthermore, epidemiological studies on human populations have shown an increase in the number of circulating white blood cells (Tan et al., 2000), and increased clotting and inflammation indicators in the blood (Gilmour et al., 2005). These are all observations that support the theory put forward by Seaton and colleagues in 1995 that PM_{10} exposure leads to low-grade, body-wide inflammation.

The second mechanism centers on the dysfunction of the autonomic nervous system resulting in changes in heart rate, heart rhythm and blood pressure. Epidemiological studies on human populations provide evidence that PM_{10} exposure results in a decrease in heart rate variability (Pope et al., 1999), and an increase in heart rate (Pope et al., 1999), cardiac arrhythmias (Peters et al., 2000), systolic blood pressure, (Ibald-Mulli et al., 2001) plasma viscosity (Peters et al., 1997), and arterial vasoconstriction (Brook et al., 2002). In animal studies, exposure to PM_{10} affects heart rate and blood pressure (Cheng et al., 2003), and increases arrhythmias (Watkinson et al., 2001), and fibrinogen levels (Ulrich et al., 2002). Together this data suggests that some component of PM triggers dysfunction of the autonomic nervous system, yet what that component is and how it triggers dysfunction remains unknown.

The final proposed mechanism involves particulate induced cardiac malfunction caused by particulates in the blood stream (Nemmar et al., 2002; Oberdorster et al., 2000; Oberdorster et al., 2004) leading to local damage to the heart muscle (Park et al., 2005) as well as the liver (Oberdorster et al., 2000) and the blood vessels (Schulz et al., 2005). Of the three proposed mechanisms, the cardiac malfunction mechanism has the least research and supporting data.

Understanding what processes are involved, how these processes are initiated and what the short- and long-term consequences of PM_{10} and $PM_{2.5}$ exposure are is the focus of ongoing research. The big questions can be grossly simplified to this: how does the air we breathe cause changes in our cardiovascular system and in extreme cases lead to the rupture of atherosclerotic plaques?

Medical research investigating how exposure to particulate matter affects the cardiovascular system

Studies from the Davis Heart & Lung Research Institute at Ohio State University reported increased lipid deposits and macrophage invasion into the wall of atherosclerotic plaques in an atherosclerotic mouse model, (ApoE -/- mouse) following long-term exposure to low concentrations of $PM_{2.5}$. In these same animals they reported reduced responsiveness of the blood vessel wall, and increased area of atherosclerotic plaques (Sun et al., 2005). They also found increased tissue factor expression, which is another indicator of inflammation, following exposure to particulate matter (Sun et al., 2008). Together these observations suggest a worsening of inflammation and atherosclerosis in mice after exposure to $PM_{2.5}$.

Work done by our laboratory at the James Hogg Research Center showed structural changes in atherosclerotic plaques from Watanabe Heritable Hyperlipidemic (WHHL) rabbits exposed to PM_{10} (Suwa et al., 2002; Tranfield et al., 2010; Yatera et al., 2008) and from ApoE -/- mice exposed to diesel exhaust (Bai et al., 2011). The observed changes were consistent with atherosclerotic plaques vulnerable to rupture.

Light microscopic studies reported a trend towards larger atherosclerotic plaques, increased infiltration of inflammatory cells, recruitment of monocytes and increased amounts of lipid accumulation in the plaques from rabbits exposed to PM_{10}. These studies document greater numbers of atherosclerotic plaques classified as advanced vulnerable plaques following exposure of the rabbits to PM_{10} (Suwa et al., 2002; Yatera et al., 2008).

Our electron microscopy studies showed three critical findings: 1. an accumulation of macrophage-derived foam cells immediately below the endothelium of atherosclerotic plaque cores, 2. the separation of the endothelium from a previously undescribed reticulum of dense extracellular matrix (ECM) that serves as the supporting layer of atherosclerotic plaques, and 3. evidence of degradation or fragmentation of the dense ECM in regions of macrophage-derived foam cell accumulation (Tranfield et al., 2010). As a consequence of fragmentation of the ECM, there was increased direct contact between macrophage-derived foam cells and the endothelial cells. Furthermore, increased macrophage-derived foam cell migration was observed over the core regions of atherosclerotic plaques from PM_{10} exposed rabbits. The evidence suggests that the cells were emigrating out of the atherosclerotic plaques and into the lumen of the aorta (Tranfield et al., 2010).

In the atherosclerotic plaques of the rabbits exposed to PM_{10}, we observed an absence of the dense ECM under the endothelial cells. Rather, we observed macrophage-derived foam cells (Figure 2b) or fragmented ECM (Figure 2c) under the endothelial cells, neither of which would provide a stable attachment surface for the endothelial cells. Quantification of these observations found that in PM_{10} exposed rabbits, 21.6% of the endothelial cell contacts were with fragmented ECM, whereas only 8.4% of endothelial contacts in control rabbits were in contact with fragmented ECM ($p < 0.0001$). The number of endothelial cell contacts with macrophage-derived foam cells was found to be 13.4% in the control rabbits and increased significantly to 38.1% in PM_{10} exposed rabbits ($p = 0.0039$) (Tranfield et al., 2010).

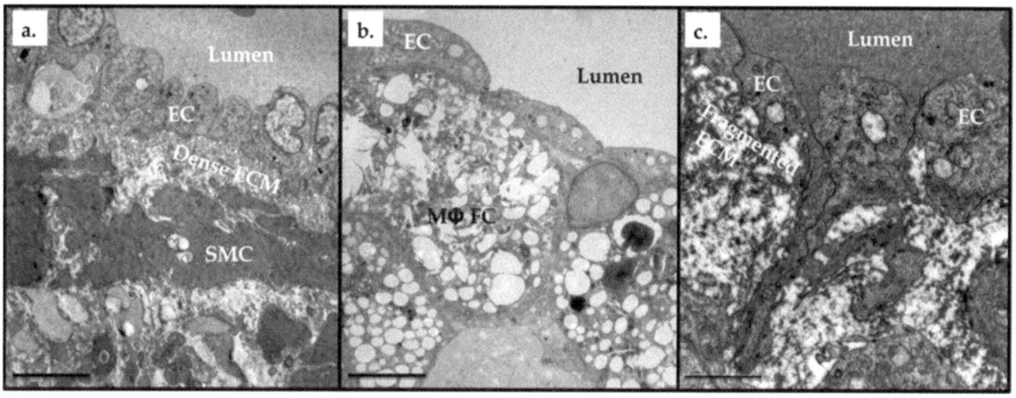

Fig. 2. The wall of an atherosclerotic plaque from a control rabbit contained smooth muscle cells (SMC) and unique dense extracellular matrix (ECM) under the endothelial cells (EC) (panel a). The wall of an atherosclerotic plaque from a rabbit exposed to PM_{10} has large lipid filled macrophage-derived foam cells (MØFC) directly under the endothelial cells (EC) (panel b) or fragmented ECM near areas of MØFC accumulation (panel c). Scale bars: a. 5 µm, b. 5 µm and c. 2 µm. Panel a and b originally published in Tranfield et al., 2010.

To better understand changes in the contact between the dense ECM and the endothelial cells, serial thin section reconstructions were done using transmission electron microscopy (Figure 3). Many contacts between the endothelial cell and the ECM were observed in the reconstructions from the control rabbits. In contrast, the endothelial cell in the reconstructions from the PM_{10} exposed rabbits had a fragmented underlying ECM and few contacts between the ECM and the endothelial cell. These observations suggest decreased stability of the endothelial cell attachments following PM_{10} exposure.

A distinction needs to be made between the core regions of an atherosclerotic plaque and the edges of an atherosclerotic plaque. In Figure 4a the edges of the plaque are outlined with white arrows whereas a white diamond marks the plaque core. Typically more stable atherosclerotic plaques grow from the edges with the center having a fibrous cap. Evidence of cell migration, lipid accumulation and plaque expansion is expected at the growing edges. As we were interested in structural indicators of instability, we focused our research on the typically-stable plaque cores well away from the active edge regions. Using a combination of transmission electron microscopy and scanning electron microscopy we observed large lipid-filled cells exiting the core regions of the atherosclerotic plaques from PM_{10} exposed rabbits (Figure 4c, d, e and f). This finding was quite unexpected.

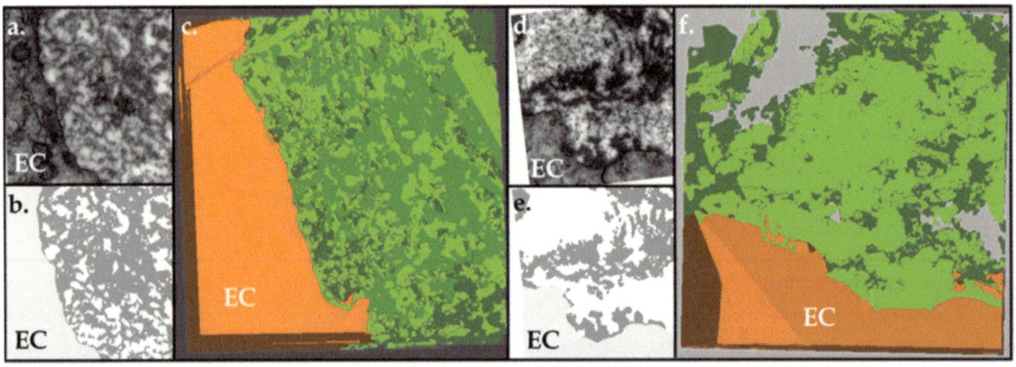

Fig. 3. Three-dimensional reconstruction of the extracellular matrix (ECM, green in c and f) under an endothelial cell (EC, orange in c and f). Panels a-c are from a control rabbit. Panels d-f are from a PM_{10} exposed rabbit. Panels a and d are a single transmission electron micrograph from the series of reconstructed images. Panels b and e are the tracing of the endothelial cell and the dense extracellular matrix shown in panel a and d respectively. Panels c and f are the full reconstruction made of 20 serial tracings from thin sections and show that the contact area between the EC and the ECM is much greater in the control reconstruction than the PM_{10} reconstruction. Methodology and further figures are published in Tranfield et al., 2010.

When all these observations are taken together we believe we have significantly contributed to the understanding of how air pollution may trigger cardiovascular events. An accumulation of macrophage-derived foam cells subtending the endothelium, decreased endothelial contact with a dense, stable reticulum of ECM material and the emigration of large leukocytes from atherosclerotic plaques are indicators of atherosclerotic plaque remodeling following PM_{10} exposure. Taken together with previous work, these findings illustrate mechanisms of remodeling following exposure to PM_{10} that may convert stable atherosclerotic plaques into unstable atherosclerotic plaques. Cardiovascular disease affects millions of people and it appears that PM_{10} exposure may be a considerable contributor to endothelial destabilization and dysfunction potentially being involved in millions of deaths annually. Although PM_{10} exposure is not usually considered an initiating risk factor for atherosclerosis, it appears to be an exacerbating risk factor, pushing existing atherosclerotic plaques to a more vulnerable phenotype.

2.2.3 At-risk groups for cardiovascular complications following PM_{10} exposure

Epidemiological investigations have identified several at-risk groups. Particulate air pollution exposure has been repeatedly linked to adverse events in individuals with a prior

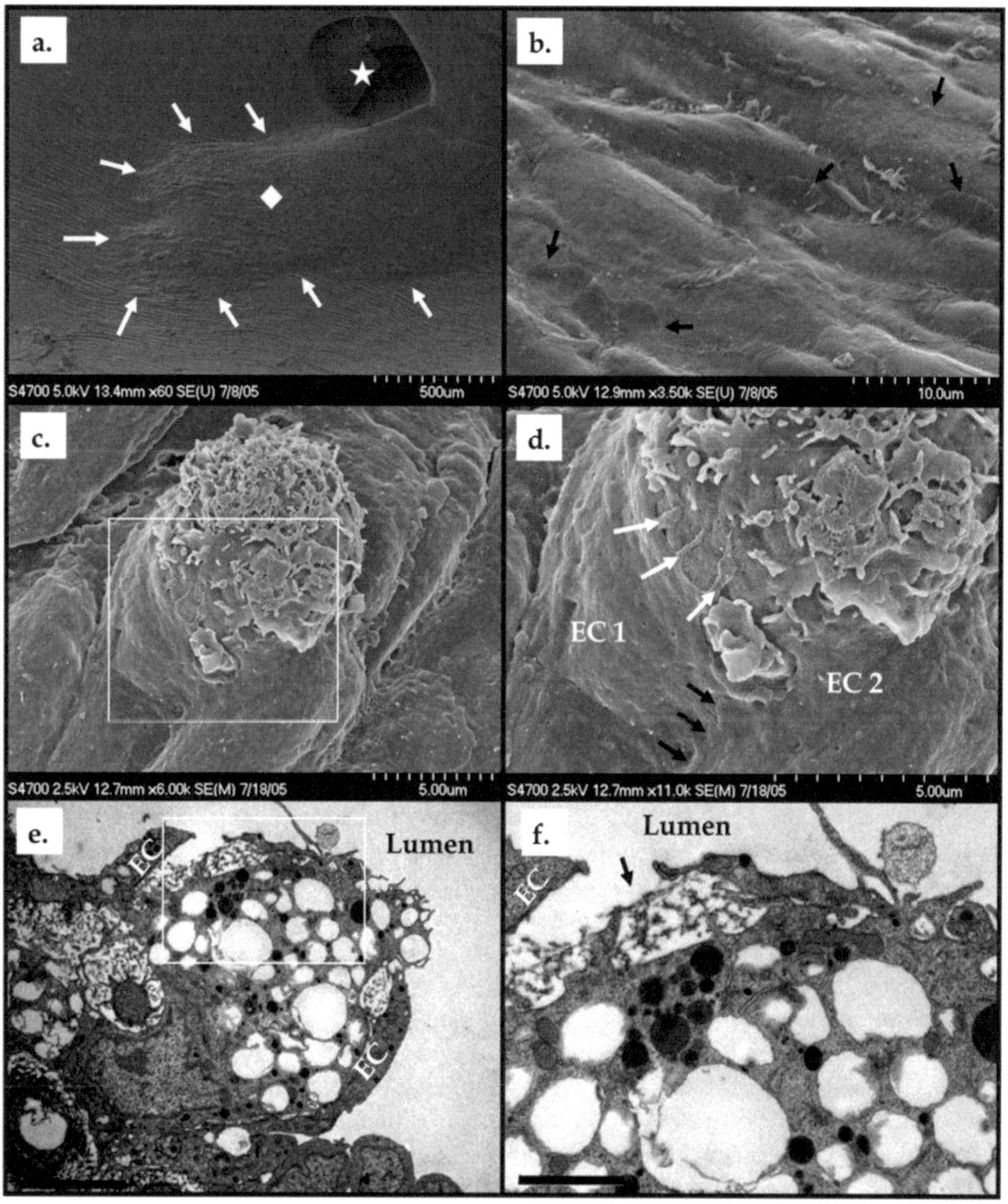

Fig. 4. Electron micrographs of the aorta. Panel a: The core region (◆) of an atherosclerotic plaque (outlined by white arrows) at a branch in the aorta (*). Panel b: Cell borders of healthy endothelium (black arrows). Panels c and d: Cell pushing between two endothelial cells into the blood vessel lumen. The border (black arrows) between the two endothelial cells (EC1 and EC2) and the EC finger-like projections up the side of the migrating cell (white arrows). Panel e and f: Transmission electron micrographs of a macrophage-derived foam cell pushing the endothelial cells aside (EC) as it emerges into the blood vessel lumen. Panel f: Extracellular matrix (arrow) caught above the migrating cell, which would only be possible if the cell is migrating out of the wall. Scale bars: e = 5 μm; f = 2 μm. All micrographs originally published in Tranfield et al., 2010.

myocardial infarction or chronic diabetes, both of which are associated with advanced atherosclerotic disease. Furthermore, exposure to $PM_{2.5}$ had a significant effect in ApoE -/- mice fed high fat chow, whereas a diminished effect was observed in ApoE -/- mice on regular chow diets. Collectively, these observations suggest that PM exposure has a negative impact in combination with high lipid diets, and existing atherosclerosis. Atherosclerotic plaque disruption with thrombus formation is the predominant mechanism leading to unstable angina, myocardial infarctions and sudden death. Therefore, it seems likely that air pollution related morbidity and mortality may also be associated with advanced atherosclerotic disease and plaque disruption.

2.2.4 PM_{10} exposure affects cardiovascular morbidity and mortality: A proposed mechanism

If you will, imagine an individual who is aging, who has at least one or two major risk factors for atherosclerosis and who has been chronically exposed to low levels of air pollution. Epidemiological investigations repeatedly link PM_{10} exposure to adverse cardiovascular events in individuals with advanced atherosclerotic disease. Medical research from our laboratory and other laboratories demonstrates that the atherosclerotic plaques in an individual undergo destabilizing structural changes as a consequence of exposure to PM_{10}. Combined, the data suggest that an individual will experience the progressive worsening and destabilization of their atherosclerotic plaques as a consequence of PM_{10} exposure. Now imagine an event that results in an increase in PM_{10} levels, such as a forest fire or a smog day in a large city. Epidemiology investigations and medical research suggest that at this point there will be a decrease in heart rate variability and an increase in circulating white cells and cytokines, and an increase in heart rate, cardiac arrhythmias, systolic blood pressure, arterial vasoconstriction, plasma viscosity, platelet activation, and fibrinogen levels. Combined, all of these factors result in an enhanced clotting (procoagulant) and enhanced inflammatory state of the circulating blood. What we have now in our hypothetical individual is vulnerable atherosclerotic plaques, increased reactivity of the blood and altered shear stress on the vasculature, a perfect deadly scenario for an acute cardiovascular event to play out as follows: as the blood pressure increases, the flow properties of the blood may change, and a vulnerable atherosclerotic plaque, whose endothelium has lost its extracellular matrix and had its surface shape and contours altered by emigrating foam cells, may rupture or break. The increased blood viscosity, fibrinogen levels and platelet activation aid in a large thrombus formation. If the thrombus does not fully fill the blood vessel and block blood flow, it may break off in the setting of increased luminal narrowing and vascular tone and be sent downstream in the progressively narrowing blood vessels. At some point this thrombus will get stuck, blocking blood flow leading to a heart attack or stroke, and potentially the death of the individual. Our hypothetical person has now become one of the 2 million people to die annually from air pollution exposure. The mechanisms involved in the death of our hypothetical person were not only the inflammatory mechanisms, but also the autonomic dysfunction mechanism. We propose that these two mechanisms are not separate; rather they are convergent processes that together lead to plaque destabilization and rupture as a consequence of chronic air pollution exposure.

3. Future actions to reduce the health consequences of air pollution

The World Health Organization predicts that there are more than 2,000,000 premature deaths every year as a consequence of air pollution exposure. This number is far too high, particularly for the friends and family who have lost a loved one. Steps can be taken on several levels to reduce this number. To begin with, through continued epidemiological and medical research scientists can continue to uncover the underlying mechanisms for the high number of deaths. Secondly, measures can be taken at local, national and international levels to reduce the global production of air pollution.

3.1 Research

Since 1952 when so many people died during the London Fog, a great deal of insight about the effects of air pollution has been uncovered. However, scientists still do not fully understand the biochemical mechanisms underlying PM related deaths. Research in this field is needed to expand scientific understanding. These efforts would be made with the hope that greater scientific knowledge can lead to medical prevention of further fatalities.

There are several overarching topics that should be investigated in further detail. The first is understanding the medical effects of individual pollutants, understanding who is at risk, what medical conditions these individual pollutants cause, or aggravate and why. Once this is better understood then efforts need to be made to understand how mixtures of pollutants act, and how mixtures of pollutants condense and modify over time. It will be important to understand if certain pollutants work synergistically to aggravate cardiopulmonary morbidity and mortality. It will be important to understand the acute and the chronic effects of the pollutants to predict subsets of the populations who are at greatest risk. Beyond this it will be important to understand the extent of the health effects of PM exposure on the otherwise healthy individuals in society.

3.2 Reduce PM creation / Increase PM reduction measures

In addition to research, measures can be taken to reduce the effects of PM by decreasing PM production and increasing PM removal from the atmosphere. To successfully accomplish a reduction in PM pollution steps can be taken at all levels of government. There is a great deal of literature already existing on this topic, but here are a few ideas to consider.

3.2.1 Local

At the local level individuals can make choices that reduce PM creation, such as purchasing locally grown food that is not transported great distances, or growing their own vegetables and fruit. Local governments can implement green programs that increase the use of bikes or carpools to reduce the use of cars for short trips. Efforts can be made to help homeowners make better choices in the selection of building materials for new homes, and help individuals make existing homes more energy efficient. Both individuals and communities can take measures to reduce energy waste, thereby reducing PM production. Taking action like bicycle commuting has multiple positive effects such as reducing a person's risk of cardiovascular disease and obesity, reducing the production of PM and saving money on fuel. However, individuals will not commute without bike lanes and safety infrastructure thus this behavioral change needs support from local government.

3.2.2 National

The contribution at the national level comes under two broad categories: financial and legal. The changes that will be required at the individual and local level will require a financial investment. Furthermore, nations should invest in research to understand the health consequences of pollution exposure as well as dedicate money to the development of less polluting technologies. Governments should consider the money they will save on health care expenses as justification for this expense.

The legal category applies to government regulation of industry. Governments need to hold polluting industries responsible for the damage being done to the environment and human health. Though industry will not be in favor of tough regulations in line with the current recommendations of the World Health Organization, the regulations need to be implemented. This may require governments to financially assist companies as they transition to less polluting business practices. The transition will be expensive and challenging, but given the impact PM pollution production is having on human health and the environment, it is a transition that must be done.

3.2.3 International/ global

The contribution at the international and global levels is similar to the contribution at the national level: financial and legal. Countries need to hold each other accountable for the pollution that is being produced. China, one of the biggest suppliers of goods in North America, is also one of the countries producing a lot of pollution. In the international arena, countries need to decide if this is an acceptable situation.

4. Conclusions

Data from epidemiological investigations and medical research strongly suggest that exposure to fine particulate matter air pollution results in deposition of particulates in the lungs, activation of a systemic inflammatory response and alteration of the ultrastructure of atherosclerotic plaques. Air pollution levels can be controlled if individuals make efforts to reduce their pollution production, and governments at the local, national and international levels invest in green infrastructure, and green technology to reduce pollution production as well as invest in ongoing medical research to understand the biological mechanisms underlying air pollution related morbidity and mortality. It will take a coordinated effort to globally reduce the production of air pollution and reduce the effect air pollution has on human health.

5. Acknowledgement

The authors wish to thank Ron Biggs for his editorial guidance.

6. References

Australian Government. (2009, 16/09/2009). Air Quality Standards. Retrieved July 13, 2011, from http://www.environment.gov.au/atmosphere/airquality/standards.html.

Bai, N., T. Kido, H. Suzuki, G. Yang, T. J. Kavanagh, J. D. Kaufman, M. E. Rosenfeld, C. van Breemen & S. F. Eeden (2011). Changes in atherosclerotic plaques induced by inhalation of diesel exhaust. *Atherosclerosis* 216(2): 299-306.

Brain, J. D., J. Godleski & W. Kreyling (1994). In vivo evaluation of chemical biopersistence of nonfibrous inorganic particles. *Environ Health Perspect* 102 Suppl 5: 119-125.

Brook, R. D., J. R. Brook, B. Urch, R. Vincent, S. Rajagopalan & F. Silverman (2002). Inhalation of fine particulate air pollution and ozone causes acute arterial vasoconstriction in healthy adults. *Circulation* 105(13): 1534-1536.

Canadian Council of Ministers of the Environment (2000). Canada -Wide Standards for Particulate Matter (PM) and Ozone. C. C. o. M. o. t. Environment. Quebec City.

Cheng, T. J., J. S. Hwang, P. Y. Wang, C. F. Tsai, C. Y. Chen, S. H. Lin & C. C. Chan (2003). Effects of concentrated ambient particles on heart rate and blood pressure in pulmonary hypertensive rats. *Environ Health Perspect* 111(2): 147-150.

Dockery, D. W. & C. A. Pope, 3rd (1994). Acute respiratory effects of particulate air pollution. *Annu Rev Public Health* 15: 107-132.

Dockery, D. W., C. A. Pope, 3rd, X. Xu, J. D. Spengler, J. H. Ware, M. E. Fay, B. G. Ferris, Jr. & F. E. Speizer (1993). An association between air pollution and mortality in six U.S. cities. *N Engl J Med* 329(24): 1753-1759.

European Commission Environment. (2011, 14/04/2011). Air Quality Standards. Retrieved July 13, 2011, from http://ec.europa.eu/environment/air/quality/standards.htm.

Evelyn, J. (1965). Fumifugium or, the inconvenience of the aer. and smoake of London dissipated. *J Chronic Dis* 18(12): 1235-1258.

Finlayson-Pitts, B. J. & J. N. Pitts (2000). *Chemistry of the upper and lower atmosphere : theory, experiments and applications*. San Diego, Calif. ; London, Academic Press.

Gamble, J. (2010). Lung cancer and diesel exhaust: a critical review of the occupational epidemiology literature. *Crit Rev Toxicol* 40(3). 189-244.

Gauderman, W. J., H. Vora, R. McConnell, K. Berhane, F. Gilliland, D. Thomas, F. Lurmann, E. Avol, N. Kunzli, M. Jerrett & J. Peters (2007). Effect of exposure to traffic on lung development from 10 to 18 years of age: a cohort study. *Lancet* 369(9561): 571-577.

Gilmour, P. S., E. R. Morrison, M. A. Vickers, I. Ford, C. A. Ludlam, M. Greaves, K. Donaldson & W. MacNee (2005). The procoagulant potential of environmental particles (PM_{10}). *Occup Environ Med* 62(3): 164-171.

Goto, Y., J. C. Hogg, C. H. Shih, H. Ishii, R. Vincent & S. F. van Eeden (2004). Exposure to ambient particles accelerates monocyte release from bone marrow in atherosclerotic rabbits. *Am J Physiol Lung Cell Mol Physiol* 287(1): L79-85.

Harmsen, A. G., B. A. Muggenburg, M. B. Snipes & D. E. Bice (1985). The role of macrophages in particle translocation from lungs to lymph nodes. *Science* 230(4731): 1277-1280.

Hinds, W. C. (1999). *Aerosol technology : properties, behavior, and measurement of airborne particles*. New York, Wiley.

Holland, W. W., A. E. Bennett, I. R. Cameron, C. V. Florey, S. R. Leeder, R. S. Schilling, A. V. Swan & R. E. Waller (1979). Health effects of particulate pollution: reappraising the evidence. *Am J Epidemiol* 110(5): 527-659.

Hong, Y. C., J. T. Lee, H. Kim & H. J. Kwon (2002). Air pollution: a new risk factor in ischemic stroke mortality. *Stroke* 33(9): 2165-2169.

Hong, Y. C., J. H. Leem & E. H. Ha (1999). Air pollution and daily mortality in Inchon, Korea. *J Korean Med Sci* 14(3): 239-244.

Ibald-Mulli, A., J. Stieber, H. E. Wichmann, W. Koenig & A. Peters (2001). Effects of air pollution on blood pressure: a population-based approach. *Am J Public Health* 91(4): 571-577.

Kelly, F. J. & J. C. Fussell (2011). Air pollution and airway disease. *Clin Exp Allergy*.

Kendall, M., T. D. Tetley, E. Wigzell, B. Hutton, M. Nieuwenhuijsen & P. Luckham (2002). Lung lining liquid modifies PM(2.5) in favor of particle aggregation: a protective mechanism. *Am J Physiol Lung Cell Mol Physiol* 282(1): L109-114.

Knox, E. G. (2008). Atmospheric pollutants and mortalities in English local authority areas. *J Epidemiol Community Health* 62(5): 442-447.

Ko, F. W. & D. S. Hui (2009). Outdoor air pollution: impact on chronic obstructive pulmonary disease patients. *Curr Opin Pulm Med* 15(2): 150-157.

Laumbach, R. J. (2010). Outdoor air pollutants and patient health. *Am Fam Physician* 81(2): 175-180.

Lin, M., D. M. Stieb & Y. Chen (2005). Coarse particulate matter and hospitalization for respiratory infections in children younger than 15 years in Toronto: a case-crossover analysis. *Pediatrics* 116(2): e235-240.

Ling, S. H. & S. F. van Eeden (2009). Particulate matter air pollution exposure: role in the development and exacerbation of chronic obstructive pulmonary disease. *Int J Chron Obstruct Pulmon Dis* 4: 233-243.

Lipfert, F. W. & R. E. Wyzga (1995). Air pollution and mortality: issues and uncertainties. *J Air Waste Manag Assoc* 45(12): 949-966.

Liu, Y., K. Lee, R. Perez-Padilla, N. L. Hudson & D. M. Mannino (2008). Outdoor and indoor air pollution and COPD-related diseases in high- and low-income countries. *Int J Tuberc Lung Dis* 12(2): 115-127.

Logan, W. P. (1953). Mortality in the London fog incident, 1952. *Lancet* 1(7): 336-338.

Mackay, J. & G. Mensah (2004). *Atlas of Heart Disease and Stroke*. Geneva, World Health Organization.

Mamane, Y. (1987). Air Pollution Control in Israel during the First and Second Century. *Atmos. Environ.* 21(8): 1861-1863.

Morris, R. D., E. N. Naumova & R. L. Munasinghe (1995). Ambient air pollution and hospitalization for congestive heart failure among elderly people in seven large US cities. *Am J Public Health* 85(10): 1361-1365.

Mukae, H., J. C. Hogg, D. English, R. Vincent & S. F. van Eeden (2000). Phagocytosis of particulate air pollutants by human alveolar macrophages stimulates the bone marrow. *Am J Physiol Lung Cell Mol Physiol* 279(5): L924-931.

Naga, S., A. K. Guptaa & U. K. Mukhopadhyay (2005). Size Distribution of Atmospheric Aerosols in Kolkata, India and the Assessment of Pulmonary Deposition of Particle Mass. *Indoor Built Environ* 14(5): 381-389.

Nemery, B., P. H. Hoet & A. Nemmar (2001). The Meuse Valley fog of 1930: an air pollution disaster. *Lancet* 357(9257): 704-708.

Nemmar, A., P. H. Hoet, D. Dinsdale, J. Vermylen, M. F. Hoylaerts & B. Nemery (2003). Diesel exhaust particles in lung acutely enhance experimental peripheral thrombosis. *Circulation* 107(8): 1202-1208.

Nemmar, A., P. H. Hoet, B. Vanquickenborne, D. Dinsdale, M. Thomeer, M. F. Hoylaerts, H. Vanbilloen, L. Mortelmans & B. Nemery (2002). Passage of inhaled particles into the blood circulation in humans. *Circulation* 105(4): 411-414.

Oberdorster, G. (2001). Pulmonary effects of inhaled ultrafine particles. *Int Arch Occup Environ Health* 74(1): 1-8.

Oberdorster, G., J. Ferin & B. E. Lehnert (1994). Correlation between particle size, in vivo particle persistence, and lung injury. *Environ Health Perspect* 102 Suppl 5: 173-179.

Oberdorster, G., J. N. Finkelstein, C. Johnston, R. Gelein, C. Cox, R. Baggs & A. C. Elder (2000). Acute pulmonary effects of ultrafine particles in rats and mice. *Res Rep Health Eff Inst*(96): 5-74; disc 75-86.

Oberdorster, G., Z. Sharp, V. Atudorei, A. Elder, R. Gelein, W. Kreyling & C. Cox (2004). Translocation of inhaled ultrafine particles to the brain. *Inhal Toxicol* 16(6-7): 437-445.

Park, S. K., M. S. O'Neill, P. S. Vokonas, D. Sparrow & J. Schwartz (2005). Effects of air pollution on heart rate variability: the VA normative aging study. *Environ Health Perspect* 113(3): 304-309.

Peng, R. D., F. Dominici, R. Pastor-Barriuso, S. L. Zeger & J. M. Samet (2005). Seasonal analyses of air pollution and mortality in 100 US cities. *Am J Epidemiol* 161(6): 585-594.

Peters, A., A. Doring, H. E. Wichmann & W. Koenig (1997). Increased plasma viscosity during an air pollution episode: a link to mortality? *Lancet* 349 (9065): 1582-1587.

Peters, A., E. Liu, R. L. Verrier, J. Schwartz, D. R. Gold, M. Mittleman, J. Baliff, J. A. Oh, G. Allen, K. Monahan & D. W. Dockery (2000). Air pollution and incidence of cardiac arrhythmia. *Epidemiology* 11(1): 11-17.

Peters, A., B. Veronesi, L. Calderon-Garciduenas, P. Gehr, L. C. Chen, M. Geiser, W. Reed, B. Rothen-Rutishauser, S. Schurch & H. Schulz (2006). Translocation and potential neurological effects of fine and ultrafine particles a critical update. *Part Fibre Toxicol* 3: 13.

Peters, A., S. von Klot, M. Heier, I. Trentinaglia, A. Hormann, H. E. Wichmann & H. Lowel (2004). Exposure to traffic and the onset of myocardial infarction. *N Engl J Med* 351(17): 1721-1730.

Pope, C. A., 3rd (1989). Respiratory disease associated with community air pollution and a steel mill, Utah Valley. *Am J Public Health* 79(5): 623-628.

Pope, C. A., 3rd, R. T. Burnett, G. D. Thurston, M. J. Thun, E. E. Calle, D. Krewski & J. J. Godleski (2004). Cardiovascular mortality and long-term exposure to particulate air pollution: epidemiological evidence of general pathophysiological pathways of disease. *Circulation* 109(1): 71-77.

Pope, C. A., 3rd, M. J. Thun, M. M. Namboodiri, D. W. Dockery, J. S. Evans, F. E. Speizer & C. W. Heath, Jr. (1995). Particulate air pollution as a predictor of mortality in a prospective study of U.S. adults. *Am J Respir Crit Care Med* 151(3 Pt 1): 669-674.

Pope, C. A., 3rd, R. L. Verrier, E. G. Lovett, A. C. Larson, M. E. Raizenne, R. E. Kanner, J. Schwartz, G. M. Villegas, D. R. Gold & D. W. Dockery (1999). Heart rate variability associated with particulate air pollution. *Am Heart J* 138(5 Pt 1): 890-899.

Pope, C. A. r., D. W. Dockery, R. E. Kanner, G. M. Villegas & J. Schwartz (1999). Oxygen saturation, pulse rate, and particulate air pollution: A daily time-series panel study. *Am J Respir Crit Care Med* 159(2): 365-372.

Samet, J. M., F. Dominici, F. C. Curriero, I. Coursac & S. L. Zeger (2000). Fine particulate air pollution and mortality in 20 U.S. cities, 1987-1994. *N Engl J Med* 343(24): 1742-1749.

Schrenk, H. H., H. Heimann, G. D. Clayton, W. M. Gafafer & H. Wexler (1949). *Air pollution in Donora, Pennsylvania: epidemiology of the unusual smog episode of October 1948.* Washington, DC, Public Health Service.

Schulz, H., V. Harder, A. Ibald-Mulli, A. Khandoga, W. Koenig, F. Krombach, R. Radykewicz, A. Stampfl, B. Thorand & A. Peters (2005). Cardiovascular effects of fine and ultrafine particles. *J Aerosol Med* 18(1): 1-22.

Schwartz, J. (1994). What are people dying of on high air pollution days? *Environ Res* 64(1): 26-35.

Schwartz, J. (1995). Short term fluctuations in air pollution and hospital admissions of the elderly for respiratory disease. *Thorax* 50(5): 531-538.

Seaton, A., W. MacNee, K. Donaldson & D. Godden (1995). Particulate air pollution and acute health effects. *Lancet* 345(8943): 176-178.

Seaton, A., A. Soutar, V. Crawford, R. Elton, S. McNerlan, J. Cherrie, M. Watt, R. Agius & R. Stout (1999). Particulate air pollution and the blood. *Thorax* 54(11): 1027-1032.

Semmler, M., J. Seitz, F. Erbe, P. Mayer, J. Heyder, G. Oberdorster & W. G. Kreyling (2004). Long-term clearance kinetics of inhaled ultrafine insoluble iridium particles from the rat lung, including transient translocation into secondary organs. *Inhal Toxicol* 16(6-7): 453-459.

Sheppard, L., D. Levy, G. Norris, T. V. Larson & J. Q. Koenig (1999). Effects of ambient air pollution on nonelderly asthma hospital admissions in Seattle, Washington, 1987-1994. *Epidemiology* 10(1): 23-30.

Sioutas, C., R. J. Delfino & M. Singh (2005). Exposure assessment for atmospheric ultrafine particles (UFPs) and implications in epidemiologic research. *Environ Health Perspect* 113(8): 947-955.

Stieb, D. M., S. Judek & R. T. Burnett (2002). Meta-analysis of time-series studies of air pollution and mortality: effects of gases and particles and the influence of cause of death, age, and season. *J Air Waste Manag Assoc* 52(4): 470-484.

Sun, Q., A. Wang, X. Jin, A. Natanzon, D. Duquaine, R. D. Brook, J. G. Aguinaldo, Z. A. Fayad, V. Fuster, M. Lippmann, L. C. Chen & S. Rajagopalan (2005). Long-term air pollution exposure and acceleration of atherosclerosis and vascular inflammation in an animal model. *Jama* 294(23): 3003-3010.

Sun, Q., P. Yue, R. I. Kirk, A. Wang, D. Moatti, X. Jin, B. Lu, A. D. Schecter, M. Lippmann, T. Gordon, L. C. Chen & S. Rajagopalan (2008). Ambient air particulate matter exposure and tissue factor expression in atherosclerosis. *Inhal Toxicol* 20(2): 127-137.

Suwa, T., J. C. Hogg, K. B. Quinlan, A. Ohgami, R. Vincent & S. F. van Eeden (2002). Particulate air pollution induces progression of atherosclerosis. *J Am Coll Cardiol* 39(6): 935-942.

Tan, W. C., D. Qiu, B. L. Liam, T. P. Ng, S. H. Lee, S. F. van Eeden, Y. D'Yachkova & J. C. Hogg (2000). The human bone marrow response to acute air pollution caused by forest fires. *Am J Respir Crit Care Med* 161(4 Pt 1): 1213-1217.

Tranfield, E. M., S. F. van Eeden, K. Yatera, J. C. Hogg & D. C. Walker (2010). Ultrastructural changes in atherosclerotic plaques following the instillation of airborne particulate matter into the lungs of rabbits. *Can J Cardiol* 26(7): e258-269.

Ulrich, M. M., G. M. Alink, P. Kumarathasan, R. Vincent, A. J. Boere & F. R. Cassee (2002). Health effects and time course of particulate matter on the cardiopulmonary system in rats with lung inflammation. *J Toxicol Environ Health A* 65(20): 1571-1595.

United States Environmental Protection Agency. (2011, 07/07/2011). National Ambient Air Quality Standards. Retrieved July 13, 2011, from http://www.epa.gov/air/criteria.html.

Virmani, R., A. P. Burke, A. Farb & F. D. Kolodgie (2002). Pathology of the unstable plaque. *Prog Cardiovasc Dis* 44(5): 349-356.

Wang, G., L. Huang, S. Gao, S. Gao & L. Wang (2002). Measurements of PM10 and PM2.5 in urban area of Nanjing, China and the assessment of pulmonary deposition of particle mass. *Chemosphere* 48(7): 689-695.

Watkinson, W. P., M. J. Campen, J. P. Nolan & D. L. Costa (2001). Cardiovascular and systemic responses to inhaled pollutants in rodents: effects of ozone and particulate matter. *Environ Health Perspect* 109 Suppl 4: 539-546.

West, J. B. & J. B. West (2003). *Pulmonary pathophysiology : the essentials*. Philadelphia, PA. ; Baltimore, Lippincott Williams & Wilkins.

Wichmann, H. E., W. Mueller, P. Allhoff, M. Beckmann, N. Bocter, M. J. Csicsaky, M. Jung, B. Molik & G. Schoeneberg (1989). Health effects during a smog episode in West Germany in 1985. *Environ Health Perspect* 79: 89-99.

World Health Organization (2005). *WHO Air quality guidelinesfor particulate matter, ozone, nitrogen dioxide and sulfur dioxide: Global update 2005*, WHO, Regional Office for Europe, Copenhagen.

Yatera, K., J. Hsieh, J. C. Hogg, E. Tranfield, H. Suzuki, C. H. Shih, A. R. Behzad, R. Vincent & S. F. van Eeden (2008). Particulate matter air pollution exposure promotes recruitment of monocytes into atherosclerotic plaques. *Am J Physiol Heart Circ Physiol* 294(2): H944-953.

Traffic-Related Air Pollution: Legislation *Versus* Health and Environmental Effects

Klara Slezakova[1,2], Simone Morais[2]
and Maria do Carmo Pereira[1]
[1]*LEPAE, Departamento de Engenharia Química, Faculdade de Engenharia, Universidade do Porto,*
[2]*REQUIMTE, Instituto Superior de Engenharia do Porto, Portugal*

1. Introduction

Ambient air quality is a very topical issue as it has an important influence on human health. Exposure to atmospheric pollutants may result in various adverse health effects. The impacts of air pollution are not confined only to human health but also to the environment as a whole. In that regard, vehicular traffic emissions are especially important, because its volume is increasing every year. Consequently pollutants, such as nitrogen oxides (NOx), carbon monoxide (CO), particulate matter (PM), and polycyclic aromatic hydrocarbons (PAHs) are emitted into the atmosphere causing a significant decline of air quality across Europe, which results in hundreds of thousands of premature deaths every year. In order to improve the situation, the European Union has been defining legislation on ambient air quality with limits of the respective pollutants and aiming to increase the levels of public health protection. Despite reductions in emissions, concentrations of these pollutants remain high – often above existing targets – exposing populations to levels that reduce life expectancy, cause premature death and widespread aggravation to health.

In this chapter, various aspects of air pollution are discussed with specific emphasis on vehicular road traffic. An overview of the current legislation related to air quality is given. The work then focuses on the health impacts of important traffic related pollutants, with particular focus on polycyclic aromatic hydrocarbons (PAHs). The general description of PAHs is presented with further discussion on their health and environmental impacts.

2. Air pollution

Air quality is a very topical issue at the moment. Ultimately we are all surrounded by air both indoors and outdoors and we need air to live; the daily human requirement for air is around 15 kg. Generally air is freely available and we have come to regard access to air of acceptable quality as a fundamental human right.

Primary air pollutants are emitted directly into the atmosphere, whilst secondary pollutants are formed in it. Primary air pollutants include nitrogen oxides, sulfur dioxide, volatile organic compounds, and particles that are released into the atmosphere from road transport emissions, stationary combustion sources, and from natural emissions. Secondary air pollutants are formed from chemical reactions of primary pollutants in the atmosphere and include ground level ozone and secondary particulates. The total emissions of the main air pollutants in 27 Member States of the European Union are presented in Table 1 (EEA, 2010).

Pollutant	Units	1990	2008	Change (%) 1990-2008
Nitrogen oxides (NOx)	Gg	17 152	10 397	- 39
Carbon monoxide (CO)	Gg	64 526	27 228	- 58
Sulphur oxides (SOx)	Gg	26 208	5 867	- 78
Particles ($PM_{2.5}$)	Gg	1 612[a]	1 403	- 13
Particles (PM_{10})	Gg	2 299[a]	2 126	- 8
Mon-methane volatile organic compounds (NMVOC)	Gg	16 807	8 296	- 51
Total polycyclic aromatic hydrocarbons (PAHs)	Mg	3 416	1 359	- 60
Amonium (NH_3)	Gg	4 997	3 799	- 24
Lead (Pb)	Mg	22 398	2 293	- 90
Cadmium (Cd)	Mg	281	118	- 58
[a]data of 2000, once information for previous years is not available				

Table 1. Emissions of the main air pollutants during 1990-2008 in 27 Member States of European Union

Table 1 clearly demonstrates that among the main air pollutants, the largest reductions across 27 Member States of the European Union have been achieved for lead and SOx, which have decreased since 1990 by 90% and 78%, respectively. The implementation of regulations setting limits of lead and sulfur dioxide levels in urban areas has contributed to these significant reductions. Other parallel political actions devoted to the control of urban atmospheric emissions include a ban of the use of lead additives in gasoline (Directive 98/70/EC), sulfur abatement technologies in industrial facilities (EEA, 2011a) and the introduction of fuels with reduced levels of sulfur (Directive 98/70/EC; EN 590/2004). These initiatives have all contributed to a sharp decrease of the emitted amounts of sulfur dioxide. Emissions of other key air pollutants also decreased since 1990. It is noteworthy that these significant reductions include emissions of the three air pollutants primarily responsible for the formation of harmful ground-level ozone in the atmosphere, namely carbon monoxide (58% reduction), non-methane volatile organic compounds (51% reduction) and nitrogen oxides (39% reduction). The concentrations of particulate matter have not shown significant improvement since 1997. Emission trends compiled for the period 2000–2008 indicate that PM_{10} emissions decreased by 8%, while $PM_{2.5}$ was reduced by 13%. Fine particulate matter is now generally recognized as one the main threats to human health from air pollution, with transport being a significant source (EEA, 2011b). Data available on cadmium reveal that since 1990 significant emission reductions have occurred for this toxic heavy metal (around 60%). These reductions were due to improved abatement technologies for combustion facilities and in the metal refining and smelting industries (EEA, 2009). However, despite the emissions reductions, concentrations of many of these pollutants remain high, often above existing standards (EEA, 2005).

Sources of air pollutants may be classified as stationary (fossil fuel power plants, petrochemical plants, petroleum refineries, food processing plants, other large and small industries, and home heating) or mobile (automobiles, industrial vehicles, trains, all types of vessels, and airplanes) (Godish, 2004). Among these, emissions from vehicle road transport are especially important as they are a significant source of pollution within urban areas throughout the world. Some authors (Fischer et al., 2000; Martuzevicius et al., 2008) reported twofold differences in the concentrations of several traffic-related primary pollutants (black carbon, fine particulate matter, benzo[a]pyrene, and benzene) in locations with high and low traffic activity.

In Europe emissions of some road transport-related pollutants, such as nitrogen oxides or non-methane volatile organic compounds have decreased since 1990 (EEA, 2010), mainly due to the introduction of new technologies (i.e. three way catalytic converters on passenger cars) and stricter regulation of emissions from heavy duty vehicles (Regulation 595/2009). Despite these decreases the Member States of the European Union still have difficulty complying with the legislative limits of traffic related pollutants (EEA, 2008), mainly due to the fact that the demand for road transport has been growing much faster than anticipated. Transport volumes are growing about 1.9% annually for passenger and 2.7% for freight transport (EEA, 2011b). Road transport remains the most important source of the ozone precursors, namely of nitrogen oxides and carbon monoxide in Europe, in 2008 contributing 40% and 34% of total European emissions, respectively (Table 2; EEA, 2008, 2010). Whereas passenger cars and heavy duty vehicles contribute the majority of road transport nitrogen oxide emissions, for carbon monoxide passenger cars alone contribute around 4/5 of the emissions from the road transport sector. Road transport is also a significant source of non-methane volatile organic compounds (Table 2) and of $PM_{2.5}$ and PM_{10} emissions (EEA, 2008, 2010).

Increases in urbanization and motor vehicle use have raised questions about the health effects of exposure to traffic pollutants. Kunzli et al. (2000) estimated that in European countries France, Switzerland and Austria, with a total population of 74 million inhabitants, 3% of total mortality per year (i.e. 20 000 deaths) are due to traffic emissions alone; hypothetically total omission of traffic emissions would lead to prolonged life expectancy of 0.35 years. Other studies indicate that living near roads with heavy traffic may considerably increase the risks of adverse health effects (Beelen et al., 2009; Heinrich et al., 2005; Janssen et al., 2001). Some of those studies also provided evidence of effects related to the distance from major roads and traffic density (Hoek et al., 2002). Recently, Brunekreef et al. (2009) reported results from a very comprehensive European cohort study on the effects of long-term exposure to traffic pollutants and cause-specific mortalities. Specifically, the authors observed effects of particulate matter ($PM_{2.5}$), nitrogen oxides and sulfur dioxides with relative risks estimated for concentration change of 10 $\mu g/m^3$ of $PM_{2.5}$, 30 $\mu g/m^3$ of NO_2, and 20 $\mu g/m^3$ of SO_2. The largest risk estimates were found for respiratory mortalities for which the relative risks were 1.37 (95 CI, 1.00–1.87) for $PM_{2.5}$, 1.07 (0.75–1.52) for NO_2, and 0.88 (0.64–1.22) for SO_2. For cardiovascular deaths the authors reported relative risks of 1.07 (95 CI, 0.94–1.21), 1.04 (0.90–1.21), and 0.94 (0.82–1.06) for $PM_{2.5}$, NO_2, and SO_2, respectively.

As it can be seen there was no association between SO_2 concentrations and mortalities as there was no traffic contribution to this pollutant. In view of this and other research studies the European Union recognizes road transport as significant pollution source and considers the reduction of its emissions fundamental in order to protect public health.

	Contribution of various sources (%)					
Pollutant	Passenger cars	Heavy duty vehicles	Light duty vehicles	Other road transport emissions	Total road transport	Other sources
Nitrogen oxides (NOx)	19	18	3		40	60
Carbon monoxide (CO)	28	2	2	2	34	66
Sulfur oxides (SOx)	-	-	-	-	0	100
Particles (PM_{10})	4	3	2	5	14	86
Particles ($PM_{2.5}$)	5	4	3	3	15	85
Mon-methane volatile organic compounds (NMVOC)	11	2	1		14	86
Total polycyclic aromatic hydrocarbons (PAHs)	8	1			9	91
Amonium (NH_3)	2	-	-	-	2	98
Lead (Pb)	4			4	4	96
Cadmium (Cd)	1	1			2	98

Table 2. Source contribution of air pollutants in 2008 in 27 Member States of European Union (EEA, 2008, 2010)

3. European standards for ambient air

Humans can be adversely affected by exposure to hazardous air pollutants in ambient air. Since the early 1970s, the European Union has made efforts to improve air quality by controlling emissions of harmful substances into the atmosphere, improving fuel quality, and by integrating environmental protection requirements into the transport and energy sectors. Thirty years of environment policy has led to a comprehensive system of environmental controls. In order to protect public health, the European Union has established and implemented a large number of health-based standards of pollutants in ambient air. Current European standards of pollutants in ambient air are summarized in Table 3.

Pollutant	Averaging period of time	Limit/Target value	Number of exceedances	Date of enforcement
Carbon monoxide	Maximum daily 8 hour mean	10 mg/m³	n/a	Limit value entered into force 1.1.2005
Nitrogen dioxide	1 hour	200 µg/m³	18	Limit value entered into force 1.1.2010
	1 year	40 µg/m³	n/a	Limit value entered into force 1.1.2010
*Ozone	Maximum daily 8 hour mean	120 µg/m³	25 days averaged over 3 years	Target value entered into force 1.1.2010
Sulfur dioxide	1 hour	350 µg/m³	24	Limit value entered into force 1.1.2005
	24 hours	125 µg/m³	3	Limit value entered into force 1.1.2005
Particles PM_{10}	24 hours	50 µg/m³	35	Limit value entered into force 1.1.2005
	1 year	40 µg/m³	n/a	Limit value entered into force 1.1.2005
Particles $PM_{2.5}$	1 year	25 µg/m³	n/a	Target value entered into force 1.1.2010. Limit value enters into force 1.1.2015
Benzene	1 year	5 µg/m³	n/a	Limit value entered into force 1.1.2010
*Polycyclic aromatic hydrocarbons	1 year	1 ng/m³	n/a	Target value entered into force 31.12.2012
*Arsenic	1 year	6 ng/m³	n/a	Target value enters into force 31.12.2012
*Cadmium	1 year	5 ng/m³	n/a	Target value enters into force 31.12.2012
*Nickel	1 year	20 ng/m³	n/a	Target value enters into force 31.12.2012
Lead	1 year	0.5 µg/m³	n/a	Limit value entered into force 1.1.2005 (or in 1.1.2010 in the immediate vicinity of the specific industrial sources situated on sites contaminated by decades of industrial activities; and a 1.0 µg/m³ limit value applied from 1.1.2005 to 31.12.2009)

n/a not available; *Target value

Table 3. European air quality standards (Directive 2008/50/EC; Directive 2004/107/EC)

With exception to so-called "fourth daughter directives" (Directive 2004/107/EC) most of the existing European legislation on ambient air (Directive 96/62/EC, daughter Directives 1999/30/EC, 2000/69/EC, 2002/3/EC, and Council Decision 97/101/EC) have been merged into a single directive in 2008 when a new Directive 2008/50/EC on ambient air quality entered into force.

As can be seen the standards apply over different periods of time, as it was estimated that health impacts associated with these pollutants occur over different exposure times. In terms of suspended particles, the directive 2008/50/EC represents a significant step forward as for the first time air quality objectives for $PM_{2.5}$ (i.e. fine particles) were set. Except for the annual $PM_{2.5}$ limit value (Table 3), the directive also introduced additional parameters that target the exposure of the population to fine particles. These parameters are exposure concentration obligations and national exposure reduction targets (Table 4). Both parameters are based on the average exposure indicator (AEI), which represents a 3-year running annual mean of $PM_{2.5}$ concentration averaged over the selected monitoring stations in agglomerations and larger urban areas, set in urban background locations to best assess the $PM_{2.5}$ exposure of the general population (Directive 2008/50/EC).

Parameter	Averaging period of time	Value	Number of exceedances	Date of enforcement
$PM_{2.5}$ Exposure concentration obligation	Based on 3 year average	20 μg/m³ (AEI)	n/a	Legally binding in 2015 (years 2013, 2014, 2015)
$PM_{2.5}$ Exposure reduction target	Based on 3 year average	Percentage reduction + all measures to reach 18 μg/m³ (AEI)	n/a	Reduction to be attained where possible in 2020, determined on the basis of the value of exposure indicator in 2010

Table 4. European $PM_{2.5}$ exposure parameters (Directive 2008/50/EC)

To meet the $PM_{2.5}$ exposure concentration obligation, AEI in 2015, should be less than 20 μg/m³. The national exposure reduction target stipulates that between 2010 and 2020 Member States should reduce their $PM_{2.5}$ concentrations by certain percentages (0, 10, 15, or 20%), depending on the level of their AEI in 2010 (Directive 2008/50/EC). If AEI in 2010 is assessed to be over 22 μg/m³, all appropriate measures need to be taken to achieve 18 μg/m³ by 2020. The reduction is not necessary in cases where AEI in 2010 was equal to, or below 8.5 μg/m³. There is no explanation given for this value, nevertheless, some authors observed (Brunekreef & Maynard, 2008) that in studies that evaluated relationships between $PM_{2.5}$ exposure and respective health responses, concentrations of 8.5 μg/m³ represented $PM_{2.5}$ levels associated with lower risks (Laden al., 2000; Pope et al., 2002). The national exposure reduction target is provisionary. Depending on the outcome of the 2013 review it should be replaced by legally binding national exposure reduction obligations.

Other significant changes of the Directive 2008/50/EC include the possibility for Member States to discount natural sources of pollution when assessing compliance against limit values. The Member states can also apply for possible time extensions of three years (for PM_{10}) or up to five years (for NO_2, benzene) for complying with the set limit values, based on conditions and the assessment by the European Commission.

Even though the regulatory efforts of the last decade, the levels of some health hazardous pollutants in ambient air, namely particulate matter and ozone have not shown any significant improvements despite the decrease of their respective emissions (Table 1). A number of countries are also likely to miss one or more legally binding 2010 emission ceilings. As many European citizens still live in cities where air quality limits set for the protection of human health are exceeded, the need to reduce exposure to air pollution remains an important issue.

4. Health effects of main traffic pollutants

4.1 Particulate matter

Particulate air pollution was one of the first types of pollution that demonstrated evidence of health effects even at low ambient levels. Thus there is a wealth of consistent evidence of particulate matter related health effects that include morbidity and mortality outcomes, both general and cause-specific. The evidence from numerous epidemiological studies on long-term responses indicated that an increase of 10 $\mu g/m^3$ in daily PM_{10} average concentration is associated with approximate risks of 1.013 and 1.009 for respiratory and cardiovascular deaths (WHO, 2006). Also increased hospitalizations and related health care visits are significant for various respiratory diseases and, to a lesser extent, for cardiovascular disease (Medina-Ramon et al., 2006; Vigotti et al., 2010). Increased symptom prevalence includes lower respiratory system symptoms, asthma, and cough (WHO, 2006). Although the mechanisms of underling respiratory morbidity and mortality due to PM exposure are not clear, it is thought that the fine particles (i.e. $PM_{2.5}$) are of greatest concern to health. Due to their smaller sizes these fine particles are breathed into the deepest parts of lungs. Thus the scientific attention has been focused on these fine particles. Studies on long-term exposure to $PM_{2.5}$, showed an association with different cardiac and pulmonary health effects. Recent studies have also reported very high associations between the atmospheric concentrations of $PM_{2.5}$ and daily mortality rates. Total mortality appears to increase approximately 2 to 4% for every 5 $\mu g/m^3$ increase in $PM_{2.5}$, associated in a higher extent with cardiopulmonary system (WHO, 2006). Furthermore, epidemiological studies have reported that there was a clear association between episodes of $PM_{2.5}$ and increases in respiratory disease (bronchitis), impaired lung function, coughing, infections of the lower respiratory tract, and respiratory symptoms in asthmatics (WHO, 2006).

4.2 Polycyclic aromatic hydrocarbons

PAHs represent a class of organic compounds with two or more fused aromatic rings. They originate from a wide variety of natural and anthropogenic sources. The largest releases of PAHs are due to the incomplete combustion of organic matter, such as coal, oil and gas (Shibamoto, 1998) during the course of industrial processes and other human activities. Forest fires, which may or may not be the consequence of human activity, are also a significant and usually unpredictable source of PAHs. In urban atmospheres, PAHs are mainly of anthropogenic origin; road vehicle traffic is one of the most important anthropogenic emission sources, in urban areas contributing by as much as 74% of PAH emissions (Omar et al., 2002). Polycyclic aromatic hydrocarbons are also emitted from a variety of stationary sources, burning of domestic fuels are a significant source of PAHs (WHO, 1998).

In general, PAHs are ubiquitous compounds with low solubility in water, high melting and boiling points, and low vapor pressures. The physical-chemical properties of PAHs are greatly influenced by their molecular structure, i.e. by number of rings and molecular weight. While the physical-chemical properties of PAHs vary considerably, the semi-volatile properties of some PAHs make them highly mobile throughout the environment, with deposition and re-volatilization processes distributing them between air, soil and water; some PAHs are subject to long-range transport through the atmosphere making them a transboundary environmental problem. PAHs, whether dissolved in water or present in the air, can undergo photodecomposition in the presence of the ultra violet light from solar radiation (Park et al., 2002).

PAHs exist as many different isomers. Out of the currently identified compounds, the United States Environmental Protection Agency (US EPA) has recommended sixteen PAHs as "priority pollutants", due to their potential carcinogenic and mutagenic properties. Table 5 summarizes the physical-chemical properties of the priority PAHs (WHO, 1998); as demonstrated in Fig. 1 all compounds are parental PAHs, i.e. aromatic rings without any alkyl substitution.

Compound	Molecular weight	Melting point	Boiling point	Vapor pressure at 25 °C	Solubility in water at 25 °C
	g/mol	(°C)	(°C)	(Pa)	(µg/L)
Naphthalene	128.17	81	218	10.4	3.17×10^4
Acenaphthylene	152.19	92-93	265	8.9×10^{-1}	3.93×10^3
Acenaphthene	154.21	95	279	2.9×10^{-1}	3.4×10^3
Fluorene	166.22	115-116	295	8.0×10^{-2}	1.98×10^3
Anthracene	178.23	216	342	8.0×10^{-4}	73
Phenanthrene	178.23	100	340	1.6×10^{-2}	1.29×10^3
Fluoranthene	202.25	109	375	1.2×10^{-3}	260
Pyrene	202.25	150	393	6.0×10^{-4}	135
Benz[a]anthracene	228.29	161	400	2.8×10^{-5}	14
Chrysene	228.29	254	448	8.4×10^{-5}	2.0
Benzo[b]fluoranthene	252.31	167	357	------------	1.2
Benzo[k]fluoranthene	252.31	216	480	1.3×10^{-7}	0.76
Benzo[a]pyrene	252.31	178	496	7.3 × 10-7	3.8
Dibenz[a,h]anthracene	278.35	267	524	1.3×10^{-8} (20 °C)	0.5 (27 °C)
Indeno[1,2,3-cd]pyrene	276.33	164	536	1.3×10^{-8} (20 °C)	62
Benzo[ghi]perylene	276.33	278	545	1.4×10^{-8}	0.26

Table 5. Physical-chemical properties of the priority PAHs (WHO, 1998)

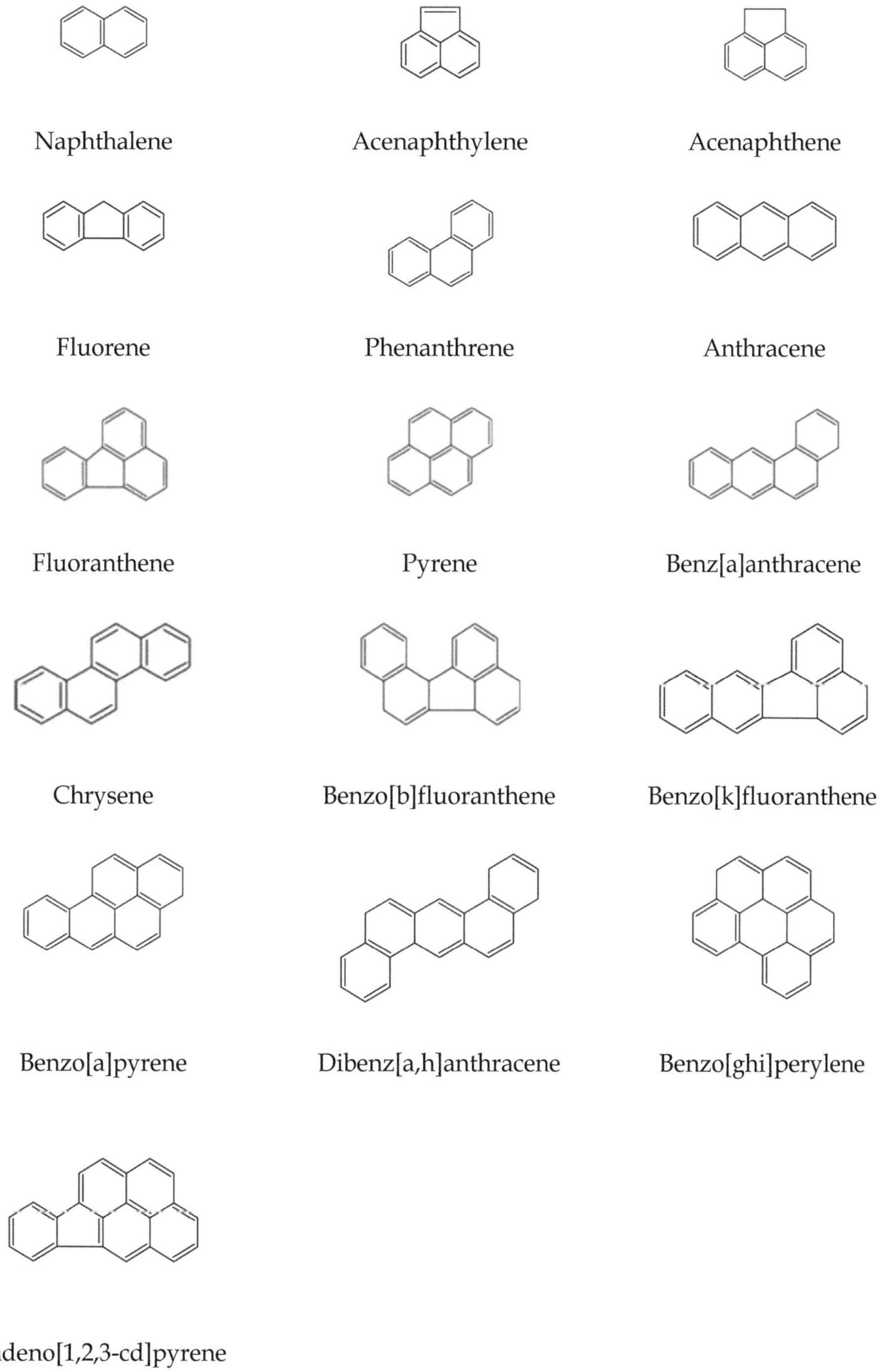

Fig. 1. Molecular structures of 16 PAHs listed as priority pollutants by U.S. Environmental Protection Agency (Shibamoto, 1998)

In the ambient air PAHs are present both in the vapor phase as well as bound to particles. PAHs with low molecular weight are usually found more in the vapor phase, but the majority of compounds with four or more rings are mainly particulate-bound (Slezakova et al., 2011; Srogi, 2007). The series of related studies performed in Oporto, Portugal (Castro et al., 2009; Slezakova et al., 2010, 2011) showed that in urban environments with major influences of vehicular traffic emissions, on average 5 to 8% of total particulate PAH content was associated with bigger particles (i.e. $PM_{2.5-10}$) whereas 92–95% of total PAH content was present in $PM_{2.5}$; in a remote site 95 % of PAHs were $PM_{2.5}$-bound (Slezakova et al., 2010). When PAHs are adsorbed onto a particle, its size is then the key parameter influencing transport of the compounds within the atmosphere. Larger particles are removed from the air by gravitational settling or impaction, but generally PAHs are not adsorbed onto these large particles. The residence time of a particle smaller than 1 µm is between 4 and 40 days, and from 0.4 till 4 days for a particle with an aerodynamic diameter of 1–10 µm (Smith, 1984). Without wet deposition the residence time of a particle can be longer, consequently PAHs adsorbed on a particle surface can travel long distances before deposition from the atmosphere (Kiss et al., 1996). Hence distribution, residence time, transport, and wet and dry deposition of PAHs in the atmosphere are mainly influenced by the nature of particulate matter. However, the persistence of PAHs in the atmosphere also depends on atmospheric conditions, such as solar radiation intensity, temperature, relative humidity; precipitation is considered to be the dominant sink for atmospheric PAHs. Temperature is probably the most important physical parameter that influences distribution of PAHs between particulate and gaseous phases. Temperature increase promotes vaporization of PAHs and gaseous PAHs are more likely to be subjected to transformation and reduction by photochemical degradation (Fang et al., 2006; Tsapakis & Stephanou, 2005). PAH decay under low outdoor humidity conditions was slower than at high humidity (Kamens et al., 1988; Tsapakis & Stephanou, 2007). In the presence of sunlight PAHs can undergo a photo-oxidation reaction that is recognized as one of the important removal process of PAHs from the atmosphere (Fang et al., 2006). Finally, the levels of other pollutants also influence the transformation of PAHs in the atmosphere and the reaction of ozone and PAHs is considered as a degradation process of these compounds, reducing their atmospheric concentrations (Park et al., 2002; Tham et al., 2008).

PAHs are typically found in a mixture of many compounds. In studies that estimate human cancer risk from exposure to complex mixtures of PAHs, benzo[a]pyrene has been commonly used as a substitute for other compounds, due to its strong carcinogenicity. However, some authors have questioned the appropriateness of this approach (Pufulete et al., 2004). The concerns are related to the variability of the compositions of different PAH mixtures. For example it was observed that benzo[a]pyrene represented less than 3% of the total PAH content in emissions originated from combustion sources (Castro et al., 2011). In various mixtures, low-potency PAHs, such as phenanthrene may occur in high concentrations (Slezakova et al., 2011) or, as recently discovered, some PAH compounds could be present in minor amounts, nevertheless possessing higher carcinogenic potency (such as dibenzo[a,l]pyrene with potency two orders of magnitude higher than benzo[a]pyrene; Castro et al., 2010, 2011; Slezakova et al., 2009). The concept of Toxicity Equivalency Factor (TEF) estimates the human cancer risk from exposure to complex PAHs using TEF for each compound in a PAH mixture, thus allowing for the aggregation of all concentrations, weighted for their carcinogenetic potency relative to that of benzo[a]pyrene.

However, the studies evaluating toxic effects of PAH mixtures do not recognize interactions between the individual PAH compounds in mixtures, which could lead to significant increases of health risks. At this moment complete understanding of these interactions is not possible as the current knowledge is still limited, thus these problems are yet to be solved by the scientific community.

4.2.1 Health impacts

Individual PAHs are extremely hazardous to human health. Many of them are cytotoxic and mutagenic (WHO, 1998) and they constitute the largest group of known carcinogens. The carcinogenic potency of individual PAHs is widely varying. Out of sixteen PAHs recommend by US EPA as priority pollutants benzo[a]pyrene has been classified by the International Agency for Research on Cancer (IARC) as an known carcinogen to humans (Group 1; IARC, 2010), whereas other PAHs have been considered as probable (Group 2A) and possible (Group 2B) human carcinogens (IARC, 2002, 2010). Table 6 shows the carcinogenicity of 16 US EPA PAHs and dibenzo[a,l]pyrene using different classification systems of IARC, US EPA and the TEF concept.

Because of their hazardous properties there has been widespread interest in analyzing and evaluating human exposure to PAHs in ambient air. Nevertheless, for obvious reasons, there are no studies in which the humans were deliberately exposed to PAHs. The information on the effects of inhaled PAHs comes only from epidemiological biomarker studies of humans exposed to PAHs in work places or in urban environments. The first PAH studies were conducted in the 1990s in the heavily polluted northern region of the Czech Republic with high ambient concentrations of benzo[a]pyrene up to tens of ng/m^3 (Binkova et al., 1996; Dejmek et al., 2000). A significant correlation between individual exposures to carcinogenic PAHs and DNA adducts was found, this effect being significant especially for non-smokers (Binkova et al., 1995). Since then, other studies were performed in less polluted areas (concentrations of benzo[a]pyrene lower then 5 ng/m^3) around the world (Jung et al., 2010; Liao et al., 2011; Novotna et al., 2007; Palli et al., 2008). Although the results of all these studies were not completely consistent, they indicated that exposure to levels of PAHs present in urban air, even at relatively low concentrations, resulted in high levels of health risks.

The health concerns of PAHs have been traditionally focused on their potential carcinogenicity in humans, which seems to be beyond dispute. PAHs are genotoxic compounds and their carcinogenicity is probably mediated by their ability to damage the DNA (Irigaray & Belpomme, 2010; Novotna et al., 2007; Palli et al., 2008). Even exposure to low doses of PAHs might be associated with various cancers, indicating that there is no safe threshold. However, regarding the PAH carcinogenicity due to exposure to polluted air, it is important to point out that there is no epidemiological evidence showing that at levels present in urban air PAHs cause cancer. Until now the only evidence of PAH carcinogenicity in humans exists for long-term exposure (of many years) to polluted air of work places with high concentrations of PAHs, which exceed those in ambient air by orders of magnitude (Bostrom et al., 2002; Peluso et al., 2001; Srogi, 2007). Due to the lack of useful, good-quality data, the quantitative cancer risk estimates of PAHs as air pollutants are very uncertain, because they are based on extrapolation from substantially higher occupational concentrations, which makes it difficult to draw conclusions (Bostrom et al., 2002).

Compound	Classification			
	IARC[a]	US EPA[b]	TEF[c]	Unit risk[d] (µg/m³)$^{-1}$
Naphthalene	2B	C	0.001	-
Acenaphthylene	not available	D	0.001	-
Acenaphthene	3	not available	0.001	-
Fluorene	3	D	0.001	-
Phenanthrene	3	D	0.001	-
Anthracene	3	D	0.01	-
Fluoranthene	3	D	0.001	2.8×10^{-4}
Pyrene	3	D	0.001	-
Chrysene	2B	B_2	0.1	8.7×10^{-4}
Benz[a]anthracene	2A	B_2	0.1	4.0×10^{-3}
Benzo[b]fluoranthene	2B	B_2	0.1	1.0×10^{-2}
Benzo[k]fluoranthene	2B	B_2	0.1	2.8×10^{-3}
Benzo[a]pyrene	1	B_2	1	8.7×10^{-2}
Dibenz[a,h]anthracene	2A	B_2	5	1.8×10^{-1}
Benzo[g,h,i]perylene	3	D	0.01	-
Indeno[1,2,3-c,d]pyrene	2B	B_2	0.1	1.1×10^{-2}
Dibenzo[a,l]pyrene	2A	not available	100[e]	8.7×10^{-0}

[a](IARC, 2002, 2010): Group 1 - carcinogenic to humans; Group 2A - probably carcinogenic to humans; Group 2B - possible carcinogenic to humans; Group 3 - unclassifiable as to carcinogenetic in humans; Group 4 - probably not carcinogenic to humans

[b](USEPA, 1986, 2005): Group A - human carcinogens; Group B - probable human carcinogens (B1: based on limited evidence of carcinogenicity in humans and sufficient evidence of carcinogenicity in animals; B2: based on sufficient evidence of carcinogenicity in animals);Group C - possible human carcinogens; Group D - not classifiable as to human carcinogenicity; Group E - evidence of non-carcinogenicity for humans

[c]Toxicity Equivalency Factor (TEF): estimation based on the relative potency to benzo(a)pyrene (Nisbet & LaGoy, 1992)

[d]Unit risk (WHO, 1998).

[e](Pufulete et al., 2004; Okona-Mensah et al., 2005)

Table 6. Classification of selected PAHs

Furthermore humans are never exposed only to a single PAH compound in ambient air, and the coexistence of PAHs in various mixtures implies further difficulties. To fully understand the carcinogenesis of PAHs and their role as air pollutants, these issues need to be correctly addressed by further research.

4.2.2 Environmental impacts

From a global point of view, the largest emissions of PAHs are found in the atmosphere. However, apart from release into air, PAHs can be also transferred directly to water, soil and sediments. Marine pollution by crude oil causes appreciable quantities of PAHs (Grueiro-Noche et al., 2010; Martins et al., 2011). Improper waste disposal and biomass burning have also caused serious PAH pollution of land in some localities (Chrysikou et al., 2008; Chung et al., 2007; Liu et al., 2010).

The most common effects of organisms that occur with long-term exposure to PAHs are bioaccumulation, behavioral alternation in some species, reduction in growth, reduced reproduction and deformities, and increased mortalities (Khanal, 2003). Tumor development has also been reported in fish exposed to benzo[a]pyrene (WHO, 1998) as well as various acute effects (Tintos et al., 2008; Viera et al., 2008). Some PAHs (naphthalene, phenanthrene, and fluoranthene) are acutely toxic to aquatic organisms and the toxicity is affected by metabolism and photosynthesis (Khanal, 2003); in the presence of ultraviolet light the toxicity of PAHs gets more intense (Arsften et al., 1996; WHO, 1998).

The effects of air pollution are not confined only to human health or environment but also to buildings and historical monuments. These impacts can have permanent consequences that might lead to potential losses of these, principally irreplaceable historical structures forever. One of the most important building deterioration phenomena is the deposition of pollutants on surfaces (Marioni et al., 2003) which consequently affects façades of buildings and monuments (Gaviño et al., 2004). Eventually the particles, together with dry-deposited gases such as SO_2 result in the formation of hard, grey - black crusts, in which airborne organic pollutants, such as PAHs and a wide range of particulate matter (including dust, pollen, and spores) are entrapped (Fig. 2). The pressure from the crystal growth breaks off small areas of stone thus exposing a more vulnerable surface. Recent studies showed that deposition of these pollutants is important also from a health hazard perspective. Historical monuments and buildings in urban areas can act as passive repositories for air pollutants present in the surrounding atmosphere and may lead to higher human exposures thus representing additional risks for human health (Slezakova et al., 2011).

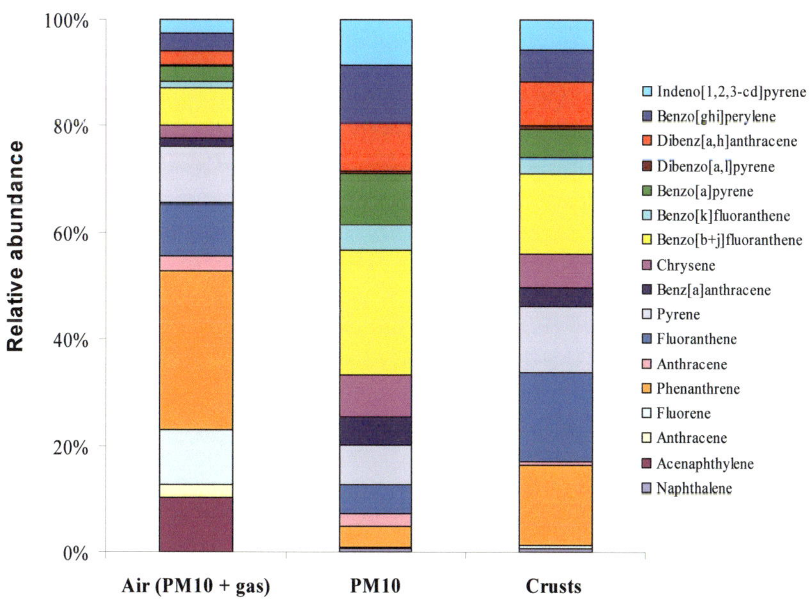

Fig. 2. Selected PAHs in Oporto, Portugal. The graph demonstrates the abundance of PAHs during the winter of 2008 in air (i.e. sum of both gas and particulate phase), in PM_{10}, and in black crusts of a selected historical monuments situated in an urban site. The similarity of the contribution profiles between PAHs in black crusts and in PM_{10} is obvious.

4.3 Nitrogen dioxide

Nitrogen monoxide is almost instantaneously oxidized to nitrogen dioxide. Of the two gases, nitrogen dioxide is much more toxic to humans. Nitrogen dioxide is less soluble than sulfur dioxide, so that a much higher proportion penetrates into the deep lung. Approximately 70–90% of nitrogen dioxide inhaled can be absorbed from the respiratory tract of humans (Tiwary & Colls, 2009). In human studies, nitrogen dioxide has been associated with adverse health effects even at low ambient concentrations. Exposure to high nitrogen dioxide levels from occupational exposure may have adverse effects such as pulmonary edema (Godish, 2004; WHO, 2006). Asthmatics appear to be the most reactive group upon exposure to nitrogen dioxide, although controlled studies on the effects of short-term exposure on the symptoms and severity of asthma have not led to clear findings (WHO, 2006). Short-term exposure studies have shown that asthma sufferers may experience enhanced sensitivity after exposure to nitrogen dioxide, and that those with normal respiratory function may experience increased airway resistance (WHO, 2006).

4.4 Ozone

Ozone is a colorless gas. As mentioned previously it differs from the other pollutants because of its secondary origin (i.e. formed in the atmosphere rather than being emitted). It is formed through a series of complex reactions in the atmosphere involving solar radiation and anthropogenic pollutants, such as non-methane volatile organic compounds and carbon monoxide, in the presence of nitrogen dioxide (Alvim-Ferraz et al., 2006). The concentration of ozone in the atmosphere depends on several factors: sunshine intensity, atmospheric convection, the height of the thermal inversion layer, and concentrations of nitrogen oxides and other precursors (WHO, 2006). As a consequence of anthropogenic activities, ground-level ozone represents a major concern because of its concentration increase. In densely populated areas of Europe and USA the levels of ozone can reach up to 200 $\mu g/m^3$ (1-hour mean; WHO, 2006). Much higher levels of ozone (up to 400 $\mu g/m^3$ during several days) can be observed in developing countries, where the combination of mega-cities with significant emissions of ozone precursors and a climate that favors photochemical reactions of ozone formation (WHO, 2006) is found. Exposure to ozone is almost exclusively by inhalation and has been associated with both acute and chronic effects. Short-term exposure to high ozone concentrations includes effects on the pulmonary and cardiovascular systems with evidence of both morbidity and mortality (WHO, 2006). Long-term exposure to relatively low levels is also of concern; it can lead to the development of atherosclerosis and asthma, reduction in lung function, and life expectancy (Sousa et al., 2009; WHO, 2006).

4.5 Carbon monoxide

Exposure to carbon monoxide may be lethal; however poisoning is typically caused in confined spaces (indoors, cars) by exposures to carbon monoxide at levels considerably higher than those existent in ambient air. Generally, the mechanism of carbon monoxide toxicity is tissue hypoxia. Carbon monoxide combines with blood haemoglobin about 200 times more readily than oxygen (Colls, 2003). The resulting carboxyhaemoglobin molecules can no longer transport oxygen from the lungs around the body, and hence the oxygen supply to the brain and other organs is reduced. The reaction is reversible, and exposure to clean air removes most of the gas from the body with a half-life of 3–4 h. Effects are particularly severe at tissues where partial pressures of oxygen are already low. The quantity of carboxyhaemoglobin formed depends on a variety of factors, such as, the concentration of carbon monoxide in the air, duration of exposure, temperature, health status, and the activity of the individual and metabolism of the individual exposed (Tiwary & Colls, 2009). At lower concentrations carbon monoxide may cause headache, fatigue, nausea, and, in some cases, vomiting.

In general there has been little research into the potential health effects of exposure to ambient concentrations of carbon monoxide (Godish, 2004). Few authors reported associations between exposure to carbon monoxides and health outcomes (mortality rates, cardiovascular disease, hospital admissions, prenatal development; Maynard & Waller, 1999) that should not be underestimated. Further research, including time-series studies, is needed.

4.6 Metals

Metals gained the attention of the scientific community because they are an important class of human carcinogen. Five transition metals—arsenic, cadmium, chromium VI, beryllium, and nickel—are accepted as human carcinogens in one form or another or in particular routes of exposure (IARC, 2011). Exposures to small doses of these metals (Goyer et al., 2004) can result in diffuse or spotted hyper-pigmentation of the skin, and if continued for years can produce benign skin lesions (hyperkeratosis) and cancer of the skin. Chronic exposure to low doses of cadmium (through cigarette smoking) can cause kidney tubular dysfunction and osteoporosis in susceptible populations. Lung cancer also occurs with chronic inhalation exposure of arsenic and cadmium (Goyer et al., 2004). Almost all metals that occur in the atmosphere are associated with particles. Breathing heavy metal particles can have serious health effects. Virtually all aspects of human immune system function are compromised by the inhalation of heavy metal particulates. Nevertheless, the epidemiological evidence for health effects associated with inhalation exposure to particulate metals is far from comprehensive. In most environments particulate-bound metals exist in low concentrations and it has not been fully established if those quantities are sufficient/significant to cause the adverse health effects (Dominici et al., 2007). However, some studies showed lung injuries and inflammation associated with exposure to metal particles (Hirshon et al., 2008; Prieditis & Adamson, 2002).

5. Conclusion

Road transport presents one of the paradoxes of modern society. While the volume of road transport has been continually growing in European countries, the amounts of road emissions of air pollutants continue to decline in member States of the European Union. These decreases are due to technical developments as well as the implementation of various regulations. However, despite the significant reductions of road transport exhaust emissions across Europe, there have not been proportional improvements in concentrations of the respective pollutants in ambient air.

Emissions from road transport are the primary source of health hazardous pollutants, such as nitrogen oxides and carbon monoxide, and a significant source for fine particulate pollution. Exposures to these emissions are typically non voluntary and represent serious risks to human heath. In order to protect public health it is necessary to reduce the levels of these exposures and to do so adequately a deeper understanding of health effects is needed. Characterizing the magnitude of those exposures and quantifying the average exposure burden imposed by living near traffic are among the problems that need to be addressed.

6. Acknowledgment

The authors would like to thank to Fundação para Ciência e Tecnologia for the financial support with grant number SFRH/BPD/65722/2009.

7. References

Alvim-Ferraz, M.C.M., Sousa, S.I.V., Pereira, M.C. & Martins, F.G. (2006). Contribution of Anthropogenic Pollutants to the Increase of Tropospheric Ozone Levels in the Oporto Metropolitan Area, Portugal since the 19th Century. *Environmental Pollution*, Vol. 140, No. 3, (April 2006), pp. 516-524, ISSN 0269-7491

Arfsten, D.P., Schaeffer, D.J. & Mulveny, D.C. (1996). The Effects of Near Ultraviolet Radiation on the Toxic Effects of Polycyclic Aromatic Hydrocarbons in Animals and Plants: A Review. *Ecotoxicology and Environmental Safety*, Vol. 33, No. 1, (February 1996), pp. 1-24, ISSN 0147-6513

Beelen, R., Hoek, G., Houthuijs, D., van den Brandt, P.A., Goldbohm, R.A., Fischer, P., Schouten, L.J., Armstrong, B. & Brunekreef, B. (2008). The Joint Association of Air Pollution and Noise from Road Traffic with Cardiovascular Mortality in a Cohort Study. *Occupational and Environmental Medicine*, Vol. 66, No. 4, (April 2009), pp. 243-50, ISSN 1351-0711

Binkova, B., Lewtas, J., Miskova, I., Lenicek, J. & Sram, R.J. (1995). DNA Adducts and Personal Air Monitoring of Carcinogenic Polycyclic Aromatic Hydrocarbons in an Environmentally Exposed Population. *Carcinogenesis*, Vol. 16, No. 5, (May 1995), pp. 1037-1046, ISSN 0143-3334

Binkova, B., Lewtas, J., Miskova, I., Rössner, P., Cerna, M., Mrackova, G., Peterkova, K., Mumford, J., Meyer, S. & Sram, R.J. (1996). Biomarker Studies in Northern Bohemia. *Environmental Health Perspective*, Vol. 104, No. 3, (May 1996), pp. 591-597, ISSN 0091-6765

Bostrom, C.E., Gerde, P., Hanberg, A., Jernstrom, B., Johansson, C., Kyrklund, T., Rannug, A., Tornqvist, M., Victorin, K. & Westerholm, R. (2002). Cancer Risk Assessments, Indicators, and Guidelines for Polycyclic Aromatic Hydrocarbons in the Ambient Air. *Environmental Health Perspective*, Vol. 110, Suppl. 3, (June 2002), pp. 451-488, ISSN 0091-6765

Brunekreef, B. & Maynard, R.L. (2008). A Note on the 2008 EU Standards for Particulate Matter. *Atmospheric Environment*, Vol. 42, No. 26, (August 2006), pp. 6425-6430, ISSN 1352-2310

Brunekreef, B., Beelen, R., Hoek, G., Schouten, L., Bausch-Goldbohm, S., Fischer, P., Armstrong, B., Hughes, E., Jerrett, M. & van den Brandt, P. (2009). Effects of Long-term Exposure to Traffic-related Air Pollution on Respiratory and Cardiovascular Mortality in the Netherlands: the NLCS-AIR Study. *Research Report (Health Effects Institute)*, Vol. 139, (March 2009), pp. 5-71

Castro, D., Slezakova, K., Delerue-Matos, C., Alvim-Ferraz, M.C., Morais, S. & Pereira, M.C. (2011). Polycyclic Aromatic Hydrocarbons in Gas and Particulate Phases of Indoor

Environments Influenced by Tobacco Smoke: Levels, Phase Distributions, and Health Risks. *Atmospheric Environment*, Vol. 45, No. 10, (March 2011), pp. 1799-1808, ISSN 1352-2310

Castro, D., Slezakova, K., Delerue-Matos, C., Alvim-Ferraz, M.C., Morais, S. & Pereira, M.C. (2010). Contribution of Traffic and Tobacco Smoke in the Distribution of Polycyclic Aromatic Hydrocarbons on Outdoor and Indoor PM2.5. *Global Nest Journal*, Vol.12, No. 1, (March 2010), pp. 3-11, ISSN 1790-7632

Castro, D., Slezakova, K., Oliva-Teles, M.T., Delerue-Matos, C., Alvim-Ferraz, M.C., Morais, S. & Pereira, M.C. (2009). Analysis of Polycyclic Aromatic Hydrocarbons in Atmospheric Particulate Samples by Microwave-Assisted Extraction and Liquid Chromatography. *Journal of Separation Science*, Vol. 32, No. 4, (February 2009), pp. 501-510, ISSN 1615-9306

Chrysikou, L., Gemenetzis, P., Kouras, A., Manoli, E., Terzi, E. & Samara, C. (2008). Distribution of Persistent Organic Pollutants, Polycyclic Aromatic Hydrocarbons and Trace Elements in Soil and Vegetation Following a Large Scale Landfill Fire in Northern Greece. *Environment International*, Vol. 34, No. 2, (February 2008), pp. 210-225, ISSN 60-4120

Chung, M.K., Hu, R., Cheung, K.C. & Wong, M.H. (2007). Pollutants in Hong Kong Soils: Polycyclic Aromatic Hydrocarbons. *Chemosphere*, Vol. 67, No. 3, (March 2007), pp. 464-473, ISSN 0045-6535

Colls, J. (2003). *Air Pollution* (2nd ed.), Taylor & Francis e-Library, ISBN 0-203-47602-6, London, United Kingdom

Council Decision 97/101/EC. (1997). Council Decisions Establishing a Reciprocal Exchange of Information and Data from Networks and Individual Stations Measuring Ambient Air Pollution within the Member States. *Official Journal of the European Communities*, L35, (February 1997), pp. 14–22

Dejmek, J., Solansky, I., Benes, I., Lenicek, J. & Sram, R.J. (2000). The Impact of Polycyclic Aromatic Hydrocarbons and Fine Particles on Pregnancy Outcome. *Environmental Health Perspective*, Vol. 108, No. 12, (December 2000), pp. 1159-1164, ISSN 0091-6765

Directive 1999/30/EC. (1999). Directive of the Council Relating to Limit Values of Sulphur Dioxide, Nitrogen Dioxide and Oxides of Nitrogen, Particulate Matter and Lead in Ambient Air. *Official Journal of the European Communities*, L163, (June 1999), pp. 41-60

Directive 2000/69/EC. (2000). Directive of the European Parliament and the Council Relating to Limit Values for Benzene and Carbon Monoxide in Ambient Air. *Official Journal of the European Communities*, L313, (December 2002), pp. 12–21

Directive 2002/3/EC. Directive of the European Parliament and the Council Relating to Ozone in Ambient Air. *Official Journal of the European Communities*, L67, (March 2002), pp. 14–30

Directive 2004/107/EC. (2005). Directive of the European Parliament and of the Council Relating to Arsenic, Cadmium, Mercury, Nickel and Polycyclic Aromatic Hydrocarbons in Ambient Air. *Official Journal of the European Union*, L23, (January 2005), pp. 3-16

Directive 2008/50/EC. (2008). Directive of the European Parliament and of the Council on Ambient Air Quality and Cleaner Air for Europe. *Official Journal of the European Union*, L152, (June 2006), pp. 1-44

Directive 96/62/EC. (1996). Council Directive on Ambient Air Quality Assessment and Management. *Official Journal of the European Union*, L296, (November 1996), pp. 55-63

Directive 98/70/EC. (1998). Directive of the European Parliament and of the Council Relating to the Quality of Petrol and Diesel Fuels. *Official Journal of the European Communities*, L350, (December 1998), pp. 58–68

Dominici, F., Peng, R.D., Ebisu, K., Zeger, S.L., Samet, J.M. & Bell, M.L. (2007). Does the Effect of PM10 on Mortality Depend on PM Nickel and Vanadium Content? A Reanalysis of the NMMAPS data. *Environmental Health Perspective*, Vol. 115, No. 12, (December 2007), pp. 1701-1703, ISSN 0091-6765

EN Standard 590/2004. (2004). *Automotive Fuels. Diesel. Requirements and Test methods,* European Committee for Standardization, ISBN 05-8044-119-9, Brussels, Belgium

Environmental European Agency (EEA). (2005). *The European Environment: State and Outlook* 2005. Office for Official Publications of the European Union, ISBN 92-9167-776-0, Luxemburg

Environmental European Agency (EEA). (2008). *Annual European Community LRTAP Convention Emission Inventory Report 1990–2006*, EEA Technical report No. 7/2008, Office for Official Publications of the European Union, ISBN 978-92-9167-366-7, Luxemburg

Environmental European Agency (EEA). (2010). *European Union Emission Inventory Report 1990–2008 under the UNECE Convention on Long-range Transboundary Air Pollution (LRTAP)*, EEA Technical Report No. 7/2010, Office for Official Publications of the European Union, ISBN 978-92-9213-102-9, Luxemburg

Environmental European Agency (EEA). (2011a). *European Union Emission Inventory Report 1990–2009 under the UNECE Convention on Long-range Transboundary Air Pollution (LRTAP)*, EEA Technical Report No. 9/2011, Office for Official Publications of the European Union, ISBN 978-92-9213-216-3, Luxemburg

Environmental European Agency (EEA). (2011b). *About Transport*, available from <http://www.eea.europa.eu/themes/transport/about-transport>, accessed 20.7.2011

Fang, G.C., Wu, Y.S., Chen, J.C., Chang, C.N. & Ho, T.T. (2006). Characteristic of Polycyclic Aromatic Hydrocarbon Concentrations and Source Identification for Fine and Coarse Particulates at Taichung Harbor near Taiwan Strait during 2004–2005. *Atmospheric Environment*, Vol. 366, No. 2-3, (August 2006), pp. 729-738, ISSN 1352-2310

Fischer, P.H., Hoek, G., van Reeuwijk, H., Briggs, D.J., Lebret, E., van Wijnen, J.H., Kingham, S. & Elliott, P.E. (2000). Traffic-Related Differences in Outdoor and Indoor Concentrations of Particles and Volatile Organic Compounds in Amsterdam. *Atmospheric Environment*, Vol. 34, No. 22, pp. 3713–3722, ISSN 1352-2310

Gaviño, M., Hermosin, B., Vergès-Belmin, V., Nowik, W. & Saiz-Jimenez, W. (2004). Composition of the Black Crust from the Saint Denis Basilica, France, as Revealed by Gas Chromatography-Mass Spectrometry. *Journal of Separation Science,* Vol. 7, No. 7-8, (May 2004), pp. 513-523, ISSN 1615-9306

Godish, T. (2004). *Air Quality* (4th ed.), Lewis Publishers, ISBN 978-15-6670-586-8, London, United Kingdom

Goyer, R., Golub, M., Choudhury, H., Hughes, M., Kenyon, E. & Stifelman, M. (2004). *Issue Paper on the Human Health Effects of Metals, accessed* 25.6.2011, available from

<http://www.epa.gov/raf/publications/pdfs/HUMANHEALTHEFFECTS81904.PDF>

Grueiro-Noche, G., Andrade, J.M., Muniategui-Lorenzo, S., López-Mahía, P. & Prada-Rodríguez, D. (2010). 3-Way Pattern-Recognition of PAHs from Galicia (NW Spain) Seawater Samples after the Prestige's Wreck. *Environmental Pollution*, Vol. 158, No. 1, (January 2010), pp. 207-214, ISSN 0269-7491

Heinrich, J., Topp, R., Gehring, U. & Thefeld, W. (2005). Traffic at Residential Address, Respiratory Health, and Atopy in Adults: The National German Health Survey 1998. *Environmental Research*, Vol. 98, No. 2, (June 2005), pp. 240-249, ISSN 0013-9351

Hirshon, J.M., Shardell, M., Alles, S., Powell, J.L., Squibb, K., Ondov, J. & Blaisdell, C.J. Elevated Ambient Air Zinc Increases Pediatric Asthma Morbidity. *Environmental Health Perspective*, Vol. 116, No. 6, (June 2008), pp. 826-31, SSN 0091-6765

Hoek, G., Brunekreef, B., Goldbohm, S., Fischer, P. & van den Brandt, P.A. (2002). Association between Mortality and Indicators of Traffic-related Air Pollution in the Netherlands: A Cohort Study. *The Lancet*, Vol. 360, No. 9341, (October 2002), pp. 1203-1209, ISSN 0140-6736

International Agency for Research on Cancer (IARC). (2002). Some Traditional Herbal Medicines, Some Mycotoxins, Naphthalene and Styrene. *IARC Monographs on the Evaluation of Carcinogenic Risks to Humans*, Vol. 82, (February 2002), pp. 367, ISSN 1017-1606

International Agency for Research on Cancer (IARC). (2010). Some non-Heterocyclic Polycyclic Aromatic Hydrocarbons and Some Related Exposures. *IARC Monographs on the Evaluation of Carcinogenic Risks to Humans*, Vol. 92, (October 2010), pp. 773, ISSN 1017-1606

International Agency for Research on Cancer (IARC). (2011). *Agents Classified by the IARC Monographs*, accessed 24.6.2011, available from <http://monographs.iarc.fr/ENG/Classification/ClassificationsAlphaOrder.pdf>

Irigaray, P. & Belpomme, D. (2010). Basic Properties and Molecular Mechanisms of Exogenous Chemical Carcinogens. *Carcinogenesis*, Vol. 31, No. 2, (February 2010), pp. 135-48, ISSN 0143-3334

Janssen, N.A., van Vliet, P., Aarts, F., Harssema, H. & Brunekreef, B. (2001). Assessment of Exposure to Traffic Related Air Pollution of Children Attending Schools near Motorways. *Atmospheric Environment*, Vol. 35, No. 22, (August 2001), pp. 3875-3884, ISSN 1352-2310

Jung, K.H., Yan, B., Chillrud, S.N., Perera, F.P., Whyatt, R., Camann, D., Kinney, P.L. & Miller, R.L. (2010). Assessment of Benzo(a)pyrene-Euivalent Carcinogenicity and Mutagenicity of Residential Indoor versus Outdoor Polycyclic Aromatic Hydrocarbons Exposing Young Children in New York City. *International Journal of Environmental Research and Public Health*, Vol. 7, No. 5, (May 2010), pp. 1889 900, ISSN 1660-4601

Kamens, R.M., Guo, Z., Fulcher, J.N. & Bell, D. (1988). Influence of Humidity, Sunlight, and Temperature on the Daytime Decay of Polyaromatic Hydrocarbons on Atmospheric Soot Particles. *Environmental Science and Technology*, Vol. 22, No. 1, (January 2008), pp. 103-108, ISSN 0013-936X

Khanal, O. (2003). *Organics in Atmospheric Particulates*. PhD Thesis, University of Auckland, New Zealand

Kiss, I.B., Koltay, E. & Szabo, G. (1996). Elemental Composition of Urban Aerosol Collected in Debrecen, Hungary. *Nuclear Instruments and Methods in Physics Research B*, Vol. 109/110, (April 1996), pp. 445-449, ISSN 0168-583X

Kunzli, N., Kaiser, R., Medina, S., Studnicka, M., Chanel, O., Filliger, P., Herry, M., Horak, J. F. & Puybonnieux-Texier, V. (2000). Public-health Impact of Outdoor and Traffic-Related Air Pollution: a European Assessment. *The Lancet*, Vol. 356, No. 9232, (September, 2000), pp. 795-801, ISSN 0140-6736

Laden, F., Neas, L.M., Dockery, D.W. & Schwartz, J. (2000). Association of Fine Particulate Matter from Different Sources with Daily Mortality in Six U.S. Cities. *Environmental Health Perspective*, Vol. 108, No. 10, (October 2000), pp. 941-947, ISSN 0091-6765

Liao, C.M., Chio, C.P., Chen, W.Y., Ju, Y.R., Li, W.H., Cheng, Y.H., Liao, V.H., Chen, S.C. & Ling, M.P. (2011). Lung Cancer Risk in Relation to Traffic-related Nano/Ultrafine Particle-bound PAHs Exposure: A Preliminary Probabilistic Assessment. *Journal of Hazardous Materials*, Vol. 190, No. 1-3, (June 2011), pp. 150-158, ISSN 0304-3894

Liu, S., Xia, X., Yang, L., Shen, M. & Li, R. (2010). Polycyclic Aromatic Hydrocarbons in Urban Soils of Different Land Uses in Beijing, China: Distribution, Sources and Their Correlation with the City's Urbanization History. *Journal of Hazardous Materials*, Vol. 177, No. 1-3, (May 2010), pp. 1085-1092, ISSN 0304-3894

Marioni, N., Birelli, M.P., Rostagno, C. & Pavese, A. (2003). The Effects of Atmospheric Multipollutants on Modern Concrete. *Atmospheric Environment*, Vol. 37, No. 33, (October 2003), pp. 4701-4712, ISSN 1352-2310

Martuzevicius, M., Grinshpun, S.A., Lee, T., Hu, S., Biswas, O., Reponen, T. & LeMasters, G. (2008). Traffic-Related PM2.5 Aerosol in Residential Houses Located Near Major Highways: Indoor versus Outdoor Concentrations. *Atmospheric Environment*, Vol. 42, No. 27, (September 2008), pp. 6575-6585, ISSN 1352-2310

Maynard, R.L. & Waller, R. (1999). Carbon Monoxide. In: *Air Pollution and Health*, S.T. Holgate, J.M. Samet, H.S. Koren, R.L. Maynard, (Eds.), pp. 749-796, Academic Press, ISBN 0-12-352335-4, London, United Kingdom

Medina-Ramon, M., Zanobetti, A. & Schwartz J. (2006). The Effect of Ozone and PM10 on Hospital Admissions for Pneumonia and Chronic Obstructive Pulmonary Disease: a National Multicity Study. *American Journal of Epidemiology*, Vol. 163, No. 6, (March 2006), pp. 579–588, ISSN 0002-9262

Nisbet, L.T.K. & LaGoy, P.K. (1992). Toxic Equivalency Factors (TEFs) for Polycyclic Aromatic Hydrocarbons (PAHs). *Regulatory Toxicology and Pharmacology*, Vol. 16, No. 3, (December 1992), pp. 290-300, ISSN 0273-2300

Novotna, B., Topinka, J., Solansky, I., Chvatalova, I., Lnenickova, Z. & Sram, R.J. (2007). Impact of Air Pollution and Genotype Variability on DNA Damage in Prague Policemen. *Toxicology Letters*, Vol. 172, No. 1-2, (July 2007), pp. 37-47, ISSN 0378-4274

Okona-Mensah, K.W., Battershill, J., Boobis, A. & Fielder, R. (2005). An Approach to Investigating the Importance of High Potency Polycyclic Aromatic Hydrocarbons (PAHs) in the Induction of Lung Cancer by Air Pollution. *Food and Chemical Toxicology*, Vol. 43, No. 7, (July 2005), pp. 103-1116, ISSN 0278-6915

Omar, N.Y.M.J., Abas, M.R.B., Ketuly, K.A. & Tahir, N.M. (2002). Concentrations of PAHs in Atmospheric Particles (PM10) and Roadside Soil Particles Collected in Kuala Lumpur, Malaysia. *Atmospheric Environment*, Vol. 36, No. 2, (January 2002), pp. 247-254, ISSN 1352-2310

Palli, D., Saieva, C., Munnia, A., Peluso, M., Grechi, D., Zanna, I., Caini, S., Decarli, A., Sera, F. & Masala, G. (2008). DNA Adducts and PM(10) Exposure in Traffic-exposed Workers and Urban Residents from the EPIC-Florence City Study. *Science of the Total Environment*, Vol. 403, No. 1-3, (September 2008), pp. 105-112, ISSN 0898-6924

Park, S.S., Kim, Y.J. & Kang, C.H. (2002). Atmospheric Polycyclic Aromatic Hydrocarbons in Seoul, Korea. *Atmospheric Environment*, Vol. 36, No. 17, (June 2002), pp. 917-2924, ISSN 1352-2310

Peluso, M., Ceppi, M., Munnia, A., Puntoni, R. & Parodi, S. (2001). Analysis of 13 32P-DNA Postlabeling Studies on Occupational Cohorts Exposed to Air Pollution. *American Journal of Epidemiology*, Vol. 153, No. 6, (March 2001), pp. 543-558, ISSN 0002-9262

Pope, C.A.III., Burnett, R.T., Thun, M.J., Calle, E.E., Krewski, D., Ito, K. & Thurston, G.D. Lung Cancer, Cardiopulmonary Mortality, and Long-term Exposure to Fine Particulate Air Pollution. *Journal of the American Medical Association*, Vol. 287, No. 9, (March 2002), pp. 1132-1141, ISSN 0098-7484

Prieditis, H. & Adamson, I.Y.R. (2002). Comparative Pulmonary Toxicity of Various Soluble Metals Found in Urban Particulate Dusts. *Experimental Lung Research*, Vol. 28, No. 7, (October-November 2002), pp. 563-76, ISSN 0190-2148

Pufulete, M., Battershill, J., Boobis, A. & Fielder, R. (2004). Approaches to Carcinogenic Risk Assessment for Polycyclic Aromatic Hydrocarbon: a UK Perspective. *Regulatory Toxicology and Pharmacology*, Vol. 40, No. 1, (August 2004), pp. 54-56, ISSN 0273-2300

Regulation 595/2009. (2009). Regulation of the European Parliament and the Council on Type-Approval of Motor Vehicles and Engines with Respect to Emissions from Heavy Duty Vehicles (Euro VI) and on Access to Vehicle Repair and Maintenance Information and Amending Regulation. *Official Journal of the European Communities*, L 188, (July 2009), pp. 1-13

Shibamoto, T. (1998). *Chromatographic Analysis of Environmental and Food Toxicants*, Marcel Dekker, INC., ISBN 0-8247-0145-3, New York, United States of America

Slezakova, K., Castro, D., Delerue-Matos, C., Alvim-Ferraz, M.C., Morais, S. & Pereira, M.C. (2011). Air Pollution from Traffic Emissions in Oporto, Portugal: Health and Environmental Implications. *Microchemical Journal*, Vol. 199, No. 1, (September 2011), pp. 51-59, ISSN 0026-265X

Slezakova, K., Castro, D., Pereira, M.C., Morais, S., Delerue-Matos, C. & Alvim-Ferraz, M.C.M. (2010). Influence of Traffic Emissions on the Carcinogenic Polycyclic Aromatic Hydrocarbons in Outdoor Breathable Particles. *Journal of the Air & Waste Management Association*, Vol. 66, No. 4, (April 2010), pp. 393-401, ISSN 1047-3289

Slezakova, K., Castro, D., Pereira, M.C., Morais, S., Delerue-Matos, C. & Alvim-Ferraz, M.C.M. (2009). Influence of Tobacco Smoke on Carcinogenic PAH Composition in Indoor PM10 and PM2.5. *Atmospheric Environment*, Vol. 43, No. 40, (December 2009), pp. 6376-6382, ISSN 1352-2310

Smith, I.M. (1984). *PAH from Coal Utilisation - Emission and Effects*. International Energy Agency (IEA), ICTIS/TR29, London, United Kingdom

Sousa, S.I.V., Alvim-Ferraz, M.C.M, Martins, F.G. & Pereira, M.C. (2009). Ozone Exposure and Its Influence on the Worsening of Childhood Asthma. *Allergy*, Vol. 64, No. 9, (July 2009), pp. 1046-1055, ISSN 1398-9995

Srogi, K. (2007). Monitoring of Environmental Exposure to Polycyclic Aromatic Hydrocarbons: a Review. *Environmental Chemistry Letters*, Vol. 5, No. 4, (March 2007), pp. 169-195, ISBN 1610-3661

Tham, Y.W.F., Takeda, K. & Sakugawa, H. (2008). Polycyclic Aromatic Hydrocarbons (PAHs) Associated with Atmospheric Particles in Higashi Hiroshima, Japan: Influence of Meteorological Conditions and Seasonal Variations. *Atmospheric Research*, Vol. 88, No. 3-4, (June 2008), pp. 224-233, ISSN 0169-8095

Tintos, A., Gesto, M., Míguez, J.M. & Soengas, J.L. (2008). β-Naphthoflavone and Benzo(a)pyrene Treatment Affect Liver Intermediary Metabolism and Plasma Cortisol Levels in Rainbow Trout Oncorhynchus Mykiss. *Ecotoxicology and Environmental Safety*, Vol. 69, No. 2, (February 2008), pp. 180-186, ISSN 0147-6513

Tiwary, A. & Colls, J. (2009). *Air Pollution* (3rd ed.), Taylor & Francis, ISBN 978-04-1547-933-2, London, United Kingdom

Tsapakis, M. & Stephanou, E.G. (2005). Occurrence of Gaseous and Particulate Polycyclic Aromatic Hydrocarbons in the Urban Atmosphere: Study of Sources and Ambient Temperature Effect on the Gas/Particle Concentration and Distribution. *Environmental Pollution*, Vol. 133, No. 1, (January 2005), pp. 147-156, ISSN 0269-7491

Tsapakis, M. & Stephanou, E.G. (2007). Diurnal Cycle of PAHs, nitro-PAHs, and oxy-PAHs in a High Oxidation Capacity Marine Background Atmosphere. *Environmental Science and Technology*, Vol. 41, No. 23, (December 2007), pp. 8011–8017, ISSN 0013-936X

United States Environmental Protection Agency (US EPA). (2005). *Guidelines for Carcinogen Risk Assessment*, EPA/630/P-03/001F, US Environmental Protection Agency, Washington, DC, United States of America, accessed 12.07.2011,available from <http://www.epa.gov/raf/publications/pdfs/CANCER_GUIDELINES_FINAL_3-25-05.pdf>

United States Environmental Protection Agency (USEPA). (1986). *Guidelines for Carcinogen Risk Assessment*, Federal Register 51(185):33992-34003, EPA/630/R-00/004, Washington, DC, accessed 18.07.2011, available from <http://www.epa.gov/raf/publications/pdfs/CA%20GUIDELINES_1986.PDF>

Vieira, L.R., Sousa, A., Frasco, M.F., Lima, I., Morgado, F., Guilhermino L. (2008). Acute Effects of Benzo[a]pyrene, Anthracene and a Fuel Oil on Biomarkers of the Common Goby Pomatoschistus Microps (Teleostei, Gobiidae). *Science of the Total Environment*, Vol. 395, No. 2-3, (June 2008), pp. 87-100, ISSN 0048-969

Vigotti, M.A., Serinelli, M. & Marchini, L. (2010). Urban Air Pollution and Children Respiratory Hospital Admissions in Pisa (Italy): A Time Series and a Case-Crossover Approach. *Epidemiologia e Prevenzione*, Vol. 34, No. 4, (July-August 2010), pp. 143-149, ISSN 1120-9763

World Health Organization (WHO), (1998). *Environmental Health Criteria 202: Selected Non-Heterocyclic Polycyclic Aromatic Hydrocarbons*, World Health Organization Publication, Geneva, Switzerland, accessed 19.07.2011, available from <http://www.inchem.org/documents/ehc/ehc/ehc202.htm#SectionNumber:1.3>

World Health Organization (WHO). (2006), *Air Quality Guidelines, Global Update 2005*. WHO Regional Office for Europe, ISBN 92-890-2192-6, Copenhagen, Denmark

6

Indoor Air Pollutants: Relevant Aspects and Health Impacts

Klara Slezakova[1,2], Simone Morais[2]
and Maria do Carmo Pereira[1]
[1]*LEPAE, Departamento de Engenharia Química, Faculdade de Engenharia, Universidade do Porto,*
[2]*REQUIMTE, Instituto Superior de Engenharia do Porto, Portugal*

1. Introduction

During the last three decades, many efforts have been made to protect populations from harmful exposure to outdoor pollutants. Networks of air monitoring stations have been located in strategic places and these provide information on the outdoor pollutant concentrations to which populations are exposed. However, people spend about 80-90% of their time in various indoor ambiences (i.e. homes, offices, restaurants, etc.) and the quality of indoor air, is an important factor influencing human health. Indoor air quality is characterized by multiple determinants, such as physical parameters, chemical emissions and biological contaminations. It is a common belief that while indoors, one is safe from harmful pollutants. However, the scientific evidence has shown that indoor air at homes can be more seriously polluted than outdoor air of the largest and most industrialized cities (WHO, 2006; Franklin, 2007). Furthermore, people who constantly stay indoors, thus being chronically exposed to indoor pollution, are often the most susceptible individuals (infants, children and seniors). To understand the relationship between indoor air quality and health, it is important to further study the indoor pollutants that have the most significant effects on human health.

Tobacco smoke is one of the most significant indoor sources of air pollution. There is no doubt that tobacco smoke causes various adverse health effects; voluminous literature has been dedicated to this topic. The adverse effects of smoking have been widely recognized for several decades, but only recently public concerns have focused on indirect exposures to tobacco smoke.

From the chemical point of view, tobacco smoke is a very complex mixture of gaseous phase and particles of different sizes. To this date more than 5000 different chemicals have been identified in tobacco smoke (Perfetti & Rodgman, 2008, 2011). Many of these, namely N-nitrosamines, polycyclic aromatic hydrocarbons, and heavy metals are known or suspected carcinogens.

Considering the importance of this topic, this chapter is dedicated to indoor air pollution and its health impacts. A brief historical perspective of the problem is presented. A general discussion on the aspects of indoor quality is given, covering indoor pollutants, their main sources, and impacts on human health. The chapter then focuses on tobacco smoke with particular emphasis on indoor particles.

2. Historical overview of indoor air pollution

Indoor air pollution has a much longer history than usually thought. Archaeological evidences suggest that indoor pollution was widely experienced in the distant past. Mummified lung tissues, preserved by tanning, freezing or desiccation, proved to be most useful to provide information on prehistoric exposure. The samples of these tissues were re-hydrated, allowing subsequent microscopic examination to identify solid materials deposited in the lungs (Brimblecombe, 1999). Various materials (mineral and wind-blown dust) that cause pneumoconiosis and silicosis were identified in samples of lung tissues throughout many different epochs and geographical locations (i.e. from a mummy of ancient Egypt, from Peruvian miner of sixteenth century, from East Anglian flint-knappers) (Brimblecombe, 1999); the most frequent occurrence was found for anthracotic particles being a result of lifelong exposure to smoke indoors. The smoke certainly was among the first major sources of indoor pollution. The soot found on the ceilings of prehistoric caves provides further evidence of indoor pollution associated with open fires as first human habitations were poorly ventilated (Spengler & Sexton, 1983). Perhaps even then, people were able to intuitively recognize negative impacts of smoke, as in the Romano - British Period, cooking was done outdoors or away from living areas (Brimblecombe, 1999). Nevertheless, during the Dark Age primitive huts still did not have chimneys. The smoke from the central hearth simply rose and then slowly escaped through holes in the roof; such conditions led to high levels of indoor pollution. The use of chimneys in the early modern period therefore represented a particularly relevant technological change. By the Elizabethan time chimneys became far more common and effective (Burr, 1997), and thus widely used. It is important to point out that these transformations were accomplished with some skepticism and prejudice; indoor smoke was considered important in hardening the timbers of the house and warding off the diseases among its habitants (Brimblecombe, 1999). Perhaps it was the reason why stoves, another step of technological development, never really took hold in England although some attempts were made; stoves grew especially popular on the continent significantly reducing exposure to indoor smoke.

Indirectly the historical evolution of indoor pollution was also related with outdoor pollution. For example, in 1952, a major air pollution disaster in London resulted in passage of the Clean Air Act (in 1956). Consequently, changes were made to the means of heating homes. Fireplaces, typically placed in each room and the use of soft coal, were successfully replaced by central or electrical heating systems (Boubel et al., 1994).

Although interest in indoor air quality has been increasing since the beginning of the twentieth century, prior to 1970s the scientific interest in these problems was rather low. However, the last two decades represented a positive change and recently public attention has focused on the risks associated with poor indoor air quality. Furthermore, exposure levels to various harmful indoor air pollutants have been increasingly considered for the protection of human health.

3. Indoor pollution

It is a common belief that when indoors one is safe from harmful pollutants. The general perception is that levels of pollution inside buildings are lower than outside as the walls protect us from external impacts. However, confined indoor spaces may cause the concentration of pollutants to rise to unacceptable levels. Furthermore, there are many

Pollutant		Emission source
Inorganic chemical substances	Carbon dioxide	Combustion activity, metabolic activity
	Carbon monoxide	Fuel burning, tobacco smoke, stoves, gas heaters, motor vehicles in garages
	Nitrogen dioxide	Outdoor air, fuel burning, motor vehicles in garages
	Sulfur dioxide	Outdoor air, fuel combustion
	Ozone	Photochemical reaction
	Radon	Soil and bedrock under houses, building materials, ground water
Organic chemical substances	Formaldehyde	Insulation, furnishings
	Polycyclic aromatic hydrocarbons	Tobacco smoke, fuel combustions
	Polychlorinated biphenyls	Heat transfer fluids used in lamp ballasts and TV capacitors, stabilizers used in PVC wire insulation materials, additives in sealants, adhesives, paints, and floor finishes
	Volatile organic compounds	Household products (paints, aerosol sprays, cleaning supplies), building materials and furnishings, office equipments (i.e. copiers and printers)
Biological pollutants	Allergens	Domestic animals, insects, house dusts
	Fungi	Internal surfaces, soils, plants, food
	Microorganisms	Occupants - people, animals, plants, air heating, ventilation, air-conditioning systems
	Pollens	Outdoor air, indoor vegetation
Other	Asbestos	Fire retardant material, insulation
	Particles	Tobacco smoke, combustions, resuspension
	Pesticides	Commercial and residential application of insecticides and herbicides

Table 1. Indoor air pollutants and their emissions sources, adapted from Jones, 2002; Król et al., 2011

additional sources of indoor pollution. They include combustion processes for house heating, lighting and cooking, emissions from the buildings materials, decorations, and activities of the indoor occupants (Jones, 2002). Indoor pollution also originates from biological sources, such as domestic animals, plants and insects. Due to a variety of these sources, the extents of indoor pollution differ significantly among places and over times. A substantial part of indoor pollution may result from outdoors. In some cases outdoor sources, such as vehicular traffic or industrial emissions can be major contributors to indoor pollution. This is especially important for homes situated in industrial areas or in urban areas in close proximity to roads. A study performed in the Netherlands showed increased mortality rates due to the exposure of particles found indoors from vehicular emissions; a relative risk of 1.95 was estimated for people living within 50 m of a major road (or 100 m from a highway) (Hoek et al., 2002). Several other authors provided evidence of human indoor exposure to traffic pollutants in relation to distance from major roads or to traffic density (Heinrich et al., 2005; Janssen et al., 2003; Martuzevicius et al., 2008; Meíja et al., 2011). Thus, the actual extent of indoor pollution results from both outdoor and indoor sources, but also of other parameters such as building architecture, furniture position, etc. Undoubtedly, the "individuality" of each indoor environment implies further research difficulties for complete understanding of indoor pollution.

Initially indoor pollutants that received the greatest attention were pollutants that penetrated from outdoors, namely sulfur dioxide, nitrogen oxides, ozone, and particles. However, the pollutants present indoors include not only these gases and particles, but a whole range of other pollutants that only increase to significant levels in enclosed indoor environments. Thus, attention was subsequently focused on pollutants that were of particular concern indoors, i.e. formaldehyde, radon, asbestos, tobacco smoke, and volatile organic compounds (Weschler et al., 2009). Later on, pesticides and other organic compounds found indoors gained scientific attention (Weschler et al., 2009). Table 1 presents the most known indoor pollutants and their respective sources (Jones, 2002; Król et al., 2011).

Indoor air pollution has been associated with a wide range of health outcomes as most of the air pollutants directly affect the respiratory and cardiovascular systems. Table 2 gives a general overview of the mechanisms and respective health outcomes of the main pollutants from indoor combustion (Bernstein et al., 2008; Goyal & Khare, 2010).

In general there are two types of health effects arising from indoor air pollutants: short-term (acute) effects and long-term (chronic) effects. Short-term health effects, such as irritation of eyes, nose, throat, and skin, headache, dizziness, and fatigue appear after a single exposure or repeated exposures. If identified they are treatable, however, most of these effects are similar to those associated with the common cold or other viral diseases, so it is often difficult to determine if the symptoms result from exposure to indoor air pollution or another cause. Long-term health effects occur only after long or repeated periods of exposure to pollutants. For example, short-term effects of smoke inhalation from indoor fuel combustion include acute respiratory irritation and inflammation, and acute respiratory infection (Goyal & Khare, 2010). Long-term effects of smoke inhalation are chronic obstructive pulmonary disease (COPD), chronic bronchitis, adverse reproductive outcomes and pregnancy-related problems, such as stillbirths and low birth weight, and lung cancer (Goyal & Khare, 2010; Okona-Mensah & Fayokun, 2011).

Pollutant	Mechanism	Potential health effects
Carbon monoxide	Binding with hemoglobin to produce carboxyhemoglobin, which reduces oxygen delivery to key organs and developing fetus	Low birth weight Increased perinatal death
Nitrogen dioxide	Acute exposure increases bronchial reactivity Long-term exposure increases susceptibility to bacterial and viral lung infections	Wheezing, exacerbation of asthma Respiratory infection, Reduced lung function in children
Sulfur dioxide	Acute exposure increases bronchial reactivity Long term: difficult to dissociate from effects of particulates	Wheezing, exacerbation of asthma Exacerbation of COPD, cardiovascular disease
Polycyclic aromatic hydrocarbons	Carcinogenic	Lung cancer Cancer of mouth, nasopharynx, and larynx
Particles	Acute bronchial irritaion, inflammation, increased reactivity Reduced mucociliary clearance Reduced macrophage response and reduced immunity	Wheezing, exacerbation of asthma Respiratory infection Chronic bronchitis and COPD Excess mortality, including from cardiovascular disease

Table 2. Examples of health risks associated with exposures to pollutants from indoor combustion

4. Selected indoor pollutants

There have been major changes in products and building materials used indoors over the last five decades. Accompanied also by modifications in building operations these changes have led to different emission profiles for indoor pollutants. For example restrictions on use of some building materials have led to a reduction of asbestos indoors. On the other hand indoor environments are less ventilated than they were decades ago, which leads to increased levels of pollutants from biological sources, i.e. mold, allergens, and fungi (Weschler et al., 2009). Furthermore, in some parts of the world air-conditioned buildings are frequently built. All of these changes have altered the type and concentrations of chemicals that occupants are exposed to in indoor environments (Weschler et al., 2009). The personal habits of building occupants have also changed. Since tobacco smoke represents a serious risk to human health and is a major source of indoor particles, the following section focuses on this pollutant. A brief overview of other health-relevant indoor pollutants, common in all regions of the world, is then given.

4.1 Tobacco smoke

4.1.1 Tobacco smoke throughout history

A history of tobacco dates back to 5000–3000 BC when the agricultural product began to be cultivated in South America (Gately, 2001). By the arrival of Christopher Columbus in 1492 the use of tobacco reached every corner of American continent including islands such as Cuba. Tobacco was used in various ways and for various purposes. It was sniffed, chewed, eaten, drunk, smeared over bodies, used in eye drops and enemas (Gately, 2001); it was blown into the warriors faces during battle, and offered to gods. Perhaps the major use of tobacco was in medicine. Mild analgesic and antiseptic properties made tobacco useful to heal minor illness such as toothache when its leaves would be packed around the tooth (Gately, 2001). It was also believed to be a remedy for snake bites when the juice of tobacco leaves was applied directly to wound. Later, the consumption of tobacco smoke evolved into burning the plant substance either by accident or with intent of exploring other means of consumption. Tobacco is a powerful insecticide and blowing its smoke over seed corn or fruits trees was an effective way of controlling pests in some civilizations (Gately, 2001). The practice of tobacco combustion also worked its way into shamanistic rituals (Wilbert, 1987); many ancient civilizations, such as Indians and Chinese, burnt incense as a part of their religious rituals. Smoking of tobacco thus probably had its origins in these incense-burning ceremonies of shamans (Robicsek, 1979). The act of smoking was not merely a method for tobacco consumption but an integral part of the rituals. Nevertheless, later it was adopted for pleasure and as a social tool.

Tobacco was introduced to Europe in 1493 when Christopher Columbus returned from his discovery voyage to America (Thielen et al., 2008). Previously Europe did not have any precedent for tobacco smoking. In fact Europeans did even lacked the vocabulary to describe the act of smoking (Gately, 2001). The English language term "smoking" was created only in the late 18th century; before then the practice was called "drinking smoke" (Lloyd & Mitchinson, 2008). Although, Europeans reacted with horror and consternation when the returning sailors smoked, the habit spread; nowadays, it is estimated that there are 1.1×10^9 smokers around the world (IARC, 2004). The medical properties of tobacco raised European's curiosity. Originally, tobacco was planted in palace gardens where it was studied by royal physicians. The initial association of tobacco with royal society enhanced its reputation and helped its spread around the world. In Spain tobacco was populated via the Roma Catholic clergy, who developed a fondness to snuff (Gately, 2001). Frenchman Jean Nicot introduced snuff to France in 1560. Nicot (from whose name the word nicotine is derived) received tobacco cuttings from famous Portuguese botanist Damião de Goes during his official stay at Portuguese court; he later planted those in the gardens of the French embassy (Taylor, 2008). Afterwards, the use of tobacco spread to England. The first report of a smoking Englishman is of a sailor in Bristol in 1556, seen "emitting smoke from his nostrils" (Lloyd & Mitchinson, 2008). Around 1600 tobacco was introduced in what today is modern-day Gambia and Senegal. By the 1650s the Portuguese brought the commodity and the plant to southern Africa, establishing the popularity of tobacco throughout all of Africa (Gately, 2001). Tobacco, both product and plant, followed the most important trade routes to major ports and markets, and then on into the hinterlands. By the mid-17th century every major civilization had been introduced to tobacco smoking. In many cases tobacco smoking had assimilated into the native culture, despite the attempts to eliminate the practice with harsh penalties or fines (Gately, 2001). During the American Civil War in 1860s the primary labor force of tobacco production shifted from slavery to share cropping (Burns, 2006). In 1881, the industrialization of tobacco production with the cigarette followed.

4.1.2 Tobacco combustion and composition

The term "tobacco smoking" is the process where tobacco is burned and the vapors either tasted or inhaled. When smoking, air is drawn into a cigarette/cigar during each puff, and combustion takes place. This process forms tobacco mainstream smoke. Emissions produced in such manner are inhaled by smoker; burn temperature is up to 1000 °C (Colls, 1997). Although health-harmful pollutants such as N-nitrosamines are formed, they influence only the smoker.

Between the puffs, the cigarette smoulders, and from its lit end it forms sidestream tobacco smoke. The combustion temperature is lower (approximately around 400 °C; Colls, 1997), but it can lead to the formation of more toxic compounds than those found in mainstream smoke. Furthermore, before further dilution by air turbulences, the concentrations of toxicants in the sidestream smoke are extremely high. The mixture of smokes present in a room is then called "environmental tobacco smoke" (also known as second-handed tobacco smoke). Environmental tobacco smoke consists of mainstream smoke exhaled into environment and sidestream smoke, after dilution and aging (Thielen et al., 2008). The aging can last for minutes or hours, but during that time the composition of all pollutants, including particulates changes.

When tobacco combustion takes place, a large number of gaseous and particulate pollutants are produced; many of those being known or suspected carcinogens and more than 100 are considered chemical poisons (Colls, 1997). Various authors reported that over 4000 different chemical components were found in tobacco smoke. However, in their last update Perfetti and Rodgman (2011) reported 5685 components in tobacco smoke that accounted for more than 99% of the mass of whole smoke. Certainly, other tobacco smoke components are present in the mixture but the total mass of these remaining components is obviously quite small (Perfetti & Rodgman, 2011). Some of the tobacco smoke components, such as carbon monoxide, carbon dioxide, nitrogen, nitric oxide, formaldehyde, and benzene are present in gaseous phase, whereas others (e.g. phenols, cresols, and hydrogen cyanide, and light molecular weight polycyclic aromatic hydrocarbons) are portioned between both vapor and particulate phases (Castro et al., 2011; Rodgman & Perfetti, 2008). Carcinogenic metals, such as arsenic and cadmium, chromium, nickel, and lead (IARC, 2011) are mainly found in the particles (Slezakova et al., 2009a; Wu et al., 1997), as well as tobacco-specific nitrosamines (Thielen et al., 2008) and higher weight polycyclic aromatic hydrocarbons (Castro et al., 2011; Rodgman & Perfetti, 2006; Slezakova et al., 2009b). At present, as many as 570 PAHs have been identified in tobacco smoke (Perfetti & Rodgman, 2011), several of them being classified by the International Agency for Research on Cancer (IARC) as carcinogens (Rodgman & Perfetti, 2006, 2008). As most of these particulate-bound compounds have known adverse impacts on human health, the respective exposures represent a serious risk to human health (IARC, 2010; WHO, 2006).

4.1.3 Health effects

Although originally little was known about the harmful health effects of tobacco smoke, by the twentieth century these had been widely recognized. Since the 1950s the health effects of tobacco smoke have been intensively studied. Voluminous literature and public media have linked active tobacco smoking to lung and heart diseases and to cancers of various organ systems (Pasupathi et al., 2009; Shah & Cole, 2010). Smoking harms nearly every organ of the human body, but the full extent of the damage is still unknown. Even today, over 50 years after the first links between smoking and lung cancer were established, more diseases are being found to be caused by smoking. However, it is known that about half of all continuing regular smokers are killed by their smoking (EC, 2004); those smokers that die in middle age, lose approximately 22 years of life, with a larger proportion of that shortened life span being spent in ill health (EC, 2004). Over 3 million people are killed every year because they smoke, dying mostly due to lung cancer and aortic aneurysm, out of these over 650 000 are European citizens (EC, 2004).

Tobacco smoke affects not only people who smoke but also those who are somehow exposed to it. Undoubtedly, the exposure of smokers is much higher compared to those of nonsmokers. The exposure of non-voluntary smokers cannot be underestimated as it was found that higher levels of cancer-causing substances occurred in sidestream smoke than in mainstream smoke (Wu et al., 1997). Thus, the exposure to environmental tobacco smoke, also called passive smoking, has also become an important health issue and it has been established beyond any doubt that passive smoking poses hazards to human health. Among the most significant concerns associated with exposure to environmental tobacco smoke are potential respiratory and other effects associated with chronic exposures. Passive smoking increases the risk and frequency of respiratory symptoms (wheeze, cough, breathlessness and phlegm) and asthma (Horak et al., 2007; Kabir et al., 2009; Trude & Skorge, 2007), being a proven cause of respiratory diseases of the lower airways (croup, bronchitis, bronchiolitis, pneumonia) in childhood and during adulthood (Skorge et al., 2005); extended exposure to environmental tobacco smoke also induce various heart disease (Wu, 1997) as well as lung cancer for non-smokers (EC, 2004; Okona-Mensah & Fayokun, 2011). Thus in 1993, the US Environmental Protection Agency (USEPA) classified passive smoking as a "Class A" human carcinogen (USEPA, 1993); accordingly, IARC declared that exposure to environmental tobacco smoke is carcinogenic to humans (IARC, 2004). The concentrations of particles in environmental tobacco smoke can reach up to 1000 $\mu g\ m^{-3}$ compared to 1-5 $\mu g\ m^{-3}$ in clean ambient air or 100 $\mu g\ m^{-3}$ in polluted ambient air; the highest concentrations can be found in poorly ventilated and crowded pubs, clubs and coffee bars (Colls, 1997; Lee et al., 2010; Slezakova et al., 2009a). Many countries have implemented certain measures of interventions such as smoking bans or restriction in workplaces or public places in order to protect public health. However, these legislative interventions cannot apply for homes or other private indoor environments where exposure to environmental tobacco smoke has remained an important health issue. In Western countries, with an adult smoking prevalence of 30-50%, it is estimated that over 50% of homes are occupied by at least one smoker (WHO, 2000a), resulting in a high prevalence of exposure to environmental tobacco smoke. Young children, in particular, who spend most of their time at home, are at increased risks for even greater exposures to tobacco smoke if their mothers smoke; it was estimated that exposure to second-hand smoke in homes increases the risk of developing asthma by 40-200% (Bernstein et al., 2008).

The indirect exposure to tobacco smoke can also occur as a consequence of third-hand smoke (Winickoff et al., 2009). Third-hand smoke refers to the residue that is left behind on furniture, walls, and carpeting after a cigarette has been extinguished. This term first appeared in print in 2006 but it became more widely known when used in 2009 by Jonathan Winickoff (Burton, 2011). Third-hand smoke may lead to contact of harmful compounds (Rehan et al., 2011) and has several exposure routes. It can remain on surfaces as a potential source of dermal exposure or be ingested by food that has been exposed to tobacco smoke (Matt et al., 2004). It can be re-emitted as source of inhalation exposure as dust can carry third-hand smoke to the lungs (Singer et al., 2002). Furthermore, after time the smoke residue can become airborne again. Petrick et al. (2011) has recently shown that residues of nicotine can interact with indoor air pollutants (i.e. ozone) resulting in the formation of secondary organic aerosols and gas and condensed phase products. The cumulative exposures to these airborne species may be greater for an infant than an adult when both breathing rate and body weight are considered (Winickoff et al., 2009). It is however rather difficult to quantify third-hand smoke contamination, because it depends largely on the respective spaces, in small confined places like a car the deposition might be really significant (Fortmann et al., 2010); personal exposures may continue to occur on the order of hours to days (Petrick et al., 2011). Although the health implications of third-hand smoke are currently unknown, children are especially susceptible to this exposure because they breathe near, crawl and play on, touch, and mouth contaminated surfaces; at up to 0.25 g per day, the dust ingestion rate in infants is more than twice that of adults (Winickoff et al., 2009). Emphasizing that third-hand smoke harms the health of children thus may be an important element in encouraging home smoking bans.

4.2 Particles

"Indoor particles", "airborne particulates", or "aerosols", these are some of the terms once used when dealing with particles. The term "particulate matter" (with abbreviation PM) is often used as a synonym for particles in pollutants science. Particulate matter, as defined by World Health Organization (WHO) is a mixture of solid or solid/liquid particles suspended in air (WHO, 2000b). These particles vary in size, shape, origin, and chemical composition. It is usual to classify the particles by their aerodynamic characteristics. Typically these are summarized by aerodynamic diameter, i.e. a diameter of a spherical particle with a density of 1 g cm^{-3} that has the same inertial properties and settling velocity as the particle in question (Wilson et al., 2002).

When breathing, particles deposit in the human respiratory system thus causing various health effects. The deposition of particles within the human respiratory system is influenced by several parameters such as particles properties (size, density and shape, chemical composition), morphology of the respiratory tract, and breathing pattern. Among these parameters, size of the particles is especially important. During breathing, particles with an aerodynamic diameter of 10 μm or less are naturally inhaled by humans; larger particles are less likely to enter the human respiratory tract. After inhalation larger particles are deposit in the nose and mouth. Particles with 6-7 μm or less pass into the lower parts of respiratory tract where they deposit in the smaller conducting air ways and gas exchange regions of lungs. According to the entrances into the various compartments of the respiratory system, particles can be classified as (Wilson, 1998): inhalable, thoracic, and respirable. Inhalable particles refer to those that enter the respiratory system during breathing, including the head airways. Thoracic particles are those that enter the lower respiratory tract including the trachea, bronchi and the gas exchanges regions of lungs. Finally, respirable particles are those that are capable of reaching the alveolar regions of lungs. It is necessary to point out that there is a great discrepancy in the literature on the use of the terms "inhalable", "thoracic" and "respirable". Thoracic particles are often used as equivalent for PM_{10}, respirable particles are frequently used as synonym for $PM_{2.5}$ (Brunekreef & Holgate, 2002). It is important to differentiate between these terms as they are not completely identical. The term PM_x originated from sampler cutpoint classification and refers to the collection of particles below or within a specified aerodynamic size range, usually defined by the upper 50% cutpoint size. Thus PM_{10} stands for particulate matter with a 50% cutpoint at 10 μm of aerodynamic diameter, $PM_{2.5}$ are particles with a 50% cutpoint at 2.5 μm of aerodynamic diameter. However, respirable particle have 50% upper cutpoint at 4.0 μm whereas, as mentioned before it is 2.5 μm for $PM_{2.5}$ (Wilson, 1998). As for the PM_{10} and thoracic particles, they both have 50% cutpoint at 10 μm, but thoracic particles have less precise size cut (Dockery et al., 1998).

The terms "fine" and "coarse" particles are also used in indoor pollution science. These terms originated from modal classification (Whitby, 1978) being based on the size distributions and formation mechanisms (Fig. 1). The coarse mode particles are with aerodynamic diameter greater than the minimum in the particle mass distribution, which generally occurs between 1-3 μm (Wilson et al., 2002). Particles of this mode are

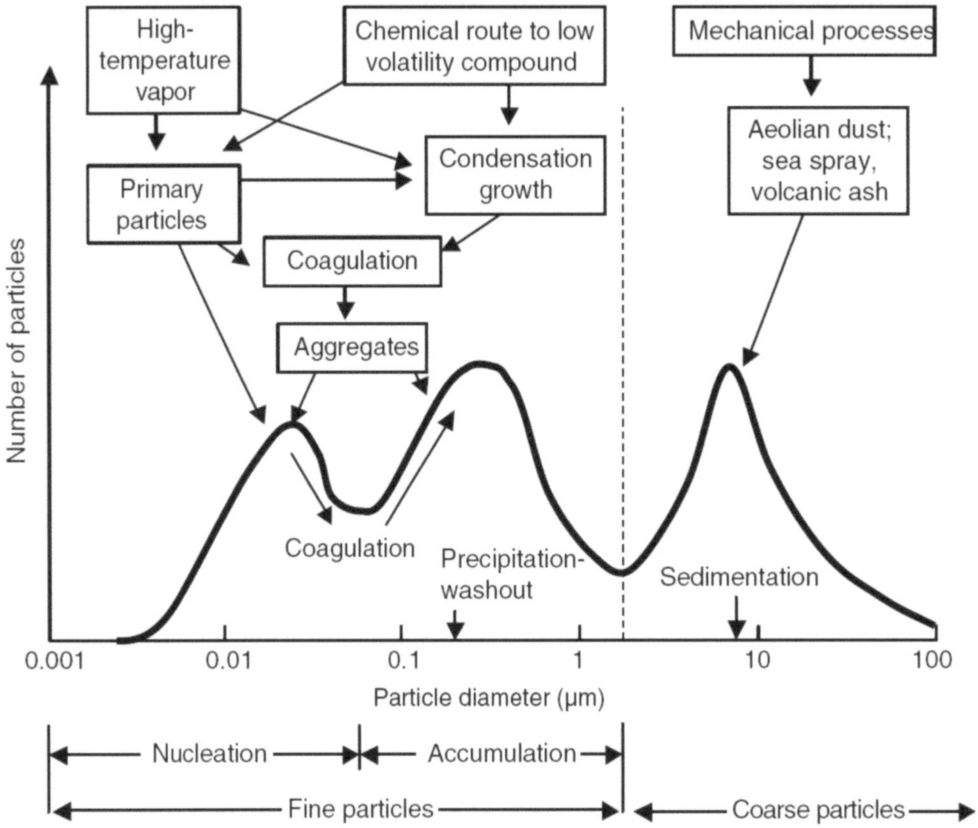

Fig. 1. Prototypical size distribution of particles, their sources and pathways of formations; dashed line corresponds approximately to 2.5 μm of diameter (Wilson et al., 2002)

mechanically produced by the break-up of larger solid particles. Pollen grains and mould spores as well as particles from plant fibers and leaves belong to this mode. The fine mode particles have an aerodynamic diameter mostly smaller than the minimum in the particle mass distribution. Based on the formation mechanisms of the particles, they are further subdivided into (WHO, 2000b): nuclei and accumulation mode particles. Nuclei (also called "ultrafine particles") particles typically have an aerodynamic diameter smaller than 0.1 μm (Oberdörster et al., 1995). These particles are directly emitted from combustion sources or formed by nucleation (i.e. condensation of low-vapor-pressure substances formed by high temperature vaporization or by chemical reactions in the atmosphere to form nuclei). Accumulation mode (Wilson et al., 2002) particles have an aerodynamic diameter between 0.1–1.0 μm. These particles are formed from nuclei-mode ones that grow by coagulation (i.e. the combination of two or more particles to form a larger particle) or by condensation (i.e. condensation of gas or vapor molecules on the surface of existing particles). Coagulation is most efficient for large numbers of particles, and condensation is most efficient for large surface areas. Over the years the terms "fine" and "coarse", as applied originally to the particle sizes, have lost their precise meaning. In many given articles the definition border is fixed by convention at 2.5 μm of aerodynamic diameter due to the measurement facilities.

4.2.1 Indoor sources

As it can be seen from Table 1 tobacco smoke and indoor combustion activities (i.e. wood and fossil fuel burning) are the main indoor sources of particles. Indoor particles are also produced by various activities, such as cleaning (vacuuming, dusting, and sweeping), cooking (broiling, baking, frying, toasting, barbecuing), by human movements, and from animals and plants (Abt et al., 2000a). In addition to these sources, emissions originated from outdoors are especially important for particulates (Castro et al., 2010; Chen & Zhao, 2010; Massey et al., 2009). Outdoor emissions are relevant particularly for fine particles as the contribution of outdoor particles indoors generally increases with decreasing particle sizes (Geller et al., 2002; Slezakova et al., 2011); it was found that outdoor 2-10 μm particles accounted for 10% to 40% of indoor emissions, whereas it was between 35% to 92% for particles smaller than 2 μm (Abt et al., 2000b; Slezakova et al., 2011).

The chemical composition of particulate matter is strongly related to its origin and sources. For example particles from combustions consist mainly of carbon and unburned or partially burned organic compounds. Except the carbonaceous materials, particles generally contain inorganic water insoluble material (i.e. various minerals) and inorganic water soluble material (i.e. sulfates, nitrates, chlorides). Although in much lower abundances, hazardous particulate components such as polycyclic aromatic hydrocarbons and heavy metals are relevant. Adsorbed onto the surface of the particles, they can contribute to adverse health effects of particulate matter. PAHs and heavy metals are predominantly found in fine particles (Castro et al., 2010, 2011; Slezakova et al., 2009a, 2009b, 2011); the large surface area of smaller particles allows them to carry greater amounts of these toxic compounds that are consequently deposit in the lower respiratory tract, thereby having a greater effect on the adverse health outcomes.

4.2.2 Health effects

The extensive epidemiological research of the last two decades has provided much evidence on the exposure to particulate air pollution and adverse health effects. However, the health impacts associated with these exposures have been much more extensively studied for outdoor particles then for indoor ones. Hence the majority of the knowledge arrives from the studies of outdoor air, whereas the number of epidemiological studies related to indoor environments is rather limited. There is still a lack of knowledge concerning health effects of different outdoor particle fractions, namely in relation to different size fractions of $PM_{2.5}$. Even more, this lack exists for indoor particles. Furthermore, the adverse effects of indoor particulate matter depend on deposition of particles in the respiratory tract, which is directly related to particle size and chemical composition. However, indoor particulates may differ substantially in composition from outdoor particulates hence their significance and contribution to the adverse health effects needs to be fully explored.

Particulate indoor air pollution has been linked to both acute and chronic health effects (Mitchell et al., 2006), including asthma, cardiac diseases, as well as impaired lung function and other conditions (Allen et al., 2008; Abbey, 1998; Pope et al., 1991; Viegi et al., 2004). Specifically fine particles have been shown to decrease forced expiratory volume in 1 second (FEV_1) in asthmatic schoolchildren (Delfino et al., 2004). Furthermore, Delfino et al. (2008) found that FEV_1 decrements were significantly associated with personal exposures to $PM_{2.5}$, but not ambient $PM_{2.5}$ levels. These results emphasize the importance of indoor exposures. The personal exposures to indoor particles are often much higher than ambient air concentrations (Brown et al., 2008). Franck et al. (2011) investigated associations between indoor particle concentrations and the risks for respiratory diseases in young children; exposures to high indoor particle concentrations were associated with increased risks for the development of obstructive bronchitis, especially for particles smaller than 1 µm. Apparently more detailed indoor measurements are necessary in order to fully understand health effects of indoor particle exposure.

4.3 Carbon monoxide

Carbon monoxide is a toxic tasteless, odorless, and colorless gas that is produced by incomplete combustion of fuels such as wood, petrol, coal, natural gas and kerosene. Indoors, carbon monoxide is produced by these combustion sources (cooking and heating) and is also introduced through the infiltration from outdoor air into the indoor environment. Exposure to high levels of carbon monoxide might be lethal. Carbon monoxide is absorbed through the lungs and diffused across the alveolar capillary membrane. Once absorbed it passes across red blood cell membranes, and enters the red blood cell stroma where it binds to hemoglobin forming carboxyhemoglobin (COHb); the affinity of carbon monoxide to hemoglobin is about 200 times higher than that of oxygen (Tiwary and Colls, 2009). Such binding reduces the capacity of blood to carry oxygen and interferes with oxygen release at the tissues; the resulting impaired delivery of oxygen can interfere with cellular respiration and cause tissue hypoxia. Health effects of carbon monoxide are generally considered in relation to carboxyhemoglobin levels in blood. Except the increased daily mortality rate, health effects of carbon monoxide include early onset of cardiovascular disease, behavioral impairment, decreased exercise performance of young healthy men, reduced birth weight and sudden infant death syndrome (Bernstein et al., 2008). The severity of poisoning is dependent on concentration, length of exposure, and the general underlying health status of the exposed individual. Acute effects of carbon monoxide poisoning are particularly severe on the organs that require a high supply of oxygen, namely the brain and heart; the latter being well documented (Jones, 2002). Chronic exposure to carbon monoxides causes symptoms that are easily misdiagnosed, such as headache, fatigue, dizziness and nausea (Jones, 2002).

4.4 Nitrogen dioxide

Nitrogen dioxide is a reddish brown gas with a characteristic pungent odor. It is a key precursor of a range of secondary pollutants whose effects on human health are well-documented (WHO, 2006). The most important indoor sources include tobacco smoke and gas-, wood-, oil-, kerosene- and coal-burning appliances such as stoves, ovens, space and water heaters and fireplaces. Outdoor nitrogen dioxide from natural and anthropogenic sources also influences indoor levels. Inhalation is the major route of exposure to nitrogen dioxide. The link between exposure to nitrogen dioxide and adverse respiratory effects in susceptible populations has been explored extensively, but results are inconclusive (Franklin, 2007; WHO, 2006). There is recent evidence suggesting that children with atopy or asthma, infants who are at risk of developing asthma, and female adults are more sensitive to the respiratory effects of nitrogen dioxide exposure (Berstein et al., 2008). An increase in indoor nitrogen dioxide of 28 $\mu g\ m^{-3}$ was associated with a 20% increased risk of lower respiratory illness in children (WHO, 2010). Indoor exposure to nitrogen dioxide may also enhance asthmatic reactions to inhaled allergens (Berstein et al., 2008).

4.5 Radon

Radon is a colorless and odorless radioactive gas that arises from the decay of radium-226. It is classified by the IARC as a human carcinogen (IARC, 2011). The main source of indoor radon is through the decay of radium in the soil subjacent to a house. Due to current construction methods, radon concentrations often become enhanced indoors. Radon itself is inert and causes little damage. However, it undergoes further radioactive decay which produces short-lived radioisotopes; the most stable of the isotopes is radon-222 which is universally referred as "radon" or "radon gas". Some of isotopes are electrically charged and can be inhaled, both directly or bound to particles. Once inhaled, they deposit in lungs causing severe health effects (WHO, 2010). There is direct evidence from residential epidemiological studies that radon causes lung cancer, even at concentrations typically found in indoor air (Al-Zoughool & Krewski, 2009). Some studies suggested also an association with other cancers, in particular leukaemia and cancers of the extra-thoracic airways (WH0, 2010).

4.6 Sulfur dioxide

Sulfur dioxide is nonflammable, nonexplosive, colorless gas with strong pungent smell. Its concentrations indoors are typically lower than those from outdoors. Inhalation is the major route of exposure to sulfur dioxide. Some studies have demonstrated that sulfur dioxide can cause bronchoconstriction (airway narrowing) in both healthy and asthmatic adults with clinical symptoms of shortness of breath, wheezing (Berstein et al., 2008), and impaired lung function (Jones, 2002). Such responses also occur at low levels of sulfur dioxide during moderate exercise, asthmatic children and adults are at higher risk. Data available from recent epidemiological study do not show any evidence of excess general and cause-specific mortalities (respiratory, cardiovascular) associated with exposures to sulfur dioxide in urban areas (Brunekreef et al., 2009).

4.7 Formaldehyde

Formaldehyde is to the general public the most know volatile organic compound that has been associated with indoor air pollution. Indoor sources include combustion processes such as smoking, heating, cooking, or candle or incense burning. Major sources in non-smoking environments are building materials and consumer products that emit formaldehyde. This applies typically to new materials and products but in conditions with high relative humidity and high indoor temperatures it can last several months (WHO, 2010). Sources of formaldehyde indoors include furniture and wooden products containing formaldehyde-based resins, insulating materials, textiles, products such as paints, wallpapers, glues, adhesives, varnishes and lacquers, household cleaning, and electronic equipment. Formaldehyde is classified as a human carcinogen (IARC, 2011) and high occupational exposures are considered as a risk for nasopharyngeal cancer (Franklin, 2007). At lower concentrations formaldehyde has mostly been associated with irritation of the eyes, nose and upper airways (Berstein et al., 2008). Several epidemiological studies reported associations between exposure to formaldehyde in homes and schools with asthma, asthma severity, allergy, and airway inflammation in children (Franklin, 2007).

4.8 Polycyclic aromatic hydrocarbons

Polycyclic aromatic hydrocarbons (PAHs) are a group of organic compounds with two or more aromatic rings. They occur in indoor air as complex mixtures, and their composition may vary from place to place. PAHs are known for their cytotoxic and mutagenic properties; although a number of PAHs are non-mutagenic, their metabolites or derivatives may be potential mutagens. PAHs also represent the largest known group of carcinogens. While some compounds are probable/possible carcinogens others are known human carcinogens (IARC, 2010). PAHs that are potent carcinogens are typically attached to particles. The primary exposure to carcinogenic PAHs found in air occurs via inhalation of these particles. Chronic exposure to PAHs may affect the pulmonary, gastrointestinal, renal and dermatological systems (Król et al., 2011). Certain PAHs can also affect the haematopoietic and immune systems, and can have teratogenic and neurological effects (Król et al., 2011). Health evaluation data suggest that lung cancer is the most serious health risk from exposure to PAHs in indoor air (WHO, 2010).

4.9 Volatile organic compounds

Volatile organic compounds (VOCs) are organic chemicals that easily vaporize at room temperature. Over 300 individual compounds have been measured in indoor environments, some of them, such as benzene, dichloromethane, and tetrachloromethane are known carcinogens (IARC, 2011). Individual compounds have been associated with a variety of health effects including irritation, neurologic and respiratory symptoms (Bernstein et al., 2008). Associations between these measures of exposure and poor respiratory health have been observed in infants, preschool and school-aged children, but the findings were not completely consistent (Franklin, 2007).

4.10 Pollutants from biological sources

As various biological materials (i.e. mold, yeasts, wood-rotting fungi, bacteria, and viruses) have been found indoors, the health impacts of inhaled biological pollutants should not be underestimated (Dales et al., 2008). Biological agents can cause diseases through atopic mechanisms, infection processes, and direct toxicity. Numerous studies conducted worldwide have reported an association between indoor pollutants from biological sources and adverse acute and chronic health effects (Bernstein et al., 2008), including rhinitis and other upper respiratory symptoms, asthma, humidifier fever, extrinsic allergic alveolitis, atopic dermitidis, high blood pressure in adults, lung and immune system adverse effects (Bernstein et al., 2008; Srikanth et al., 2008).

5. Guidelines

The fulfillment of indoor climate requirements are stated as objectives of the Directive 2002/91/EC on Energy Performance of Buildings, however no specifications on how to achieve this are provided (Jantunen et al., 2011). Portugal is the only Member State that included an Indoor Air Quality assessment in the procedure of assessing energy performance according to the Directive (Jantunen et al., 2011). In 2008 the EU commission revised the directive. The new Directive 2010/31/EC still includes the requirement for a good indoor climate, but still does not specify any actions to guarantee this goal; the directive emphasizes energy efficiency, but does not require any information on indoor air climate. However, European Union set recommendation guidelines for levels of indoor exposure to radon (Commission Recommendation 90/143/Euratom), expressed as effective dose equivalent. For existing buildings the effective dose equivalent is 20 mSv per annum (for practical purposes, may be taken as equal to an annual average concentration of radon gas of 400 Bq/m^3). For future constructions the dose is 10 mSv per annum, i.e. equivalent to an annual average concentration of 200 Bq/m^3.

Despite the efforts of information campaigns on health effects of indoor pollution and on the maintenance of a healthy indoor environment, the public is still more aware of the adverse impacts of outdoor pollution rather than indoor pollution. Improving indoor air quality is a specific action of the European Union (CEC, 2004), with two key elements: addressing environmental tobacco smoke, and developing networks and guidelines on other factors affecting indoor air quality by using research and exchange of best practice. Concurrently, the World Health Organization continues with its efforts to define conditions for healthy air. In order to encourage the relevant policy developments for ensuring healthy indoor air, guidelines for a range of chemical substances most commonly polluting indoor air have been recently set (WHO, 2010). If sensibly applied as part of policy development, indoor exposure to air hazardous pollutants should decline thus leading to a reduction in adverse effects on health.

6. Conclusion

During last few decades indoor air quality has finally received much deserved scientific attention. Although considerable progress has been made in our knowledge about indoor pollution and its sources, the problem is still not completely understood. The unique individuality of each indoor environment (i.e. construction, inhabitants habits, etc.) implies further research difficulties and indoor ambiences also differ between regions as well as between continents. Despite that, the problems of poor indoor air that modern societies face are similar for many countries around the world. It is certainly necessary to continue with research efforts. In particularly associations between indoor air quality and health impacts need to be better addressed as so far much of the knowledge is derived from outdoor exposure studies.

Much effort has been invested in the reduction of outdoor pollution. However, reducing ambient pollution does not necessarily result in a proportionate decrease in indoor air pollution - a situation which has important implications for interventions. Therefore, regulatory aspects of indoor air quality also need to be considered. As the links between indoor air quality and health effects are becoming better understood, various attempts have been made to address this issue. For example, the USA and many European countries have successfully implemented interventions to protect public health from some hazardous pollutants, such as tobacco smoke. Asian or South American countries still have a high prevalence of second-hand tobacco smoke in public places, hence the need for future smoke-free regulation in those countries. As for the indoor particles there is still lack of scientific evidence which prevents the establishment of comprehensive indoor limit values and guidelines for health protection.

To ensure the protection of public health, it is necessary to combine all our available resources including scientific knowledge and regulatory power, thus providing the healthiest indoor environments possible for this and future generations.

7. Acknowledgment

The authors would like to thank to Fundação para Ciência e Tecnologia for the financial support with grant number SFRH/BPD/65722/2009.

8. References

Abbey, D.E., Burchette, R.J., Knutsen, S.F., McDonnell, W.F., Lebowitz, M.D. & Enright, P.L. (1998). Long-Term Particulate and other Air Pollutants and Lung Function in Nonsmokers. *American Journal of Respiratory and Critical Care Medicine*, Vol. 158, No. 1, (July 1998), pp. 289-298, ISSN 1073-449X

Abt, E., Suh, H.H., Allen, G. & Koutrakis, P. (2000a). Characterization of Indoor Particle Sources: A Study Conducted in the Metropolitan Boston Area. *Environmental Health Perspective*, Vol. 108, No. 1, (January 2000), pp. 35–44, ISSN 0091-6765

Abt, E., Suh, H.H., Catalano, P. & Koutrakis, P. (2000b). Relative Contribution of Outdoor and Indoor Sources to Indoor Concentrations. *Environmental Science and Technology*, Vol. 34, No. 17, (August 2000), pp. 3579- 3587, ISSN 0013-936X

Allen, R.W., Mar, T., Koenig, J., Liu, L.J., Gould, T., Simpson, C. & Larson, T. (2008). Changes in Lung Function and Airway Inflammation among Asthmatic Children. *Inhalation Toxicology*, Vol. 20, No. 4, (February 2008), pp. 423-33, ISSN 0895-8378

Al-Zoughool, M. & Krewski, D. (2009). Health Effects of Radon: a Review of the Literature. *International Journal of Radiation Biology*, Vol. 85, No. 1, (January 2009), pp. 57-69, ISSN 0955-3002

Bernstein, J.A., Alexis, N., Bacchus, H., Bernstein, I.L., Fritz, P., Horner, E., Li, N., Mason, S., Nel, A., Oullette, J., Reijula, K., Reponen, T., Seltzer, J., Smith, S. & Tarlo, S.M. (2008). The Health Effects of Non-Industrial Indoor Air Pollution. *Journal of Allergy and Clinical Immunology*, Vol. 121, No. 3, (January 2008), pp. 585-591, ISSN 0091-6749

Boubel, R.W., Fox, D.L., Turner, D.B. & Stern, A.C. (1994). *Fundamentals of Air Pollution*, (3rd Ed.), Academic Press, ISBN 0-12-118930-0, London, United Kingdom

Brimblecombe, P. (1999). Air Pollution and Health History, In: *Air Pollution and Health*, S.T. Holgate, J.M. Samet, H.S. Koren, R.L. Maynard, (Eds.), pp. 5-21, Academic Press, ISBN 0-12-352335-4, London, United Kingdom

Brown, K.W., Sarnat, J.A., Suh, H.H., Coull, B.A., Spengler, J.D. & Koutrakis, P. Ambient (2008). Site, Home Outdoor and Home Indoor Particulate Concentrations as Proxies of Personal Exposures. *Journal of Environmental Monitoring*, Vol. 10, No. 9, (July 2008), pp. 1041-51, ISSN 1464-0333

Brunekreef, B. & Holgate, S.T. (2002). Air Pollution and Health. *Lancet*, Vol. 360, No. 9341, (October 2002), pp. 1233–1242, ISBN 0140-6736

Brunekreef, B., Beelen, R., Hoek, G., Schouten, L., Bausch-Goldbohm, S., Fischer, P., Armstrong, B., Hughes, E., Jerrett, M. & van den Brandt, P. (2009). Effects of Long-term Exposure to Traffic-related Air Pollution on Respiratory and Cardiovascular Mortality in the Netherlands: the NLCS-AIR Study. *Research Report (Health Effects Institute)*, Vol. 139, (March 2009), pp. 5-71

Burns, E. (2006). *The Smoke of the Gods: A Social History of Tobacco*, Temple University Press, ISBN 978-1-592-13480-9, Philadelphia, Pennsylvania, USA

Burr, M.L. (1997). Health Effects of Indoor Combustion Products. *Journal of the Royal Society of Health*, Vol. 117, No. 6, (December 1997), pp. 1252-1256, ISSN 0264-0325

Burton, A. (2011). Does the Smoke Ever Really Clear? Thirdhand Smoke Exposure Raises New Concerns. *Environmental Health Perspective*, Vol. 119, No. 2, (February 2011), pp. A70–A74, ISSN 0091-6765

Castro, D., Slezakova, K., Delerue-Matos, C., Alvim-Ferraz, M.C., Morais, S. & Pereira, M.C. (2011). Polycyclic Aromatic Hydrocarbons in Gas and Particulate Phases of Indoor Environments Influenced by Tobacco Smoke: Levels, Phase Distributions, and Health Risks. *Atmospheric Environment*, Vol. 45, No. 10, (March 2011), pp. 1799-1808, ISSN 1352-2310

Castro, D., Slezakova, K., Delerue-Matos, C., Alvim-Ferraz, M.C., Morais, S. & Pereira, M.C. (2010). Contribution of Traffic and Tobacco Smoke in the Distribution of Polycyclic Aromatic Hydrocarbons on Outdoor and Indoor PM2.5. *Global Nest Journal*, Vol. 12, No. 1, (March 2010), pp. 3-11, ISSN 1790-7632

Chen, C. & Zhao, B. (2010). Review of Relationship between Indoor and Outdoor Particles: I/O ratio, Infiltration Factor and Penetration Factor. *Atmospheric Environment*, Vol. 45, No. 2, (January 2011), pp. 275-288, ISSN 1352-2310

Colls, J. (1997). *Air Pollution*, (1st Ed.), Chapman & Hall, ISBN 0-419-20650-7, London, United Kingdom

Commission Recommendation 90/143/Euratom. Commission Recommendation on the Protection of the Public against Indoor Exposure to Radon. *Official Journal of the European Communities*, L80, (March 1990), pp. 26–28

Dales, R., Liu, L., Wheeler, A.J. & Gilbert, N.L. (2008). Quality of Indoor Residential Air and Health. *Canadian Medical Association Journal*, Vol. 179, No. 2 (July 2008), pp.147-52, ISSN 0820-3946

Delfino, R.J., Staimer, N., Gillen, D., Tjoa, T., Sioutas, C., Fung, K., George, S. & Kleinman, M.T. (2006). Personal and Ambient Air Pollution is Associated with Increased

Exhaled Nitric Oxide in Children with Asthma. *Environmental Health Perspective*, Vol. 114, No. 11, (November 2006), pp. 1736–1743, ISSN 0091-6765

Delfino, R.J., Staimer, N., Tjoa, T., Gillen, D., Kleinman, M.T., Sioutas, C. & Cooper, D. (2008). Personal and Ambient Air Pollution Exposures and Lung Function Decrements in Children with Asthma. *Environmental Health Perspective*, Vol. 116, No. 4, (April 2008), pp. 550–558, ISSN 0091-6765

Directive 2002/91/EC. Directive of the European Parliament and the Council on the Energy Performance of Buildings. *Official Journal of the European Communities*, L1, (December 2002), pp. 65–71

Directive 2010/31/EC. Directive of the European Parliament and the Council on the Energy Performance of Buildings. *Official Journal of the European Communities*, L153, (May 2002), pp. 13–35

Dockery, D.W, Pope III, A.C. & Speizer, F.E. (1998). Effects of Particulate Air Pollution Exposures, In: *Air Pollution in 21st Century – Priority Issues and Policy*, Schneider T., (Ed.), pp. 671–777, ISBN 978-0-444-82799-9, Elsevier Science, Amsterdam, Netherlands

European Community (EC). (2004). *Tobacco or Health in the European Union - Past, Present and Future*. Office for Official Publications of the European Communities, ISBN 92-894-8219-2, Luxembourg

Fortmann, A.L., Romero, R.A., Sklar, M., Pham, V., Zakarian, J., Quintana, P.J.E., Chatfield, D. & Matt, G.E. (2010). Residual Tobacco Smoke in Used Cars: Futile Efforts and Persistent Pollutants. *Nicotine and Tobacco Research*, Vol. 12, No. 10, (August 2010), pp. 1029-1036, ISSN 1462-2203

Franck, U., Herbarth, O., Röder, S., Schlink, U., Borte, M., Diez, U., Krämer, U. & Lehmann, I. (2011). Respiratory Effects of Indoor Particles in Young Children are Size Dependent. *Science of the Total Environment*, Vol. 409, No. 9, (April 2011), pp. 1621-1631, ISSN 0048-9697

Franklin, P.J. (2007). Indoor Air Quality and Respiratory Health of Children. *Pediatric Respiratory Reviews*, Vol. 8, No. 4, (October 2007), pp. 281-2866, ISSN 1526-0542

Gately, I. (2001). *Tobacco: A Cultural History of How an Exotic Plant Seduced Civilization*, Simone & Schuster, ISBN 0-8021-3960-4, London, United Kingdom

Geller, M.D., Chang, M., Sioutas, C., Ostro, B.D. & Lipsett, M.J. (2002). Indoor/Outdoor Relationship and Chemical Composition of Fine and Coarse Particles in the Southern California Deserts. *Atmospheric Environment*, Vol. 36, No. 6, (February 2002), pp. 1099-1110, ISSN 1352-2310

Goyal, R. & Khare, M. (2010). Indoor Air Pollution and Health Effects, In: *Air Pollution – Health and Environmental Impacts*, B.R. Gurjar, L.T. Molina, C.S.P. Ojha, (Eds.), pp. 109-134, CRC Press, ISBN 978-1-4398-0962-4 , Boca Raton, Florida, USA

Heinrich, J., Topp, R., Gehring, U. & Thefeld, W. (2005). Traffic at Residential Address, Respiratory Health, and Atopy in Adults: The National German Health Survey 1998. *Environmental Research*, Vol. 98, No. 2, (June 2005), pp. 240-249, ISSN 0013-9351

Hoek, G., Brunekreef, B., Goldbohm, S., Fischer, P. & van den Brandt, P.A. (2002). Association between Mortality and Indicators of Traffic-related Air Pollution in the Netherlands: A Cohort Study. *The Lancet*, Vol. 360, No. 9341, (October 2002), pp. 1203-1209, ISSN 0140-6736

Horak, E., Morass, B. & Ulmer, H. (2007). Association between Environmental Tobacco Smoke Exposure and Wheezing Disorders in Austrian Preschool Children. *Swiss Medical Weekly*, Vol. 137, No. 43-44, (November 2007), pp. 608–13, ISSN 1424-7860

International Agency for Research on Cancer (IARC). (2010). Some non-Heterocyclic Polycyclic Aromatic Hydrocarbons and Some Related Exposures, *IARC Monographs on the Evaluation of Carcinogenic Risks to Humans*, Vol. 92, (October 2010), pp. 773, ISSN 1017-1606

International Agency for Research on Cancer (IARC). (2011). *Agents Classified by the IARC Monographs*, accessed 24.6.2011, available from <http://monographs.iarc.fr/ENG/Classification/ClassificationsAlphaOrder.pdf>

International Agency for Research on Cancer, IARC. (2004). *Tobacco Smoke and Involuntary Smoke - IARC Monographs on the Evaluation of Carcinogenic Risks to Humans Vol. 83*, International Agency for Research on Cancer, ISBN 92-832-1283-5, Lyon, France

Janssen, N.A., Brunekreef, B., van Vliet, P., Aarts, F., Meliefste, K., Harssema, H. & Fischer, P. (2003). The Relationship between Air Pollution from Heavy Traffic and Allergic Sensitization, Bronchial Hyperresponsiveness, and Respiratory Symptoms in Dutch Schoolchildren. *Environmental Health Perspective*, Vol. 111, No. 12, (September 2003), pp. 1512-1518, ISSN 0091-6765

Jantunen, M., Fernandes, E., Carrer, P. & Kephalopoulos, S. (2011). *Promoting Actions for Healthy Indoor Air (IAIAQ)*, European Commission Directorate General for Health and Consumers, ISBN 978-92-79-20419-7, Luxembourg

Jones, A.P. (2002). Indoor Air Quality and Health, In: *Air Pollution Science for the 21st Century*, J. Austin, P. Brimblecombe, W. Sturges, (Eds.), pp. 57-116, Elsevier Science Ltd., ISBN 0-08-044119-X, Oxford, United Kingdom

Kabir, Z., Manning, P.J., Holohan, J., Keogan, S., Goodman, P.G. & Clancy, L. (2009). Second Hand Smoke Exposure in Cars and Respiratory Health Effects in Children. *European Respiratory Journal*, Vol. 34, No. 3, (September 2009), pp. 629–633, ISSN 0903-1936

Król, S., Zabiegała, B. & Namieśnik, J. (2011). Monitoring and Analytics of Semivolatile Organic Compounds (SVOCs) in Indoor Air. *Analytical and Bioanalytical Chemistry*, Vol. 400, No. 6, (June 2011), pp. 1751-69, ISSN 1618-2642

Lee, J., Lim, S., Lee, K., Guo, X., Kamath, R., Yamato, H., Abas, A.L., Nandasena, S., Nafees, A.A. & Sathiakumar, N. (2010). Secondhand Smoke Exposures in Indoor Public Places in Seven Asian Countries. *International Journal of Hygiene and Environmental Health*, Vol. 213, No. 5, (September 2010), pp. 348-351, ISSN 1438-4639

Lloyd, J. & Mitchinson, J. (2008). *The Book of General Ignorance*, Faber and Faber Ltd., ISBN 978-0-571-24139-2, London, United Kingdom

Martuzevicius, D., Grinshpun, S.A., Lee, T., Hu, S., Biswas, P., Reponen, T. & LeMasters, G. (2008). Traffic-related PM2.5 Aerosol in Residential Houses Located near Major Highways: Indoor versus Outdoor Concentrations. *Atmospheric Environment*, Vol. 42, No. 27, (September 2008), pp. 6575-6585, ISSN 1352-2310

Massey, D., Masia, J., Kulshrestha, A., Habil, M. & Taneja, H. (2009). Indoor/Outdoor Relationship of Fine Particles less than 2.5 μm (PM2.5) in Residential Homes Locations in Central Indian Region. *Building and Environment*, Vol. 44, No. 10, (October 2009), pp. 2037-2045, ISSN 0360-1323

Matt, G., Quintana, P., Hovell, M., Bernert, J., Song, S., Novianti, N., Juarez, T., Floro, J., Gehrman, C., Garcia, M. & Larson, S. (2004). Households Contaminated by Environmental Tobacco Smoke: Sources of Infant Exposures. *Tobacco Control,* Vol. 13, No. 1, (March 2004), pp. 29–37, ISSN 0964-4563

Mejía, J.F., Low Choy, S., Mengersen, K. & Morawska, L. (2011). Methodology for Assessing Exposure and Impacts of Air Pollutants in School Children: Data Collection, Analysis and Health Effects - A Literature Review. *Atmospheric Environment,* Vol. 45, No. 4, (February 2011), pp. 813-823, ISSN 1352-2310

Mitchell, C.S., Zhang, J., Sigsgaard, T., Jantunen, M., Lioy, P.J. & Samson, R. (2007). Current State of the Science: Health Effects and Indoor Environmental Quality. *Environmental Health Perspective,* Vol. 115, No. 6, (June 2007), pp. 958-964, ISSN 091-6765

Oberdörster, G., Gelein, R.M., Ferin, J. & Weiss, B. (1995). Association of Particulate Air Pollution and Acute Mortality: Involvement of Ultrafine Particles. *Inhalation Toxicology,* Vol. 7, No. 1, (January-February 1995) pp. 111–124, ISSN 0895-8378

Okona-Mensah, K. & Fayokun, R. (2011). Environmental Tobacco Smoke and Cancer, In: *Encyclopedia of Environmental Health,* J. Nriagu, (Ed.), pp. 528-541, Elsevier Science, ISBN 978-0-444-52272-6, London, UK

Pasupathi, P., Bakthavathsalam, G., Rao, Y.Y. & Farook, J. (2009). Cigarette Smoking—Effect of Metabolic Health Risk: A Review. *Diabetes and Metabolic Syndrome: Clinical Research and Reviews,* Vol. 3, No. 2, (June 2009), pp. 120-127, ISSN 1871-4021

Perfetti, T.A. & Rodgman, A. (2011). The Complexity of Tobacco and Tobacco Smoke. *Beiträge zur Tabakforschung International,* Vol. 24, No. 5, (May 2011), pp. 215-232, ISSN 0173-783X

Petrick, L.A., Svidovsky, A. & Dubowski, Y. (2011). Thirdhand Smoke: Heterogeneous Oxidation of Nicotine and Secondary Aerosol Formation in the Indoor Environment. *Environmental Science and Technology,* Vol. 45, No. 1, (December 2010), pp. 328–333, ISSN 0013-936X

Pope, C., Dockery, D., Spengler, J. & Raizenne, M. (1991). Respiratory Health and PM10 Pollution: a Daily Times Series Analysis. *American Review of Respiratory Disease,* Vol. 144, No. 3, (September 1991), pp. 668-674, ISSN 0003-0805

Rehan, V.K., Sakurai, R. & Torday, J.S. (2011). Thirdhand Smoke: a New Dimension to the Effects of Cigarette Smoke on the Developing Lung. *American Journal of Physiology - Lung Cellular and Molecular Physiology,* Vol. 301, No. 1, (July 2011), pp. L1-L8, ISSN 1522-1504

Robicsek, F. (1979). *The Smoking Gods: Tobacco in Maya Art, History, and Religion,* University of Oklahoma Press, ISBN 0-8061-1511-4, Norman, Oklahoma, USA

Rodgman, A. & Perfetti, T.A. (2006). The Composition of Cigarette Smoke: A Catalogue of the Polycyclic Aromatic Hydrocarbons. *Beiträge zur Tabakforschung International,* Vol. 22, No. 1, (April 2006), pp. 13-69, ISSN 0173-783X

Rodgman, A. & Perfetti, T.A. (2008). *The Chemical Components of Tobacco and Tobacco Smoke,* CRC Press, ISBN 978-1-420-07883-1, Boca Raton, Florida, USA

Shah, R.S. & Cole, J.W. (2010). Smoking and Stroke: the More you Smoke the More you Stroke. *Expert Review of Cardiovascular Therapy,* Vol. 8, No. 7, (July 2010), pp. 917-32, ISSN 1477-9072

Singer, B., Hodgson, A., Guevarra, K., Hawley, E. & Nazaroff, W.W. (2002). Gas-phase Organics in Environmental Tobacco Smoke. 1. Effects of Smoking Rate, Ventilation, and Furnishing Level on Emission Factors. *Environmental Science and Technology*, Vol. 36, No. 5, (January 2002), pp. 846–853, ISSN 0013-936X

Skorge, T.D., Eagan, T.M., Eide, G.E., Gulsvik, A. & Bakke, P.S. (2005). The Adult Incidence of Asthma and Respiratory Symptoms by Passive Smoking in Uterus or in Childhood. *Atmospheric Journal of Respiratory Critical Care Medicine*, Vol. 172, No. 1, (July 2005), pp. 61-66, ISSN 1073-449X

Slezakova, K., Castro, D., Pereira, M.C., Morais, S., Delerue-Matos, C. & Alvim-Ferraz, M.C.M. (2009b). Influence of Tobacco Smoke on Carcinogenic PAH Composition in Indoor PM10 and PM2.5. *Atmospheric Environment*, Vol. 43, No. 40, (December 2009), pp. 6376-6382, ISSN 1352-2310

Slezakova, K., Pereira, M.C. & Alvim-Ferraz, M.C. (2009a). Influence of Tobacco Smoke on the Elemental Composition of Indoor Particles of Different Sizes. *Atmospheric Environment*, Vol. 43, No. 3, (January 2009), pp. 486-493, ISSN 1352-2310

Slezakova, K., Pires, J.C.M., Martins, F.G., Pereira M.C. & Alvim-Ferraz, M.C. (2011). Identification of Tobacco Smoke Components in Indoor Breathable Particles by SEM–EDS. *Atmospheric Environment*, Vol. 45, No. 4, (February 2011), pp. 863-872, ISSN 1352-2310

Spengler, J.D. & Sexton, K. (1983). Indoor Air Pollution: A Public Health Perspective. *Science*, Vol. 221, No. 4605, (July 1983), pp. 9-17, ISSN 0036-8075

Srikanth, P., Sudharsanam, S. & Steinberg, R. (2008). Bio-aerosols in Indoor Environment: Composition, Health Effects and Analysis. *Indian Journal of Medical Biology*, Vol. 26, No. 4, (October-December 2008), pp. 302-312, ISSN 1998-3646

Taylor, R.B. (2008). *White Coat Tales - Medicine's Heroes, Heritage and Misadventures*, Springer, ISBN 978-0-387-73079-0, New York, USA

Thielen, A., Klus, H. & Müller, L. (2008). Tobacco Smoke: Unravelling a Controversial Subject. *Experimental and Toxicologic Pathology*, Vol. 60, No. 2-3, (June 2008), pp.141-156, ISSN 0940-2993

Tiwary, A. & Colls, J. (2009). *Air Pollution* (3rd ed.), Taylor & Francis, ISBN 978-04-1547-933-2, London, United Kingdom

Trude, D. & Skorge, M.D. (2007). Environmental Tobacco Smoke (ETS) in Childhood and Incidence of Respiratory Symptoms in Adulthood. *Respiratory Medicine: COPD Update*, Vol. 3, No. 4, (November 2007), pp. 125, ISSN 0954-6111

US Environmental Protection Agency, USEPA (1993). *EPA Designates Passive Smoking a "Class 1" or Known Human Carcinogen*, accessed 24.5.2011, available from: <http://www.epa.gov/history/topics/smoke/01.html>

Viegi, G., Simoni, M., Scognamiglio, A., Baldacci, S., Pistelli, F., Carrozzi, L. & Annesi-Maesano, I. (2004). Indoor Air Pollution and Airway Disease. *International Journal of Tuberculosis and Lung Disease*, Vol. 8, No. 12, (December 2004), pp. 1401–1415, ISSN 1815-7920

Weschler, C.J. (2009). Changes in Indoor Pollutants since the 1950s. *Atmospheric Environment*, Vol. 43, No. 1, (January 2009), pp. 153–169, ISSN 1352-2310

Whitby, K.T. (1978). The Physical Characteristics of Sulfur Aerosols. *Atmospheric Environment*, Vol. 12, No. 1-3, (April 2003), pp. 135–159, ISSN 1352-2310

Wilbert, J. (1987). *Tobacco and Shamanism in South America*, ISBN 0-3000-5790-3, London, United Kingdom

Wilson, W.E. (1998). Fine and Coarse Particles: Chemical and Physical Properties Important for the Standard-Setting Process, In: *Air Pollution in 21st Century – Priority Issues and Policy*, Schneider T., (Ed.), pp. 87–116, ISBN 978-0-444-82799-9, Elsevier Science, Amsterdam, Netherlands

Wilson, W.E., Chow, J.C., Claiborn, C., Fusheng, W., Engelbrecht, J. & Watson, J.C. (2002). Monitoring of Particulate Matter Outdoors. *Chemosphere*, Vol. 49, No. 9, (December 2002), pp. 1009–1043, ISSN 0045-6535

Winickoff, J., Friebely, J., Tanski, S., Sherrod, C., Matt, G., Hovell, M. & McMillen, R. (2009). Beliefs about the Health Effects of "Thirdhand" Smoke and Home Smoking Bands. *Pediatrics*, Vol. 123, No. 1, (January 2009), pp. 74–79, ISSN 0031-4005

World Health Organization (WHO), (2000a). *Air Quality Guidelines*, (2nd Edition), WHO Regional Publications, European Series No. 91, ISBN 92-890-1358-3, Copenhagen, Denmark

World Health Organization (WHO), (2000b). *Particulate Matter, Chapter 7.3*, WHO Regional Publications, Copenhagen, Denmark, accessed 17.06.2011, available at <http://www.euro.who.int/__data/assets/pdf_file/0019/123085/AQG2ndEd_7_3Particulate-matter.pdf>

World Health Organization (WHO). (2006). *Air Quality Guidelines, Global Update 2005*. WHO Regional Office for Europe, ISBN 92-890-2192-6, Copenhagen, Denmark

World Health Organization (WHO). (2010). *WHO Guidelines for Indoor Air Quality: Selected Pollutants*. WHO Regional Office for Europe, ISBN 978-92-890-0213-4, Copenhagen, Denmark

Wu, A. (1997). Cardiovascular Effects. In: *Health Effects of Exposure to Environmental Tobacco Smoke*, California Environmental Protection Agency, accessed 8.6.2011, available from: <http://www.oehha.org/air/environmental_tobacco/finalets.html>

Wu, D., Landsberger, S. & Larson, S.M. (1997). Determination of the Elemental Distribution in Cigarette Components and Smoke by Instrumental Neutron Activation Analysis. *Journal of Radioanalytical and Nuclear Chemistry*, Vol. 217, No. 1, (March 1997), pp. 77-82, ISSN 0236-573

7

The Potential Environmental Benefits of Utilising Oxy-Compounds as Additives in Gasoline, a Laboratory Based Study

Mihaela Neagu (Petre)
Petroleum-Gas University of Ploiesti, Romania

1. Introduction

Resolving the conflict between growth oriented powers, which tend to extend polluting emissions has become a focus of 21st century politics.

The growth of transportation requirements in modern society implies the consumption of large quantities of fuel. It is a fact that fossil fuel reserves have dramatically dropped and can no longer sustain the ever growing demand. The need to protect existing crude oil resources has also fuelled the search for alternative renewable energy resources that are compatible with auto fuel. Furthermore these fuels must face another challenge: through their burning in the vehicles' engines they have to reduce polluting exhaust emissions.

An innovating solution, through which the relation between transportation and the environment is reconciled, is the substitution of auto fuel with different proportions of oxygenated biocomponent. The introduction of a certain oxygen percentage in auto gasoline started in 1970, with the purpose of increasing the number of octanes of gasoline, as a replacement of tetraethyl lead (TEL). The first oxygenated compound used as an octanic additive for gasoline was methyl *tert*-butyl ether (MTBE). Shortly after introduction, it was discovered that using MTBE leads to a reduction of polluting exhaust emissions. For a gasoline with 15% MTBE, carbon monoxide emissions are reduced by 10-15%, nitric oxide by 1.0-1.7%, and total hydrocarbon emissions are reduced by 10-20% (Song et al., 2006). More than 85% of reformulated gasoline contained MTBE, because of the lowered price, low vapour pressure, total miscibility with gasoline, medium boiling point and reduction of fuel consumption (He et al., 2003). However, MTBE is 30 times more soluble in water than hydrocarbons. This undesired property has proved in time that, when MTBE, reformulated gasoline leaks from underground storage tanks or auto tanks, it moves through soil to groundwater thus contaminating it. The subsequent environmental and human health problems led to a ban on the use of MTBE in gasoline, starting with 2001, in the USA (Poulopoulos & Philippopoulos, 2001).

In Europe, the USA's point of view regarding the use of MTBE is not fully agreed upon. The benefits of using MTBE as a gasoline additive, from the point of view of improving the quality of fuel and the reduction of exhaust emissions in the atmosphere are more obvious than the drawback created by possible leaks from the storage tanks (Osman et al., 1993; Tavlarides et al., 2000; Zervas et al., 2004). Nevertheless, social pressures have determined the promotion of other oxygenated compounds. The first solution provided by researchers and accepted by refiners and the users was to revert back to use of ethanol. Tests of exhaust emissions of vehicles fuelled by gasoline oxygenated with 10% ethanol have shown a reduction of 4.7-5.8% in carbon monoxide and 5-15.3% total hydrocarbons emissions, as well as a reduction in the emitted levels of nitric oxide. The reduction of exhaust emissions also depends on the fuel burning efficiency, operating conditions of the engine (speeds and charges), ethanol content in the gasoline and the air/fuel ratio (He et al., 2003). Still, using ethanol as a biocomponent in gasoline has its set of drawbacks. The heat value of ethanol is less than that of gasoline. Consequently, the heat value of ethanol blended gasoline fuels will decrease when the proportion of ethanol increases (Hsieh et al., 2002). The most controversial aspects are related to volatility and stability on contact with water (Aakko & Nylund, 2004; Bayraktar, 2005; Cataluña et al., 2008). Recent studies and experimental research motivated by the presence of ethanol in fuel showed increases in the vapour pressure of reformulated gasoline, which is dependent upon the content of saturated hydrocarbons, the vapour pressure of the base fuel and ethanol content in the mixture (da Silva et al., 2005; Martini et al., 2007; Muzˇíková et al., 2009; Pospíšil et al., 2007; Pumphrey et al., 2000; Rosca et al., 2009). The distillation curves of gasoline blends with ethanol show a region that indicates the formation of azeotropes with minimum boiling temperature between ethanol and some light hydrocarbons in the gasoline (D'Ornellas, 2001; Hsieh et al., 2002; Neagu et al., 2010). This in turn significantly contributes to reformulated gasoline volatility, prevalence of vapour lock and the loss of emissions by evaporation and increased acetaldehyde emissions (Poulopoulos & Philippopoulos, 2001; Zervas et al., 2001, 2002). Recent studies concerning the use of superior alcohols in reformulated gasoline have shown surprising results. Isopropyl alcohol as well as the butanols can be extracted from the same renewable materials as the ethanol, through fermentation processes, but with lower capability and higher recovery costs. Although obtaining these bioalcohols seems to be uneconomical, using them in auto gasoline produces more favourable results than the addition of ethanol (Brekke, 2007). Biobutanols have the advantage of lower consumption (it has almost the same energy content as the petroleum-based gasoline: 26-27 MJ/litre of butanol and 32-33 MJ/litre gasoline), research octane number 94, has a low content of oxygen in the molecule and thus can be mixed in a bigger proportion with gasoline (up until 16%), a very low vapour pressure (VOC emissions are reduced) and much lower affinity towards water than ethanol (A r n o l d, 2008; Szulczyk, 2010).

Ethers' role as a substitute for auto gasoline has increased since the 1990s. Since ether has a lower vapour pressure than ethanol it also causes a reduction of essential organic compounds in the exhaust gases. Directly connected to the essential exhaust compounds is the level of the ozone and its role in global warming.

The position of oxygenated biocomponents as substitutes for petroleum-based gasoline consolidated with the fight for reducing the emissions of greenhouse gases (Aakko & Nylund, 2004; He et al., 2003; Szklo et al., 2007). Carbon dioxide emitted by the burning of oxygenated biocomponents can be remedied to a large extent by growing plants that can absorb the carbon dioxide. The introduction of an oxygen percentage in gasoline is legally sustained and mandatory in all countries of the European Union. At the end of 2008, the

European Parliament introduced a legislative package in the area of energy and climatic changes which sets targets for reducing greenhouse gases in the period of time following the Kyoto Protocol (2008-2012), with medium (2020) and long (2050) term targets. A part of this legislative package is the revised Fuel Quality Directive 2009/30/EC (EC, 2009). The directive appeals the gradual reduction of GHG emissions per unit of energy from fuel and energy supplied for the transportation sector with a 6% reduction target over the 2010 - 2020 time frame. Another request of the directive is to increase the percentage of oxygenated compounds in fuel, up to a total content of oxygen of 3.5 %weight. The changing of the total content of oxygenated compounds, as well as other quality specifications of fuels was stipulated by revising international standards (Table 1). The quality of commercial gasoline in Europe is set by EN 228 Standard (Dixson-Declève & Szalkowska, 2009).

Characteristic	Current specifications	Target specifications
Oxygen content, weight%	Max 2.7	3.7
Oxygen compounds content, weight%:		
-methanol	3	3
-ethanol	5	10
-iso-propyl alcohol	10	12
-iso-butyl alcohol	7	15
-tert-butyl alcohol	10	15
-ethers	15	22
-other oxygenated compounds	10	15

Table 1. EN 228 Standard specifications regarding the content of oxygenated compounds in gasoline

The quality standard of commercial gasoline predicts the growth of oxygenated compounds content, primary alcohols (methanol, ethanol, isopropyl alcohol, iso-butyl alcohol), as well as ether compounds. The role of the ether oxygenated compounds (with five or more carbon atoms in the molecule) in gasoline formulation will be decisive because their content could increase from 15 up to 22 vol.%. International experiences related to using methyl *tert*-butyl ether (MTBE) and *tert*-amyl-methyl ether (TAME) as additives for commercial gasoline suggest using other ethers as well, such as ethyl *tert*-butyl ether (ETBE) and *tert*-amyl ethyl ether (TAEE) for partial substitution of petroleum-based gasoline. Recent research has indicated as favourable the usage of ETBE as a partially renewable component because in its production process bioethanol can be used, just like in the case of TAEE synthesis.

Extensive researche on the properties of various blends of biocomponents in petroleum-based fuel has been conducted, in particular research that emphasises the advantages and disadvantages of using these products in existing vehicles' engines as well as in the new vehicles' engines. At the request of the auto manufacturers, at least until 2013, the oxygen content in gasoline will remain at a maximum 2.7 weight%.

In the first part of this research the physical-chemical properties of oxygenated compounds, primary alcohol and ethers, are presented, as well as their main properties on which petroleum-based and oxygenated gasoline are accepted as commercial products.

The second part is dedicated to a laborious experimental study on the volatility and octane properties of gasoline oxygenated with different proportions of primary bioalcohols and ether. Our research aimed, firstly, on the experimental determination of vapour pressure and distillation curves of synthetic gasoline partial substituted with 2-10% vol methanol, ethanol, isopropanol, tert-butanol and other synthetic gasoline partially substituted with 4-15 vol.% MTBE, TAME, ETBE, TAEE (Neagu et. al., 2010, 2011). Based on these properties, vapour lock indexes were calculated. By interpreting the experimental results and the calculated ones, the advantages and disadvantages of each oxygenated compound are highlighted. In the final part of this study, a comparison between the investigated properties of the oxygenated gasoline with bioalcohols and those with ethers is presented.

2. The oxy-compounds used as bio-substitutes for petroleum-based gasoline

A relatively recent classification divides biocomponents into alcohols and ethers. The main difference between the two categories is that in the alcohols, each hydroxyl functional group

Alcohol	MeOH	EtOH	IPA	TBA
CAS number	67-56-1	64-17-5	67-63-0	75-65-0
Chemical formula	CH_4O	C_2H_6O	C_3H_8O	$C_4H_{10}O$
Molecular weight, g/mol	32.04	46.07	60.10	74.12
Density (at 20 C), g/cm^3	0.792	0.789	0.786	0.781
Boiling temperature, °C	64.7	78.3	82.3	82.3
RVP, kPa	31.7	16.0	12.6	5.5
Oxygen, wt.%	49.9	34.7	26.6	21.6
Solubility in water	miscible	miscible	miscible	miscible
Blending RON/MON	122-133/92	121-130/96	117-118/95-98	105-109/94-95

Table 2. The physical and chemical properties of fuel oxygenates type alcohols as partial substitutes compounds of commercial gasoline (Lesnik, 2002; Nylund et al., 2008)

Ether	MTBE	TAME	ETBE	TAEE
CAS number	1634-04-4	994-05-8	637-92-3	919-94-8
Chemical formula	$C_5H_{12}O$	$C_6H_{14}O$	$C_6H_{14}O$	$C_7H_{16}O$
Molecular weight, g/mol	88.15	102.18	102.18	116.20
Density, g/cm^3	0.741	0.764	0.752	0.750
Boiling temperature, C	55.2	86.3	72.2	101.42
RVP, kPa	55	10	28	NA (not available)
Oxygen, wt.%	18.15	15.7	15.66	13.77
Solubility in water	4.8 g/100 g	1.2 g/100 g	1.2 g/100 g	NA
Blending RON/MON	115-118/101	109-112/ 98-99	117-119/ 102-103	NA

Table 3. The physical and chemical properties of fuel oxygenates type ethers as partial substitute compounds of commercial gasoline (Lesnik, 2002; Nylund et al., 2008).

(-OH) is bound to a carbon atom, usually connected to other carbon or hydrogen atoms, and in ethers, each oxygen atom is linked to two alkyl groups. Among the alcohols used into the formulation of commercial gasoline are the following: MeOH (methanol), EtOH (ethanol), IPA (iso-propyl alcohol) and TBA (tert-butyl alcohol). In Table 2 are included some physical and chemical properties of alcohols.

The ethers most commonly used as substitutes for gasoline are: MTBE (methyl *tert*-butyl ether), TAME (*tert*-amyl methyl ether), ETBE (ethyl *tert*-butyl ether), TAEE (*tert*-amyl ethyl ether). Among the ethers, MTBE is the most widely used oxygenate compound, followed by ETBE and TAME. In Table 3 are included some physical and chemical properties of ethers.

3. Commercial gasoline properties

Quality standards indicate a large number of properties that must be met by suppliers of fuel. Drivers are generally unaware of the complexity of fuel products, and the manufacturers' efforts to produce high quality fuel that can satisfy consumer needs whilst also generating low emissions. From the point of view of the drivers it is important only if the engine has an easy start in the cold season, warms up rapidly, the engine has adequate power without knocking, provides good fuel economy, there are no deposits or corrosion in the fuel system and last but not least, if the fuel is cheap.

Below we will present some of the most important characteristics of gasoline and how they affect driving performance.

Fuel volatility is the gasoline's tendency to vaporize. In cold weather, gasoline is blended to vaporize easily. In the warm season, the gasoline is blended to vaporise less easily in the combustion chamber of an engine in order to prevent vapour lock or other hot-fuel handling problems and to minimize evaporation, which contributes to an increase in hydrocarbon emissions. According to EN228 European standard the properties that are being used to measure gasoline volatility are: Reid vapour pressure, distillation profiles and Vapour Lock Index (VLI).

The vapour pressure of a fuel must be high enough to be able to supply a smooth start of the engine, but not too high so that it does not contribute to the appearance of a vapour lock or excessive evaporate emissions. *The distillation curve* of gasoline is a graphic representation of the variation in the boiling temperature according to the volume percentage of distillated (evaporated). The gasoline is made of a variety of chemical compounds which evaporate at different temperatures. The more volatile components evaporate at lower temperatures, while the less volatile ones evaporate at higher temperatures.

The various regions of the distillation curve can be correlated with the gasoline and driving performance:

- the starting area should provide: easier cold starting and when warm, avoid vapour plugs and have low emissions;
- the middle area should provide: rapid warm-up and smooth running, fuel economy for short-trip, good engine power;
- the final area should provide: fuel economy for long-trips, freedom from engine deposits, minimal dilution of the lubricating oil and low exhaust emissions of volatile organic compounds.

On the basis of the evaporated percentage at a temperature of 70°C (E70) and of Reid pressure vapour, a parameter used to control vapour lock and other hot-fuel handling problems, can be calculated; namely the VLI *(Vapour Lock Index)*.

$$VLI = 10 \cdot VP + 7 \cdot E70 \tag{1}$$

The European Union's EN228 gasoline specification controls the volatility of gasoline by setting limits for the vapour pressure, distillation profile (evaporated percentage at three temperatures and final boiling point), the percentage of maximum distillation residue and VLI properties (Table 4). The European Standard employs six volatility classes according to the summer, winter and transition periods.

Volatility class	Vapour pressur ekPa	Evaporated at 70°C, E70, % vol	Evaporated at 100°C, E100, % vol	Evaporated at 150°C, E150, % vol	Final boiling point, °C, max	Distillation residue, % vol, max	VLI (10VP+7E 70) Index, max
A	45-60	20-48	46-71	75	210	2	-
B	45-70	20-48	46-71	75	210	2	-
C/C1	50-80	22-50	46-71	75	210	2	C (-) C1 (1050)
D/D1	60-90	22-50	46-71	75	210	2	D (-) D1 (1150)
E/E1	65-95	22-50	46-71	75	210	2	E (-) E1 (1200)
F/F1	70-100	22-50	46-71	75	210	2	F (-) F1 (1250)

Table 4. The requirements of volatility classes according to EN 228 standard (Motor Gasolines Technical Review, 2009)

From the point of view of the six volatility classes of commercial gasoline, classes *A* (RPV for summertime: 45.0-60.0 kPa) and *D/D1* (RPV for wintertime: 60.0-90.0 kPa) are relevant.

The octane number characterises the antiknock performances of auto gasoline. There are two laboratory tests through which the number of octanes is determined: a test that is made on an engine with a single cylinder in mild-knocking conditions and low speed and which has as a result the *research octane number* (RON) and a test that is made on the same type of engine, but in high speed and high-temperature knocking conditions and which has as a result *the motor octane number* (MON) of tested gasoline. A fast way to estimate the number of octanes is using the IROX 2000 Fuel Analyzer Portable Gasoline Analysis with MID-FTIR, from Grabner Instruments.

4. Volatility and octane properties of oxygenated gasoline. Experimental and discussions

Of the primary alcohols, as biocomponents to partially substitute commercial gasoline, the most studied is bioethanol. Many experimental studies underlined that, through the combustion of bioethanol-hydrocarbons blends, emissions through evaporation and the prevalence of vapour lock increases. Both effects are due to modifications to the volatility properties of bioethanol oxygenated gasoline. Based on these drawbacks of bioethanol, we aim to develop an experimental study that addresses all of the gasoline volatility properties oxygenated with primary alcohols (1 to 4 carbon atoms in the molecule). In particular the volatility properties of iso-propyl alcohol and tert-butyl alcohol gasoline blends are investigated, because they have been less studied. In order to have a complete picture of the effect of all bio-alcohols, we have included in the experimental study other important properties of mixtures with gasoline, such as antiknock. Finally, by comparing the properties of volatility (Reid vapour pressure, distillation curves and parameters characteristic curves of distillation and vapour lock index) and the octane numbers (RON and MON) of oxygenated gasoline with each of the primary alcohols (methanol, ethanol , iso-propyl alcohol and tert-butyl alcohol), we can argue the advantages and disadvantages of using each of them as biocomponents. The interpretation of the experimental results also includes the effect of the bioalcohols over oxygenated gasoline behaviour in current vehicles, as well as some considerations relating to exhaust emissions.

The ethers synthesized from methanol (derived from natural gas) and C4 hydrocarbons, specifically MTBE or TAME, have practically demonstrated their benefits as octane additives for auto gasoline. Less studied has been their effect upon the volatility properties of gasoline blends. Over the last decade the interest in the two ethers, ETBE and TAEE has increased. Most importantly, they are considered as partially renewable, being synthesized from bioethanol and the C5 hydrocarbons fraction. Details regarding their impact over the octane and volatility properties of gasoline blends are less known. To compare, the effect of every type of ether on volatility and octane properties, an experimental was designed using MTBE, TAME, ETBE and TAEE. The experimental results highlight the advantages and disadvantages of every type of ether. Also, in the case of these oxygenated gasolines, the behaviour in vehicle engines is interpreted and assessments on the loss emissions by evaporation are made.

The first step of the experimental research was to prepare four conventional gasoline blends, noted A, B, C and D. Three components were mixed in different proportions: the catalytic cracking gasoline, the catalytic reforming gasoline and an isomerization fraction. All conventional gasoline's were analysed from the point of view of volatility (distillation curves and Reid pressure vapour), octane numbers, total aromatics, olefinic and parafinic hydrocarbons. The results of the experimental determinations of the main gasoline characteristics, as well as the lab equipment used in these experiments, are presented in table 5.

4.1 Bioalcohols or ethers gasoline mixtures volatility

The volatility properties of gasoline are very important characteristics which affects the vehicle's driveability. For any type of gasoline, these properties depend on the hydrocarbons classes, their concentration and distribution in gasoline. In the case of oxygenated gasoline, Reid pressure vapour as well as the distillation curves are greatly influenced by the type and content of the oxygenated compound.

In order to demonstrate the way in which the oxygenated compound type affects the volatility properties of gasoline, we prepared conventional gasoline blends with primary alcohols and ethers, respectively. Out of gasoline A and B blends with 2, 4, 6, 7, 10 vol% of every alcohol (methanol, ethanol, iso-propyl alcohol and tert-butyl alcohol) were prepared. Out of gasoline C and D blends with 4, 7, 10, 15 vol% of every ether (MTBE, TAME, ETBE, TAEE) were prepared.

Properties	Values and UM				Lab Equipment
	Gasoline A	Gasoline B	Gasoline C	Gasoline D	
Hydrocarbons content: -aromatic -olefinic -saturated	 40.3% vol. 8.6 % vol 51.1 % vol	 36.3 % vol. 3.2 % vol 60.5 % vol	 38.1 % vol. 12.9 % vol 49.0 % vol	 33.9 % vol. 11.5 % vol 54.6 % vol	IROX 2000 Fuel Analyzer Portable Gasoline Analysis with MID-FTIR
Reid pressure vapour	56 kPa	59.8 kPa	56 kPa	63.7 kPa	MINIVAP VPS/VPSH Vapor Pressure Tester
Distillation curves: - Initial - E70 - E100 - E150 - FBP	 44.8 ˚C 24.8 % vol 43.0 % vol 74.5 % vol 198.3 ˚C	 43.9 ˚C 25.2 % vol 45.1 % vol 75.4 % vol 196.4 ˚C	 41.1 ˚C 33.0 % vol 51.5 % vol 78.0 % vol 190.4 ˚C	 41.8 ˚C 35.0 % vol 53.0 % vol 78.0 % vol 195 ˚C	MINIDIS Analyzer Portable Minidistilattion
Octane numbers: -MON -RON	 85.0 95.6	 85.7 96.0	 85.0 95.0	 85.0 95.5	IROX 2000 Fuel Analyzer Portable Gasoline Analysis with MID-FTIR

Table 5. Conventional gasoline characterisation and experimental equipment

Each gasoline-alcohol or gasoline-ether blend was analysed from the point of view of the hydrocarbons content, the volatility properties, the octane numbers and the total amount of oxygen. In oxygenated gasoline, the oxygen content is determined with IROX 2000 Fuel Analyzer Portable Gasoline Analysis with MID-FTIR, as represented in Fig. 1 and Fig. 2. It is obvious the fact that, in the case of oxygenated gasoline, once the amount of alcohol or ether increases, the oxygen amount increases as well. EN 228 standard for commercial gasoline quality limits for now the total amount of oxygen to 2.7 weight%. According to this limit, we analysed the volatility properties of oxygenated gasoline with bioalcohols or ethers. When interpreting the experimental volatility properties, we took into consideration the criteria after which oxygenated gasoline are being framed in the specified EN228 standard volatility classes.

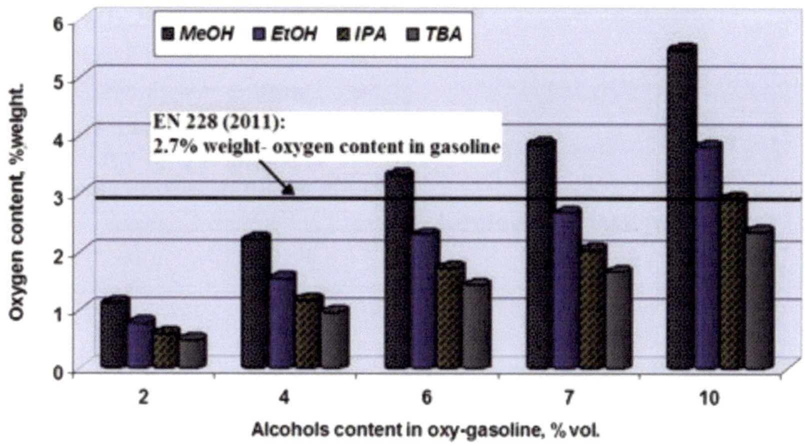

Fig. 1. The total oxygen content in oxygenated gasoline with primary alcohols

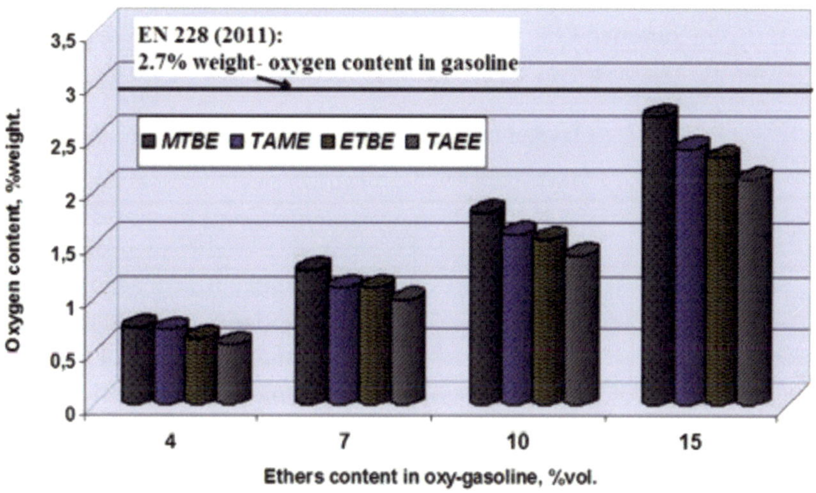

Fig. 2. The total oxygen content in oxygenated gasoline with ethers

The first volatility property analyses was the Reid pressure vapour of alcohol-gasoline and ether-gasoline blends. The experimental results are graphically represented according to the oxygen content of these blends (Figs. 3- 4).Reid pressure vapour for the two gasoline blends (A and B) with 2-10 vol.% primary alcohols are influenced by the vapour pressures of conventional gasoline, such as those of primary alcohols. Both conventional gasolines are a part of A volatility class taking into consideration the values of the vapour pressures and in accordance with EN228 European standard, whilst gasoline B is placed at the superior limit of this class (Table 5). By substituting conventional gasoline A with 4 vol% methanol or with 6 vol% ethanol, we can obtain blends that, from the point of view of Reid pressure vapour, are situated at the superior limit of usage during summer. Blending gasoline A with aprox. 8 vol% ethanol leads to obtaining a 2.7 weight% oxygen content in gasoline and a vapour pressure that makes it suitable in the cold season (Fig 3).

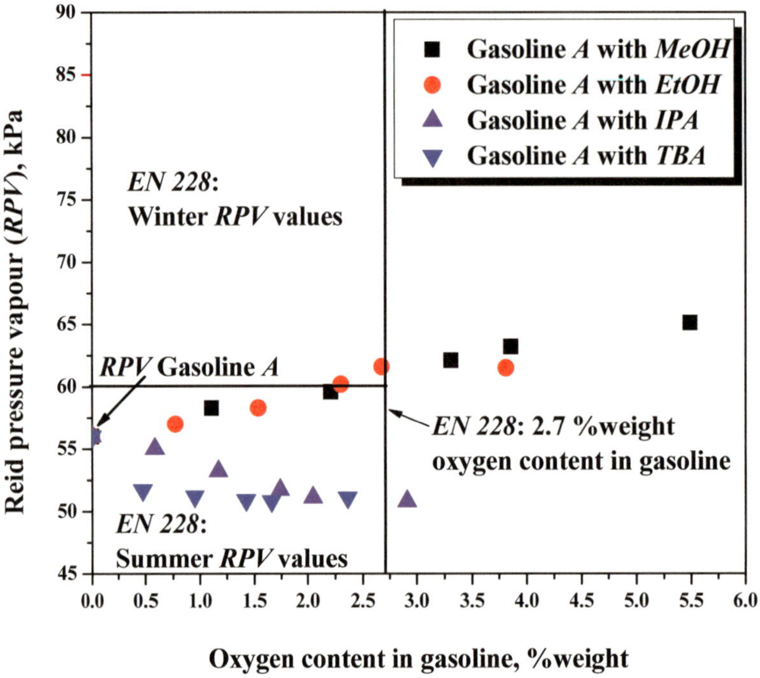

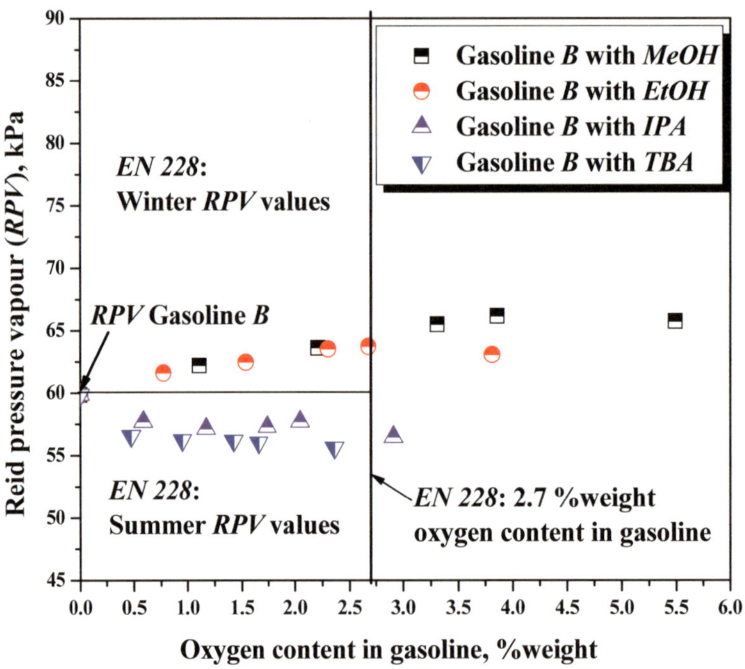

Fig. 3. Variations of Reid pressure vapour with the oxygen content of alcohol-gasoline blends

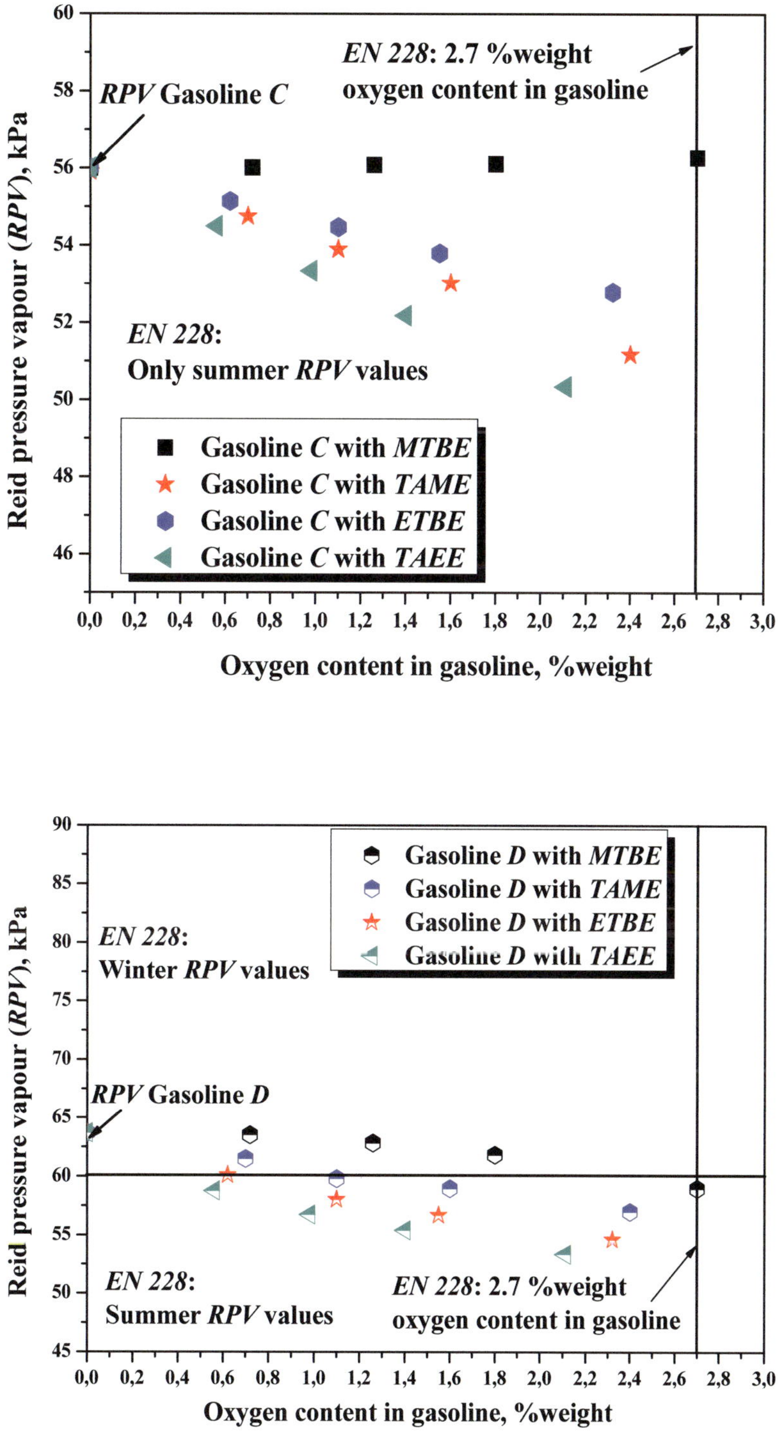

Fig. 4. Variations of Reid pressure vapour with the oxygen content of gasoline-ether blends

In contrast, by oxygenating gasoline B with methanol or ethanol (in any proportion, but without exceeding the maximum oxygen content), we only obtained gasoline with a vapour pressure over 60kPa, suitable for consumption in the cold season (Fig. 3). Therefore, in both cases, blending gasoline with methanol or ethanol causes an increase in the vapour pressure. This fact has implications in commercial gasoline formulation. In practice, conventional gasoline, with different C4 hydrocarbons proportion, are formulated just with the purpose of increasing vapour pressure. For summer blends of gasoline with methanol or ethanol, formulations with the C4 fraction must be avoided, or dealt with cautiously. In the case of substituting conventional gasoline with IPA or TBA, regardless of the oxygenated compound content, the vapour pressure decreases. Nevertheless, gasoline-IPA or gasoline-TBA blends are in the same class volatility as with conventional gasoline. This fact is favourable because substituting conventional gasoline with different IPA or TBA proportions does not replace gasoline additives with a C4 fraction, as is desired by the refiners. Another positive aspect of IPA or TBA in oxygenated gasoline is that they can substitute large proportions of conventional gasoline without exceeding the maximum oxygen content allowed in the blends. Blends of 9-10 vol.% IPA or 10 vol.% TBA can be used in the case of gasoline such as A type, and 8-9 vol.% IPA or 10 vol.% TBA in the case of gasoline similar to B type (Neagu et al., 2010).

In experimental research of the volatility of blends of hydrocarbons with ethers, gasoline C and D were used. Gasoline type C is in A volatility class (for summertime) taking into consideration the vapour pressures, whereas gasoline type D is in B volatility class. For gasoline C with 4-15 vol.% MTBE, Reid pressure vapour increases with the ether content (Fig 4). This is a consequence of the fact that pure MTBE has a similar vapour pressure as gasoline C (Tables 3 and 5). Regardless of the MTBE content, gasoline C blends are situated in the A volatility class, just like conventional gasoline. In the case of gasoline D, oxygenated with MTBE, vapour pressure decreases, and at 15 vol.% MTBE, vapour pressures falls into A volatility class (Fig 4). As a consequence of the low pressures of pure ethers, vapour pressures for gasoline C or D oxygenated with TAME, ETBE and TAEE decrease. According to EN 228 standard, judging by the vapour pressure, gasoline oxygenated with ethers are placed in summertime classes. It is beneficial to note that through adding C4 hydrocarbons, their pressure can be increased up to suitable wintertime values. Such flexibility in using ether oxygenated gasoline, especially those with ETBE or TAEE favours them in commercial gasoline producers' options. These ethers have yet another advantage: in order to achieve a maximum content of oxygen in the gasoline, larger quantities than MTBE and even larger than for primary alcohols can be used (Neagu et al., 2011).

The distillation curves were determined experimentally for all oxygenated gasoline. Out of the large number of experimental results, distillation curves for gasoline A and B, non-oxygenated and oxygenated with 10 vol.% alcohol (Fig. 5) and for gasoline C and D, non-oxygenated and oxygenated with 15 vol.% ether (Fig. 6) are graphically represented.

The distillation curves of gasoline A and B are strongly influenced by the presence, in different proportions, of primary alcohols. This observation is exemplified, in the case of gasoline oxygenated with 10% vol. primary alcohols, in Fig. 5. In these curves three distinct regions can be identified, as in the case of conventional gasoline, but with different influences and names, like: azeotropes with different minimum boiling temperature regions, transition region and dilution region.

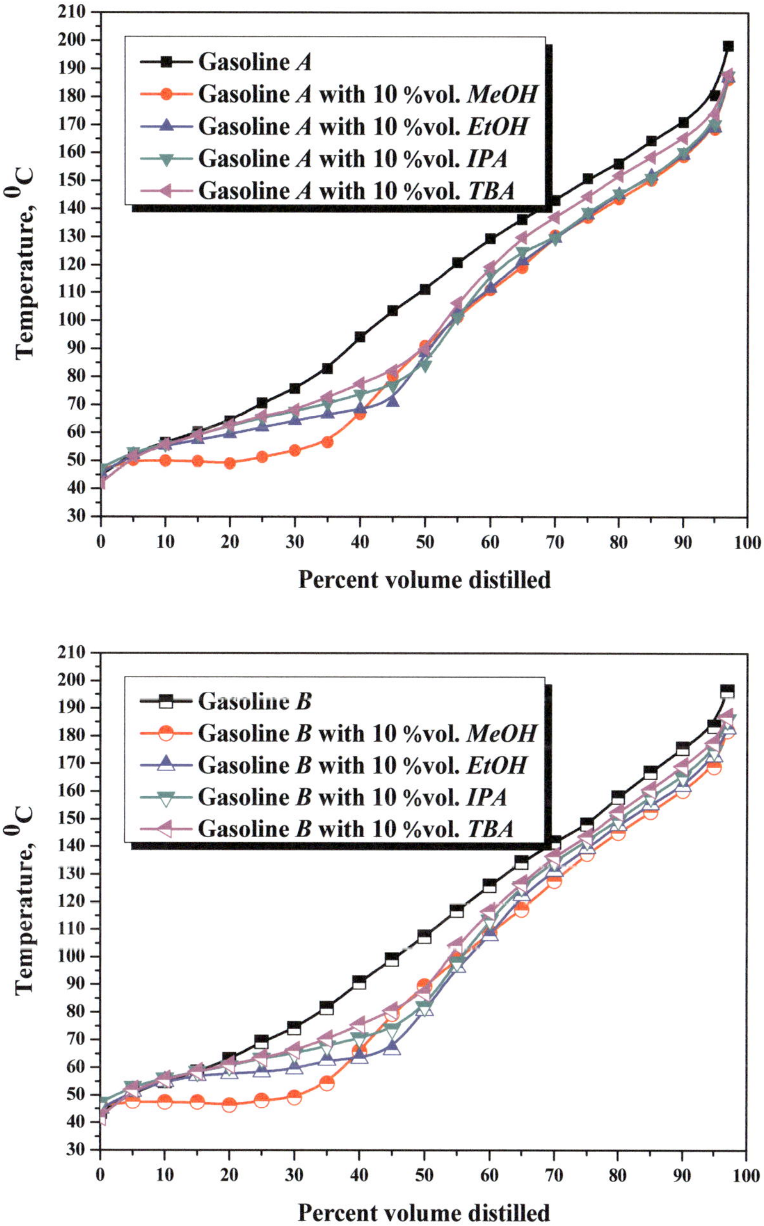

Fig. 5. The influence of alcohols over the distillation curves of oxy-gasoline A and B

The presence of azeotropes with minimum boiling temperature inside the distillation curves of gasoline-alcohol blends is explained by the fact that light hydrocarbons C5-C8 (alkanes, alkenes, aromatics) in the gasoline with polar compounds such as primary alcohols form azeotropes with a minimum boiling temperature. The decrease in the boiling temperatures of gasoline-alcohols blends boiling temperatures in the azeotrope regions has a positive effect upon the vehicle easy start, but favours the appearance of vapour locks and increase of exhaust hydrocarbons.

Between the distillation curves of oxygenated gasoline with alcohols and of oxygenated gasoline with ethers there is a major difference. The ethers do not form azeotropes with the hydrocarbons in the gasoline; they only have an influence on the temperature at which the evaporation of hydrocarbons takes place. Hence, in the distillation curves of gasoline oxygenated with ethers only the boiling temperatures of the pure ethers and the chemical composition of conventional C and D gasoline are influenced.

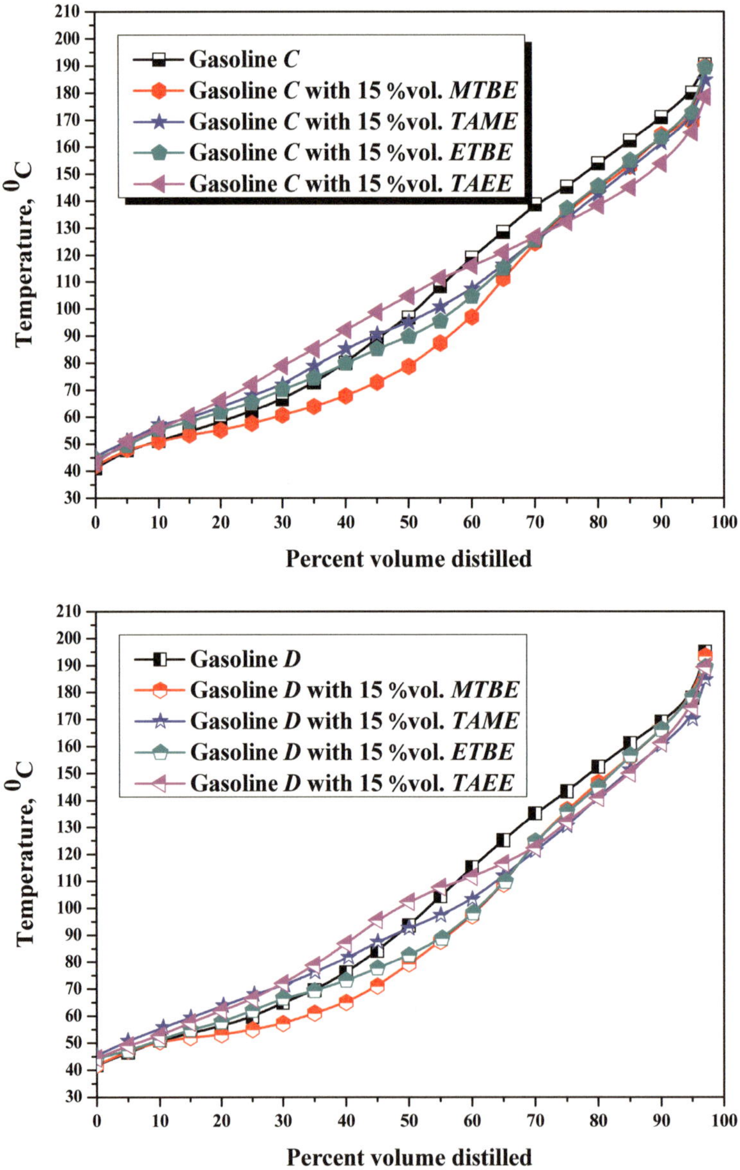

Fig. 6. The influence of ethers over the distillation curves of oxy-gasoline C and D

The difference between the behaviours of the alcohols and ethers towards the distillation curves is better highlighted by analyzing the respective values of the evaporated percentage of the fuel at certain temperatures: 70°C (E70), at 100°C (E100) and 150°C (E150). The comparison of these values that are representative for the distillation curves with the ones indicated in EN 228 standard will allow us to incorporate the oxygenated gasoline within the classes of volatility.

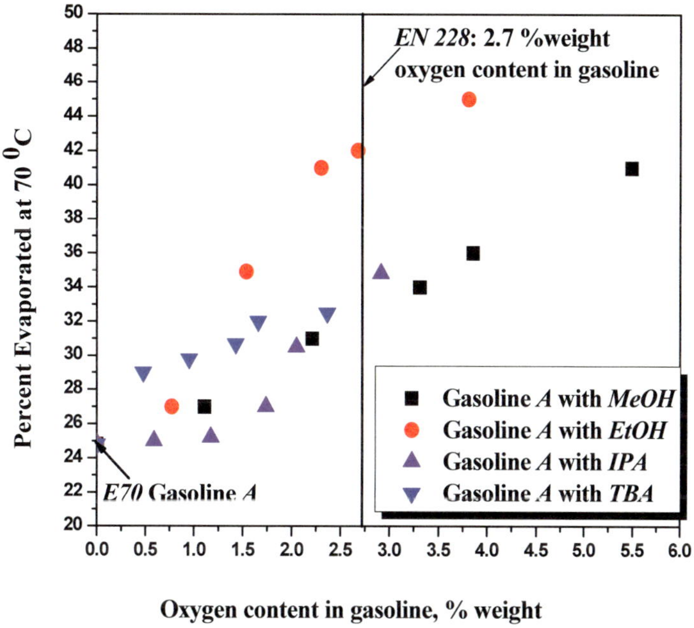

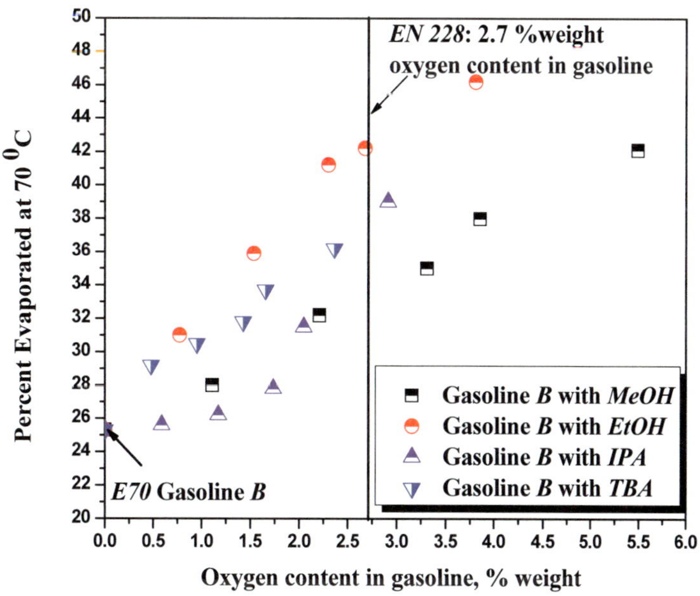

Fig. 7. The influence of alcohols over the percentage evaporated at 70°C of oxy-gasoline A and B

The type of alcohol strongly influences the E70 values of A or B gasoline mixtures (Fig. 7). The effect of the replacement of gasoline with ethanol on the E70 value is more obvious than in the cases in which gasoline is replaced with methanol. The explanation is that at 70°C the azeotropes with minimum boiling temperature of the light hydrocarbons from the ethanol gasoline evaporate. In the case of methanol, the problem of azeotropes evaporation at 70°C does not exist. But methanol, which has its boiling point at 64.7°C, favours a slight evaporation of the hydrocarbons that has boiling temperatures around 70°C. For IPA or TBA gasoline, the boiling point of the alcohols being the same (Table 2), the desired effect on the E70 value is due to the different oxygen content and chemical structures of these alcohols.

Furthermore, the type of the base gasoline influences the E70 values of the primary alcohols, as follows: for the same type and same content of alcohol, the E70 values for blends with B gasoline are higher than the ones for A gasoline because B gasoline has a higher content of saturated hydrocarbons, which influences the region of azeotropes with minimum boiling temperatures which it forms with each alcohol.

From the point of view of the values of the evaporated percentage at 70°C, all gasoline-alcohol blends are enclosed in volatility class A, i.e. in the domain of 20-48% vol. values, according to the gasoline quality standard EN 228.

In the case of the gasoline oxygenated with ethers, the evaporated percents at the temperature of 70°C increase in the presence of the MTBE and decrease in the presence of the TAME, ETBE or TAEE (Fig. 8). This behaviour is justified by the boiling temperature of ethers (Table 3). The introduction of MTBE, which has the lowest boiling point among the studied ethers (55°C), allows a light evaporation of his mixtures with hydrocarbons from the curves of the gasoline distillation region around 70°C. Instead, TAEE, which has the highest boiling point (101.42°C), like TAME, which has a boiling point at 86.3°C, will have as an effect a decrease in the hydrocarbons percentages that could evaporate at this temperature. Due to the fact that ETBE has a boiling point close to 70° C (72° C), the introduction of a high proportion of this ether (in present 15%vol., but will increase up to 22%vol. according to the Revised Fuel Quality Directive 2009/30/EC) has a minor effect on E70. From the point of view of the engine operation, the oxygenated gasoline with MTBE improved the cold ignition of the vehicle through the fact that it helps with the evaporation of the hydrocarbons from the start region of the distillation curve, but without increasing vapour lock. Instead, the gasoline oxygenated with TAEE or TAME, will evaporate harder, but the addition of a supplementary additive (C4+ light hydrocarbons) will correct this deficiency. Furthermore it was observed that gasoline oxygenated with ETBE, has a minimal influence on hydrocarbon evaporation in the start region of the distillation.

The presence of alcohols introduces a significant advantage by increasing evaporated percentages at 100°C, this signifies that the vehicle will offer an easier start-up and lower fuel consumption. Methanol, because it has the lowest boiling point among the primary alcohols, will favour less the evaporation of the gasoline hydrocarbons, at 100°C. Instead, ethanol (boiling point at 78.3°C), isopropyl alcohol and tert-butyl alcohol (boiling point 82.3°C) provide benefits in terms of hydrocarbons evaporation from the area of 100°C (Fig. 9). In the case of B oxygenated gasoline, the volatility of the base gasoline is a factor that favours hydrocarbon evaporation at a temperature of 100 °C. From the point of view of the values of the evaporated percentage at the temperature of 100°C, all the gasoline-alcohols mixtures were found to be in the domain of the 46-71% vol., according to the gasoline quality standard EN 228.

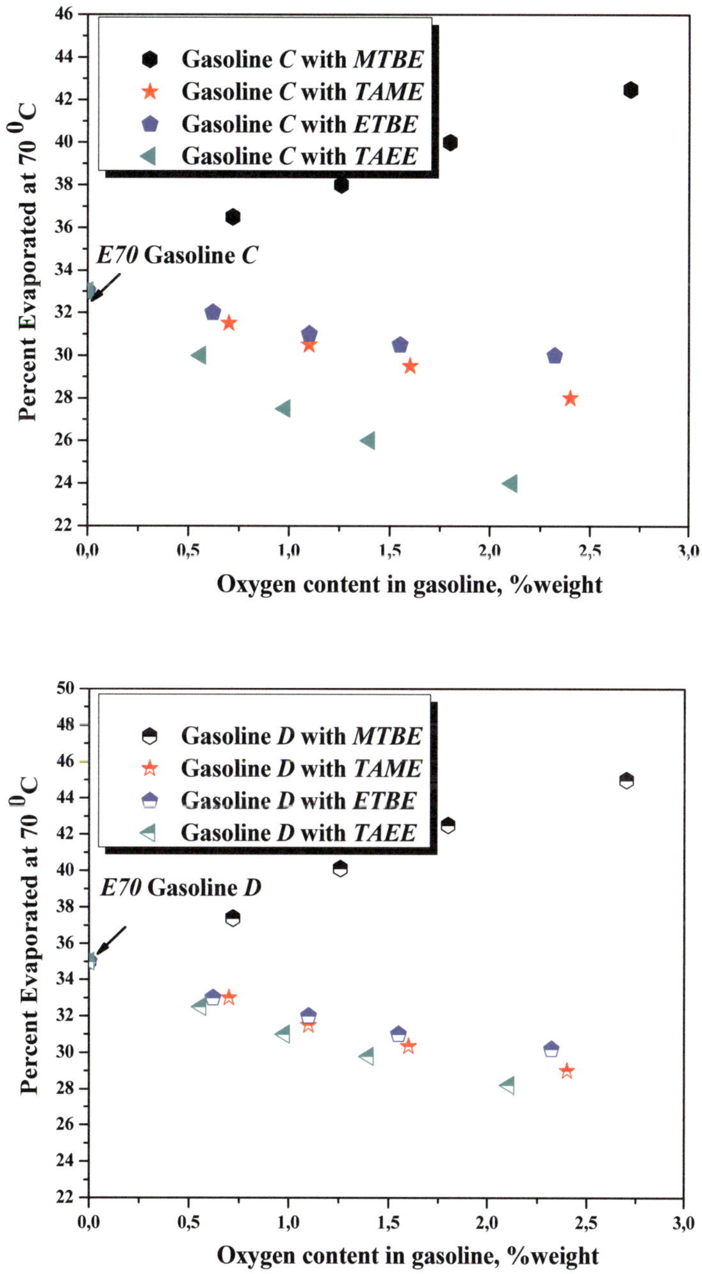

Fig. 8. The influence of ethers over the percentage evaporated at 70°C of oxy-gasoline C and D

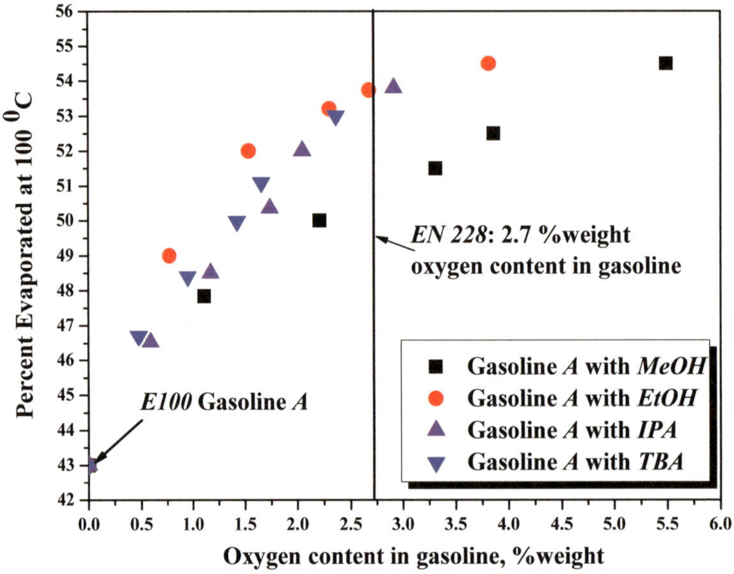

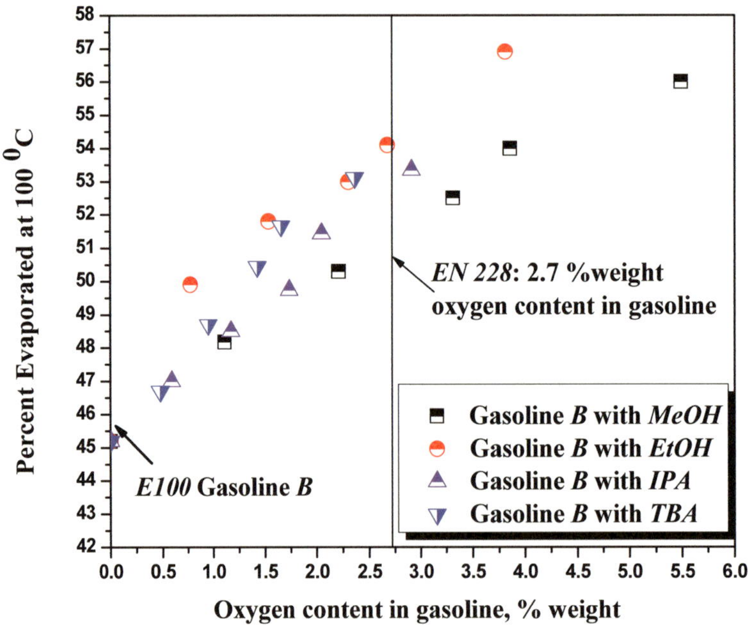

Fig. 9. The influence of alcohols over the percent evaporated at 100°C of oxy-gasoline A and B

The evaporated percents at the temperature of 100°C increase in the presence of ethers with the boiling point lower than 100°C, namely MTBE, ETBE or TAME (Fig. 10). The influence of these ethers on E100 is inversely proportional to their boiling temperatures. Instead, TAEE (the boiling point of the pure component is 101.42°C) influences in a negative way the evaporation at the temperature of 100°C. The negative effect is more marked at gasoline C, less volatile than gasoline D. The gasoline oxygenated with MTBE, ETBE or TAME, through the fact that it evaporates more readily at 100°C, as compared to conventional gasoline, means that it offers an easier start-up and lower fuel consumption.

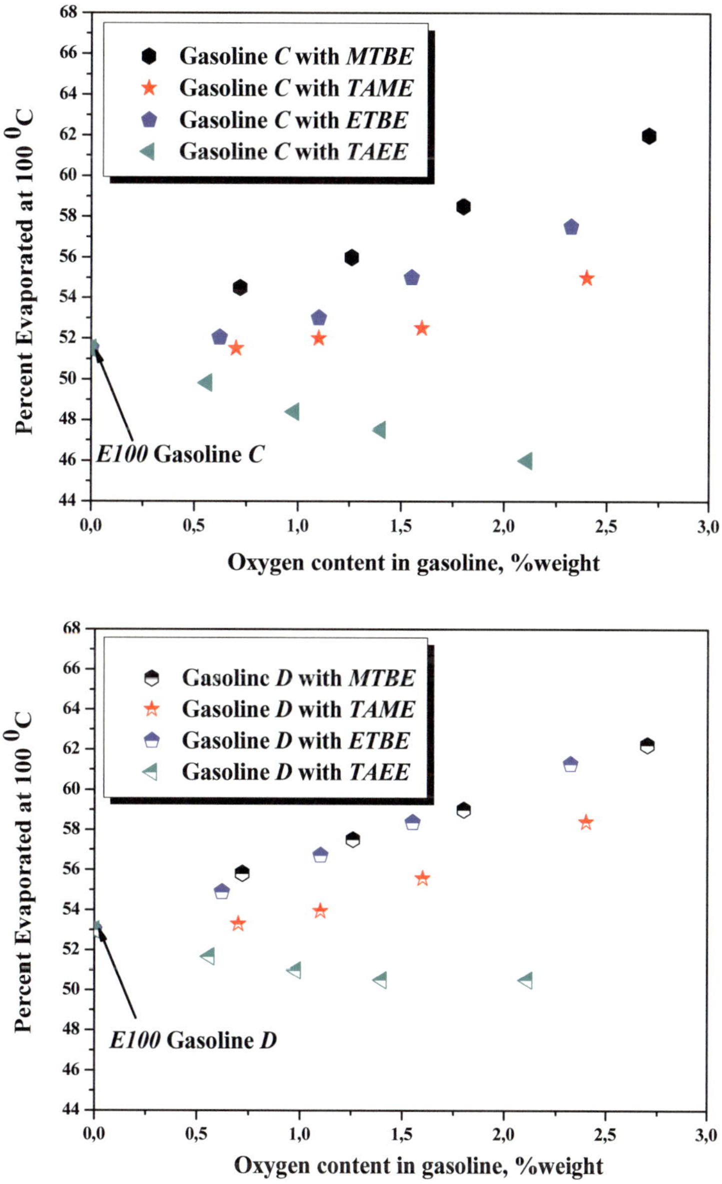

Fig. 10. The influence of ethers over the percent evaporated at 100°C of oxy-gasoline C and D.

Evaporation, at a temperature of 150°C, is favoured by the presence of primary alcohols, which translates into the following effects: a decrease in fuel consumption on long-trips, an enhancement in lubricating oil dilution and a decrease in engine deposits. The boiling temperatures of alcohols, and also their chemical structures, are the main factors that trigger the evaporation of hydrocarbons at 150°C. Adding methanol in fuels, less than 4% vol., has a rather smaller effect over the evaporation of the heavier hydrocarbons in the gasoline, which occurs at around 150°C. On the other hand, ethanol and IPA make a stronger contribution to

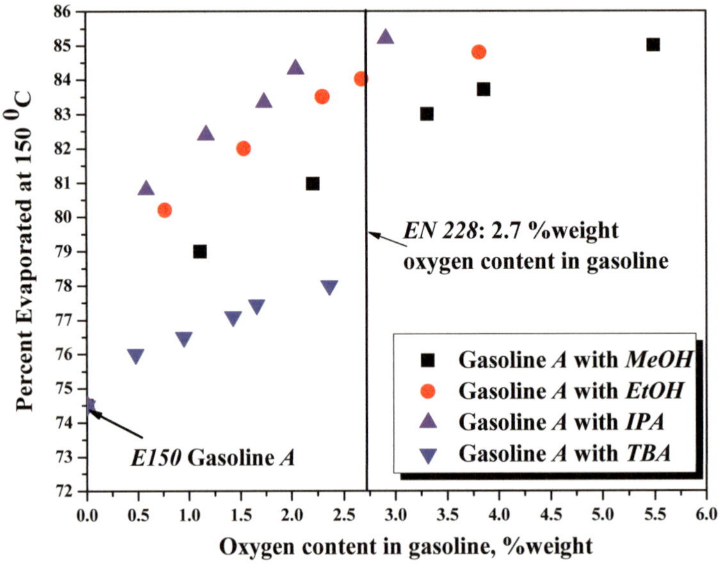

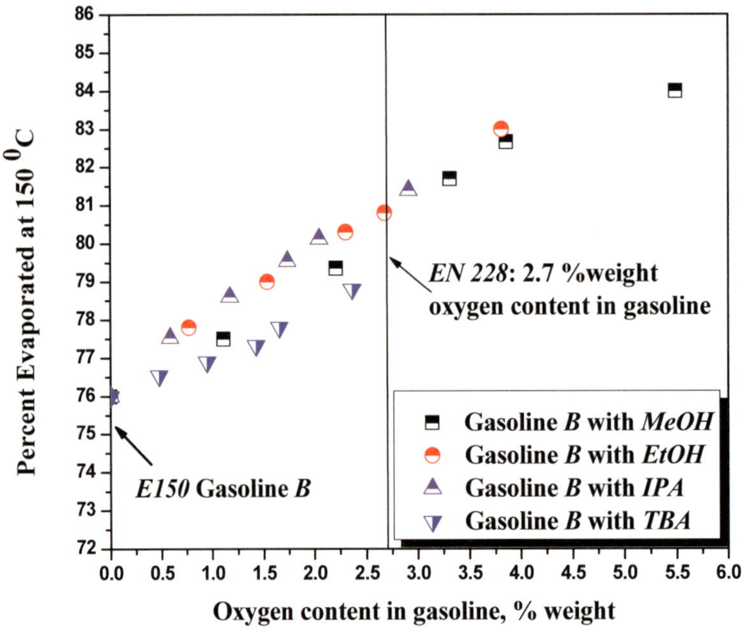

Fig. 11. The influence of alcohols over the percent evaporated at 150°C of oxy-gasoline A and B

the evaporation of the heavier hydrocarbons due to the fact that their boiling point is somewhat higher (Fig.11). One would have expected a similar effect from butanol also, but we believe that its effect is very much reduced because of its branched chemical structure. From the point of view of the quality standards of fuels EN 228, the evaporation percentage at a temperature of 150°C for all gasoline-alcohol blends is over 75.

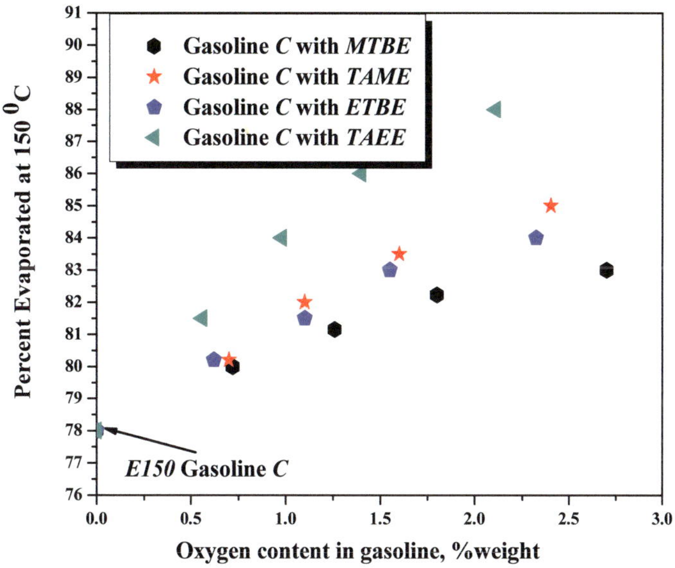

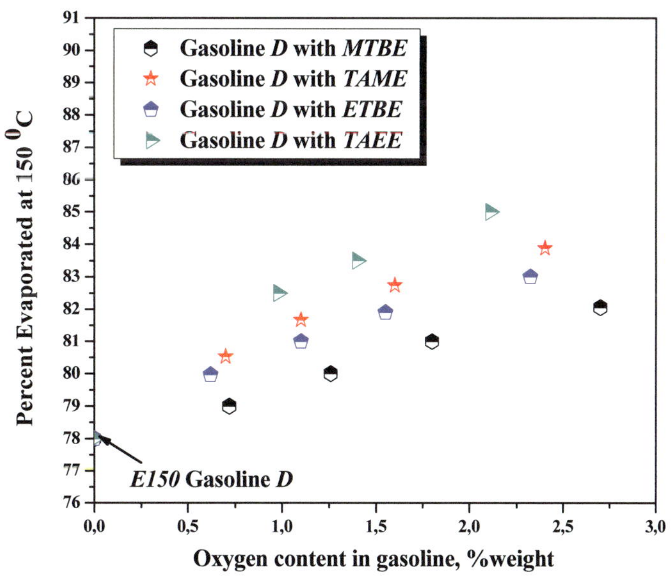

Fig. 12. The influence of ethers over the percent evaporated at 150°C of oxy-gasoline A and B

The percentages evaporated at a temperature of 150°C from oxy-gasoline with the ethers under study increase proportionally with each volume increase of each ether. The increase in E150 is proportional with the boiling points of ethers. TAEE (with boiling point at 101.42°C) provides the best contribution to the evaporation of gasoline at a temperature of 150°C - the effect is more visible with gasoline C (less volatile), rather than with gasoline D. In the case of gasoline oxygenated with ethers, the percentage evaporated at a temperature of 150°C is over 75, according to standard EN228.

Another volatility property is the vapour lock index VLI. This property is calculated with Eq. (1), based on the value of the vapour pressure experimentally determined and the evaporated percentages at a temperature of 70°C (Figs. 13 and 14).

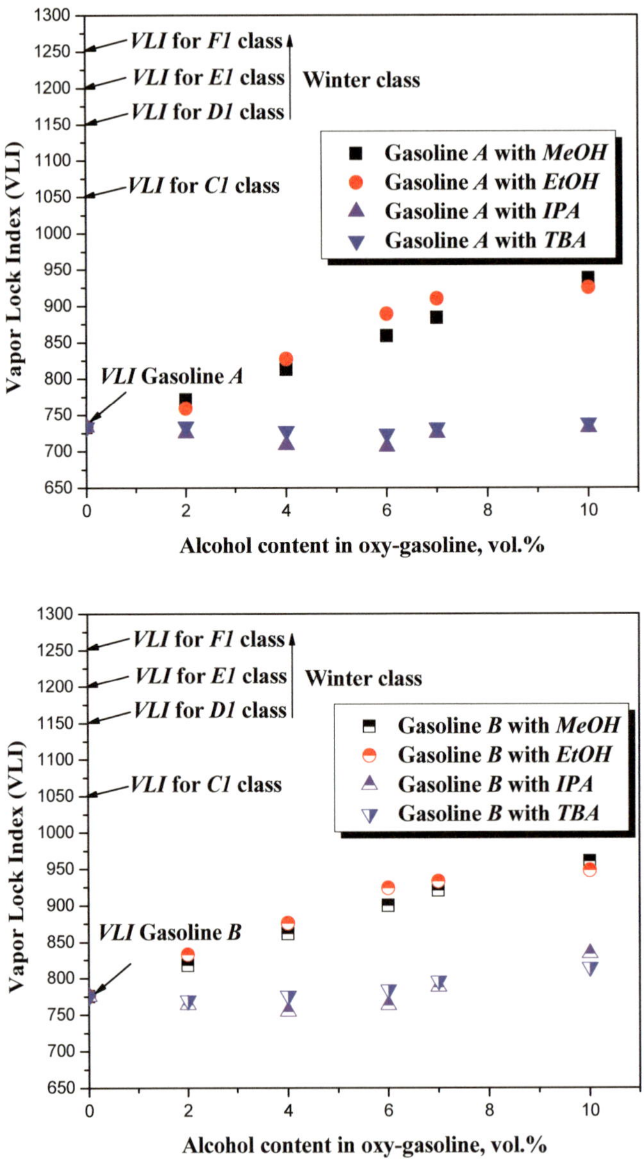

Fig. 13. Vapour lock index *(VLI)* of oxy- gasoline with alcohols

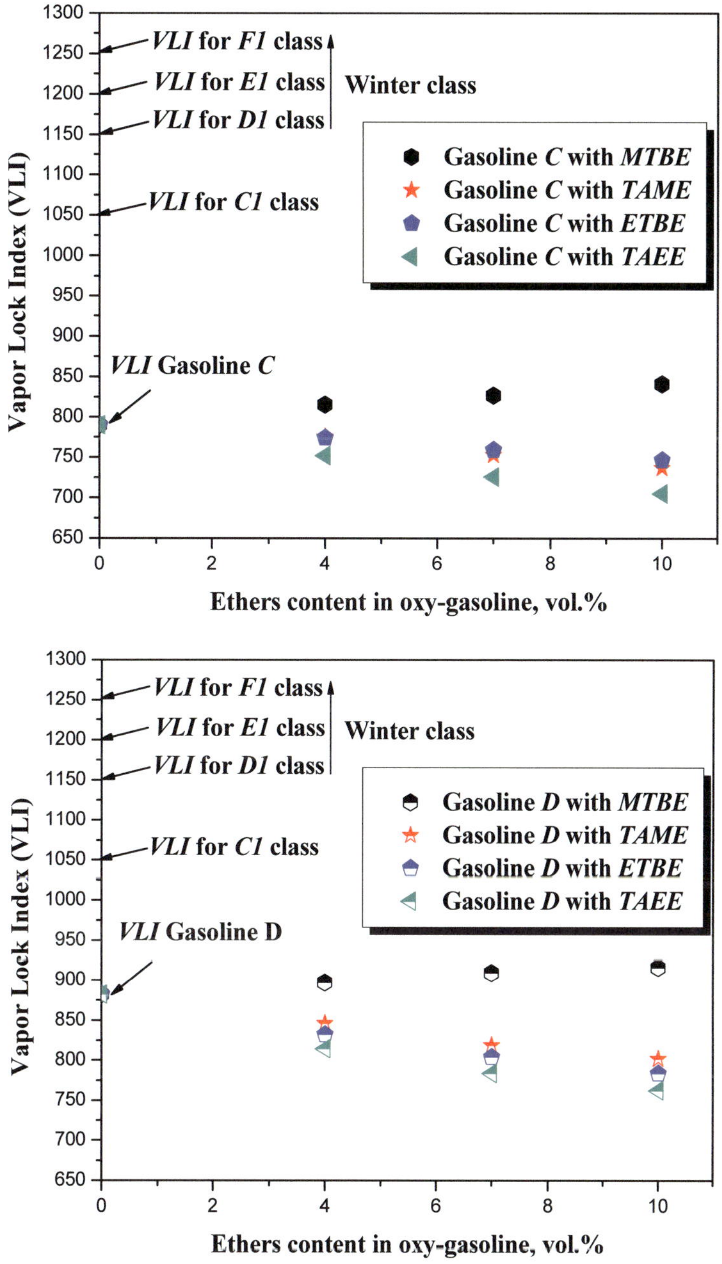

Fig. 14. Vapour lock index *(VLI)* of oxy-gasoline with ethers

From the point of view of the vapour lock index VLI, oxy-gasoline with alcohols, but also with MTBE, presents an increase in the tendency of forming vapour locks, unlike conventional gasoline. On the other hand, oxy-gasoline with TAME, TAEE or ETBE indicates a decrease in the vapour lock index, just as Reid pressure vapours and evaporated percentage at a temperature of 70°C decreased.

4.2 Octane properties of blends between gasoline and bio-alcohols or ethers

From the very beginning the introduction of a particular oxy-compound in commercial gasoline (1970 MTBE), was mainly to achieve an octane value increase. Both primary alcohols and all other ethers have an increased octane value, which may suggest that the effect of all oxy-compounds is that of having a positive in-take on octane value of blends. In order to sustain this idea, the engine octane value (MON) and Research octane value (RON) were experimentally determined using IROX 2000 Fuel Analyzer Portable Gasoline Analysis with MID-FTIR. The experimentally-determined results are correlated with the oxygen content in gasoline, as shown in the Tables 6 and 7.

Oxygen content in gasoline, % weight	Gasoline A with MeOH		Gasoline B with MeOH	
	MON	*RON*	*MON*	*RON*
1.11	0.32	0.83	0.39	0.74
2.21	0.85	1.50	0.77	1.48
3.31	1.12	2.34	1.16	2.22
3.86	1.45	2.62	1.36	2.62
5.49	1.88	3.59	1.79	3.43
Oxygen content in gasoline, % weight	Gasoline A with EtOH		Gasoline B with EtOH	
	MON	*RON*	*MON*	*RON*
0.77	0.34	0.71	0.29	0.66
1.40	0.62	1.27	0.73	1.32
2.30	0.98	1.92	0.98	1.98
2.68	1.19	2.38	1.15	2.33
3.81	1.70	3.23	1.51	3.06
Oxygen content in gasoline, % weight	Gasoline A with IPA		Gasoline B with IPA	
	MON	*RON*	*MON*	*RON*
0.59	0.18	0.49	0.14	0.38
1.17	0.46	0.81	0.39	0.74
1.74	0.78	1.34	0.63	1.26
2.05	0.86	1.44	0.73	1.50
2.91	1.30	2.28	1.12	2.07
Oxygen content in gasoline, % weight	Gasoline A with TBA		Gasoline B with TBA	
	MON	*RON*	*MON*	*RON*
0.48	0.16	0.25	0.10	0.20
0.95	0.40	0.42	0.37	0.40
1.43	0.53	0.64	0.56	0.60
1.66	0.70	0.73	0.74	0.79
2.36	0.95	0.96	0.93	1.00

Table 6. The effect of the type of alcohol and oxygen content on net increase of octane numbers in gasoline.

Table 6 shows that both motor octane numbers and research octane numbers increase with increasing alcohol content. The biggest increase is upon replacement of gasoline with methanol, followed by ethanol, isopropanol, tert-buthyl alcohol. Net increase in octane number for gasoline-alcohol blends is smaller than with conventional gasoline of higher octane number. For example: net the increase of the MON with gasoline A substituted by 10 %vol. IPA is 1.30 octane, while for gasoline B is 1.12 octane. Net increase of the RON with gasoline A substituted by 10% vol. IPA is 2.28 octane, while for gasoline B is 2.07 octane.

Oxygen content in gasoline, % weight	Gasoline C with MTBE		Gasoline D with MTBE	
	MON	*RON*	*MON*	*RON*
0.72	0.64	0.88	0.46	0.83
1.26	1.12	1.54	1.01	1.50
1.80	1.60	2.20	1.36	2.15
2.70	2.40	3.30	2.10	3.23
Oxygen content in gasoline, % weight	Gasoline C with TAME		Gasoline D with TAME	
	MON	*RON*	*MON*	*RON*
0.70	0.60	0.50	0.27	0.31
1.10	0.85	0.80	0.70	0.56
1.60	1.00	1.50	1.06	1.00
2.40	1.80	2.30	1.50	1.80
Oxygen content in gasoline, % weight	Gasoline C with ETBE		Gasoline D with ETBE	
	MON	*RON*	*MON*	*RON*
0.62	0.68	0.92	0.59	0.90
1.10	1.14	1.61	1.12	1.58
1.55	1.62	2.30	1.48	2.25
2.32	2.42	3.45	2.26	3.38
Oxygen content in gasoline, % weight	Gasoline C with TAEE		Gasoline D with TAEE	
	MON	*RON*	*MON*	*RON*
0.56	0.40	0.40	0.20	0.22
0.98	0.70	0.70	0.49	0.49
1.40	1.00	1.00	0.80	0.89
2.11	1.50	1.50	1.20	1.43

Table 7. The effect of the type of ether and oxygen content on net increase of octane values in gasoline

Both motor octane numbers and research octane numbers increase as the content of each ether increases (Table 7). Octane numbers vary as follows: ETBE>MTBE>TAME>TAEE. Net increase of octane numbers with gasoline-alcohol blends are smaller than with conventional gasoline of higher octane values and with bigger aromatics content (gasoline C). For example: net increase of MON with gasoline C substituted by 15 % vol. ETBE is 2.42 octane, while for gasoline D is 2.26 octane. Net increase of RON with gasoline C substituted by 15 % vol. ETBE is 3.45 octane, while for gasoline D is 3.38 octane.

Comparing the effects of alcohols and ethanol on octane values of oxy-gasoline, the conclusion is as follows: for motor octane numbers, it is more effective to use ether oxy-compounds, while for research octane numbers it is more effective to use ethanol, and also ETBE and MTBE.

5. Conclusion

In today's era, where various and major changes in climate emerge ever more often, and where humanity tends to offer more and more project-like solutions to using regenerable raw material, primary alcohols (with 1 or 4 carbons/molecule) and ethers (with 5 to 7 carbons/molecule) play a leading role. There are still a number of issues that need to be resolved before they will be commonly used as bio-components in gasoline for vehicles, which implies additional research and tests run on engines. Last but not least, the future of these bio-components depends essentially on legislative aid and the evolution of the automobile industry. Thus, the formulation of commercial gasoline quality to meet all quality prescriptions, and at the same time to contribute essentially to reducing air pollution, is a continuous challenge for all researchers and refiners.

A major effect on vehicle engines, and also on exhaust gas is played by the volatility and antiknock performances of oxy-gasoline. The present study is based on a very laborious experimental research design. We determined and analyzed in detail the volatility properties (Reid pressure vapour, distillation curves, and vapour lock index) and octane properties (motor octane number and research octane number) of two synthetic conventional gasoline oxygenated with 2-10% vol. primary alcohols (methanol, ethanol, iso-propyl alcohol, tert-butyl alcohol). Also, we have determined and analyzed these properties for 2 other synthetic conventional gasoline oxygenated with 4-15% vol. ethers (MTBE, TAME, ETBE, TAEE). The present study contributes to highlighting the advantages and disadvantages of using oxy-compounds (primary alcohols or ethers, as partial substitutes for petroleum-based gasoline).

The main volatility property of oxy-gasoline is the Reid pressure vapour. From the point of view of the refiners, this property makes all the difference between summer gasoline and winter gasoline. From the point of view of the vapour pressure, oxy-gasoline with methanol or ethanol is recommended during winter, as the vapour pressure is higher. Conventional gasoline, with an initial vapour pressure of 60 kPa, oxygenated with MTBE, will have an even higher vapour pressure. In this case, this gasoline can be used efficiently in winter with no need to use additives with C4+ hydrocarbon fractions. On the other hand, oxy-gasoline with IPA, TBA, TAME, ETBE, TAEE, that have low vapour pressure, can be used in summer, but if a C4 hydrocarbons fraction is used, the gasoline can reach the vapour pressure required by the quality standard of winter gasoline. Such flexibility in using oxy-gasoline with ethers, and especially with ETBE or TAEE will offer a top position in any producer's choices for gasoline. Apparently, it seems that IPA and TBA alcohols are substitutes which can ensure, for the gasoline they are oxygenating, the proper flexibility from the point of view of volatility correction. Although these alcohols are obtained from renewable material, are not, YET, beneficial. For this reason, we consider that the possibility of their being used beneficially in the future is strictly dependant on developing future technologies that can produce them in sufficient quantities and at reasonable costs. Depending on the development of the production industry, isopropanol and tert- butyl alcohol (or other butanols) may be, for example, used in a blend with bio-ethanol in order to correct the deficiencies associated with high volatility of oxy-gasoline.

Gasoline distillation curves are modified when combined with oxy-compounds. With bioalcohols, distillation curves indicate an azeotrope region. In this region, evaporation of hydrocarbons occurs much faster than with conventional gasoline. This is a beneficial aspect, as it aids the vehicle start up on ignition, even at cold temperatures. The disadvantage of this is that it increases the frequency of vapour plugs and evaporative emissions.

Ethers do not form azeotropes with gasoline hydrocarbons. Based on their boiling point, ethers influence hydrocarbon evaporation differently along distillation curves and vehicles operating in all gears. MTBE ensures evaporation along the whole distillation curve of oxy-gasoline, and especially volatile gasoline. ETBE, although it slightly affects evaporation at 70°C, has the advantage that it ensures evaporation for the rest of the distillation curve regardless of the gasoline type. TAME is not at all advantageous for evaporation at 70°C, but it is advantageous at 100°C. TAEE influences evaporation at 70°C and 100°C, but is far more advantageous for evaporation at 150°C.

Other volatility properties such as vapour lock index VLI offers an idea on the gasoline's tendency to form vapour plugs. In fact, VLI combines vapour pressure and a property for the beginning part of the distillation curve, E70. Unlike classic gasoline, oxy-gasoline with methanol or ethanol are more likely to form vapour plugs. This tendency is rather smaller with oxy-gasoline with IPA or TBA. Oxy-gasoline with ethers does not tend to form vapour plugs, and VLI values are rather smaller than VLI values for non oxy-gasoline (except those with MTBE). This behaviour is completely justifiable, as oxy-gasoline with TAME, ETBE or TAEE have E70 values and smaller vapour pressure than conventional gasoline.

In conclusion, oxy-gasoline with ethers displays more beneficial volatility properties than primary alcohols, especially than bio-ethanol.

From the point of view of antiknock properties, oxy-gasoline with ethers have higher octane numbers than alcohols. On the other hand, only MTBE and ETBE would lead to similar research octane numbers to those of oxy-gasoline with ethanol.

Ethers, specifically ETBE which is an oxy-compound partially renewable, have great potential to be used - in the future - as partial substitutes for gasoline. Alone, or combined with bio-ethanol, they enhance both volatility properties and octane numbers in gasoline for commercial use.

In the light of the information presented herein, we believe that we brought a significant contribution to the domain, clarifying a number of aspects associated with the current and potential usage of oxy-compounds in auto gasoline formulation.

6. Acknowledgement

The present study has been performed by the funding received from *CNCSIS-UEFISCSU 1291/2008 Project.*

7. References

Arnold , F. (2008). The Race for New Biofuels, Engineering & Science, No . 2, pp. 12-19

Aakko, P.& Nylund, N.-O. (2004). Technical view on biofuels for transportation-Focus on ethanol end-use aspects, *Research Report*, PRO3/5100/03 06.05.2004. Date of access:

10.10.2008, Available from: http://www.vtt.fi/inf/julkaisut/muut/2004/ EtOH_VTT5100_03.pdf

Bayraktar, H. (2005). Experimental and theoretical investigation of using gasoline–ethanol blends in spark-ignition engines, *Renewable Energy*, Vol. 30, Issue 11, pp. 1733–1747, ISSN: 0960-1481

Brekke, K. (2007, March). Butanol-An Energy Alternative?, *Ethanol Today*, pp. 36-39

Cataluña, R.; da Silva, R.; Weber de Menezes, E. & Ivanov,R.B. (2008). Specific consumption of liquid biofuels in gasoline fuelled engines, *Fuel*, Vol. 87, Issues 15-16, pp. 3362–3368, ISSN: 0016-2361

D'Ornellas, C.V. (2001). The effect of ethanol on gasoline oxidation stability. *SAE Technical Paper Series* 2001-01- 3582. 30.07.2011. Available from: http://papers.sae.org/2001-01-3582/

da Silva, R.; Catalun˜a, R.; Weber deMenezes, E; Samios, D.& Sartori Piatnicki, C.M. (2005). Effect of additives on the antiknock properties and Reid vapor pressure of gasoline, *Fuel*, Vol. 84, Issue 7-8, pp.951–959, ISSN: 0016-2361

DIRECTIVE 2009/30/EC OF THE EUROPEAN PARLIAMENT AND OF THE COUNCIL of 23 April 2009, Official Journal of the European Union, L 140/88, Available from: http://eur lex.europa.eu/LexUriServ/LexUriServ.do?uri=OJ:L:2009:140:0088:0113:EN:PDF

Dixson-Declève, S. & Szalkowska, U. (2009). Biofuel Standards & Quality Needs, *2nd International Conference on Biofuels Standards*, Brussels, March 2009, http://ec.europa.eu/energy/renewables/events

He, B-Q.; Wang, J-X.; Hao, J-M.; Yan, X-G. & Xiao, J-H. (2003). A study on emission characteristics of an EFI engine with ethanol blended gasoline fuels. *Atmospheric Environment*, Vol. 37, pp. 949–957, ISSN 1352-2310

Hsieh, W. D.; Chen, R. H.; Wu, T.L. & Lin, T. H. (2002). Engine performance and pollutant emission of an SI engine using ethanol–gasoline blended fuels. *Atmospheric Environment*, Vol. 36, pp. 403–410

Lesnik, B. (2002).Physical and Chemical Properties of the Fuel Oxygenates, *U.S. Environmental Protection Agency, ASTSWMO State Symposium on Fuel Oxygenates* , October , 2002

Martini, G.; Manfredi, U.; Mellios, G.; Mahieu, V.; Larsen, B.; Farfaletti, A.; Krasenbrink, A.; De Santi, G.; McArragher, S.; Thompson, N.; Baro, J.; Zemroch, P. J.; Rogerson, J.; Farenback-Brateman, J.; Canovas, J.; Dijs, I.; Rose, K.; Bazzani, R.; Boggio, F.; Celasco, A.; Cucchi, C. & (Barry) Cahill. G.F. (2007). *Joint EUCAR/JRC/CONCAWE Study on: Effects of Gasoline Vapour Pressure and Ethanol Content on Evaporative Emissions from Modern Cars.* 30.07.2011. Available from: http://publications.jrc.ec. europa.eu/repository/handle/111111111/585

Motor Gasolines Technical Review (FTR-1). (2009). Chevron Corporation. 11.26.2009. Available from: http://www.chevron.com/products/prodserv/fuels/documents/69083_MotorGas_Tech%20Review.pdf

Muzˇíková, Z.; Pospíšil, M. & Šebor, G. (2009).Volatility and phase stability of petrol blends with ethanol, *Fuel*, Vol. 88, Issue 8, pp. 1351–1356, ISSN: 0016-2361

Neagu (Petre), M., Rosca, P.; Dragomir, R. E. & Mihai, O. (2010). Bioalcohols - compounds for Reformulated Gasolines, Part I. The effect of alcohols on volatility properties of gasolines, *Revista de Chimie*, Vol. 67, Issue 7, pp. 706-711, ISSN 0034-7752

Neagu (Petre), M., Rosca, P.& Dragomir, R. E.. (2011). The Effect of Bio-ethers on the Volatility Properties of Oxygenated Gasoline, *Revista de Chimie*, Vol. 62, Issue 5, pp. 567-574, ISSN 0034-7752

Nylund, N.-O.; Aakko-Saksa, P.& Sipilä, K.(2008). Status and outlook for biofuels, other alternative fuels and new vehicles, Espoo 2008. VTT Tiedotteita. Research Notes 2426. Available from: http://www.task39.org/LinkClick.aspx?fileticket=HaLS1Lla19k%3D&tabid=4426&language=en-US

Osman, M.M.; Matar, M.S. & Koreish, S. (1993). Effect of methyl tertiary butyl ether (MTBE) as a gasoline additive on engine performance and exhaust emissions, *Fuel Sci. Technol. INT'L, Vol,* 11, Issue10, pp.1331-1343.

Pospíšil, M.; Mužíková, Z. & Šebor, G. (2007). Volatility and distillation properties of ethanol-petrol blends, *Svojstva goriva i maziva*, Vol. 46, Issue 4, pp: 335-353

Poulopoulos, S.G. & Philippopoulos, C.J. (2001). Comparison between methyl tertiary butyl ether and ethanol as oxygenate additives: The influence on the exhaust emissions, *7th International Conference on Environmental Science and Technology Ermoupolis*, Syros island, Greece, Sept. 2001

Pumphrey, J.A.; Brand, J.I. & Scheller, W.A. (2000). Vapour pressure measurements and predictions for alcohols–gasoline blends. *Fuel*, Vol. 79, Issue 11, pp.1405–1411, ISSN: 0016-2361

Rosca, P.; Neagu (Petre), M.; Dragomir, R. E. & Mihai, O. (2009). The Volatility of Reformulated Gasolines with Alcohols, *Proceedings of the 5th WSEAS International Conference Energy, Environment, Ecosystems, Development and Landscape Architecture*, pp. 116-121, ISBN: 978-960-474-125-0, Athens, Greece, Sept. 2009

Song, C-L.; Zhang, W-M.; Pei, Y-Q.; Fan, G-L. & Xu, G-P. (2006). Comparative effects of MTBE and ethanol additions into gasoline on exhaust emissions. *Atmospheric Environment*, Vol. 40, pp. 1957–1970, ISSN 1352-2310

Szklo, A.; Schaeffer, R. & Delgado, F. (2007). Can one say ethanol is a real threat to gasoline? *Energy Policy*, Vol. 35, pp. 5411–5421, ISSN: 0301-4215

Szulczyk, K. (2010). Which is a better transportation fuel – butanol or ethanol? *International Journal of Energy and Environment (IJEE)*, Volume 1, Issue 3, 2010, pp.501-512 ISSN 2076-2909 (Online)

Tavlarides, V.; Poulopoulos, S.G. & Philippopoulos, C.J. (2000). MTBE Addition in Gasoline: The Effect on Automotive Exhaust Emissions. *Tech. Chron. Sci. J. TCG*, V, No 1-2, pp. 26-28

Zervas, E. ; Montagne, X. & Lahaye, J. (2001). C1–C5 organic acid emissions from an SI engine: influence of fuel and air/fuel equivalence ratio. *Environmental Science and Technology*, Vol. 35, pp.2746–2751

Zervas, E.; Montagne, X. & Lahaye, J. (2002). Emission of alcohols and carbonyl compounds from a spark ignition engine. Influence of fuel and air/fuel equivalence ratio. *Environmental Science and Technology*, Vol. 36, pp. 2414–2421

Zervas, E.; Montagne, X. & Lahaye, J. (2004). Impact of Fuel Composition on the Emission of Regulated Pollutants and Specific Hydrocarbons from a SI Engine. *Tech. Chron. Sci. J. TCG*, V, No 1-2, pp. 35-44, ISSN 1352-2310.

Part 3

Food Safety

8

Studies on the Isolation of *Listeria monocytogenes* from Food, Water, and Animal Droppings: Environmental Health Perspective

Nkechi Chuks Nwachukwu[1] and Frank Anayo Orji[2]
[1]*Department of Microbiology, Faculty of Biological Sciences, Abia State University, Abia State,*
[2]*Enzyme and Genetics Division, Department of Biotechnology, Federal Institute of Industrial Research, Oshodi, Lagos State, Nigeria*

1. Introduction

Veterinarians, Medical doctors, Environmentalists and other scholars know listeriosis by various names such as tiger river disease, silage sickness, leukocytosis, cheese sickness. Interestingly, Gustav Hülphers first discovered the bacteria and named it *Bacillus hepatis*. However, he did not preserve his bacterial strains, and the bacterium was later recognized as *Listeria monocytogenes* (Vishal. 2004). Fifteen years later, Murray *et al.* (1926) also identified bacteria identical to *L. monocytogenes*, as the cause of monocytosis in rabbit and guinea pig. The scholars preserved the isolates of the bacteria (ATCC no. 15313; ATCC no. 4428) so the credit goes to Murray *et al.* for isolation of *L. monocytogenes* for the first time. In addition to the existing knowledge, Pirie finally named the species *L. monocytogenes* in 1940 and thereafter it was included in the 6th edition of Bergey`s Manual of Determinative Bacteriology (1948).

In the early 1980's Listeriosis was classified under anthropozoonoses, which was changed to amphixenoses in the late 1990s. It lacks its true definition of Zoonotic disease because of involvement of an inanimate reservoir (food and Environment) as the major cause of listeriosis. Up to 1961, *L. monocytogenes* was regarded as the one and only species of the genus *Listeria* but later other species have been identified. Listeriosis is of great public health concern because of its high mortality (20 to 30%) and its common source epidemic potential. The most important aspect of this organism in food hygiene is the ability of the bacteria to survive in a wide range of temperatures and to make biofilms on various environmental surfaces, which serve as natural habitats or reservoirs (Duggan and Phillips, 1998). Direct transmission is possible, especially among veterinarians, performing gynecological interventions with aborted animals. Animals may be diseased or asymptomatic carriers of *L. monocytogenes* shedding the organism in their faeces. Thus, earlier it was believed that *L. monocytogenes* was causing disease by direct transmission from animals to humans. Today it is generally considered that ingestion is the main mode of infection with food and water being the main vehicles of infection. A listeriosis outbreak in the Maritime Provinces of Canada (1981) was indeed related to food but it was not until the outbreak of California from January to August 1985 (Linnan *et al.*, 1988) that food was recognized as an important vehicle of *Listeria* transmission. According to Mead *et al.* (1999) food is an important vehicle of *Listeria* transmission in 99% of listeriosis cases. Risk assessments by the World Health Organisation (WHO) have estimated that 99% of all Listeriosis could be eliminated if the *L. monocytogenes* level never exceed 1000 cfu/g in food at the point of consumption. Nosocomial infection has also been described, placing physicians and other medical staff at risk.

Listeria monocytogenes is a Gram-positive rod-shaped bacterium. It is the agent of **listeriosis**, a serious infection caused by eating food contaminated with the bacteria. Listeriosis has been recognized as an important public health problem in the United States. The disease affects primarily pregnant women, newborns, and adults with weakened immune systems.

Listeriosis is a serious disease for humans; the **overt form** of the disease has mortality greater than 25 percent. The two main clinical manifestations are sepsis and meningitis. Meningitis is often complicated by encephalitis, a pathology that is unusual for bacterial infections.

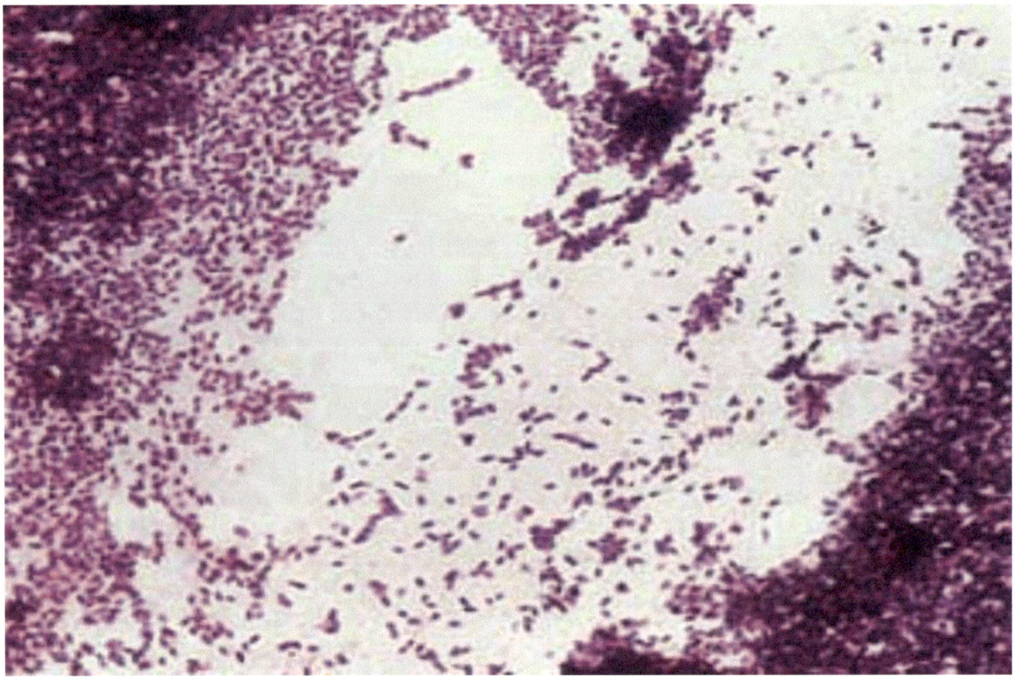

Fig. 1. *Listeria monocytogenes* Gram Stain as seen in a light Microscope (Kenneth, 2004).

Microscopically, *Listeria* species appear as small, Gram-positive rods, which are sometimes arranged in short chains. In direct smears they may be coccoid, so they can be mistaken for streptococci. Longer cells may resemble *Corynebacteria.* Flagella are produced at room temperature but not at 37°C. Hemolytic activity on blood agar has been used as a marker to distinguish *Listeria monocytogenes* among other *Listeria* species, but it is not an absolutely definitive criterion. Further biochemical characterization may be necessary to distinguish between the different *Listeria* species (Linnan *et al.*, 1988).

As Gram-positive, non- spore forming, catalase-positive rods, the genus *Listeria* was classified in the family Corynebacteriaceae through the seventh edition of Bergey's Manual. 16S rRNA cataloging studies of Stackebrandt et al. (1983) demonstrated that *Listeria monocytogenes* was a distinct taxon within the ***Lactobacillus-Bacillus*** branch of the bacterial phylogeny constructed by Woese (1981). In 2001, the Family **Listeriaceae** was created within the expanding Order **Bacillales**, which also includes Staphylococcaceae, Bacillaceae and others. Within this phylogeny there are six species of *Listeria*. The only other genus in the family is *Brochothrix*.

2. Natural habitats of *Listeria* and incidence of disease

Until about 1960, *Listeria monocytogenes* was thought to be associated almost exclusively with infections in animals, and less frequently in humans. However, in subsequent years, listeriae, including the pathogenic species *L. monocytogenes* and *L. ivanovii*, began to be isolated from a variety of sources, and they are now recognized to be widely distributed in Nature. In addition to humans, at least 42 species of wild and domestic mammals and 17 avian species, including domestic and game fowl, can harbor listeriae. *Listeria monocytogenes* is reportedly carried in the intestinal tract of 5-10% of the human population without any apparent symptoms of disease. Listeriae have also been isolated from crustaceans, fish, oysters, ticks, and flies (Doyle and Schoeni, 1986).

The term **listeriosis** encompasses a wide variety of disease symptoms that are similar in animals and humans. *Listeria monocytogenes* causes listeriosis in animals and humans; *L. ivanovii* causes the disease in animals only, mainly sheep. Encephalitis is the most common form of the disease in ruminant animals. In young animals, visceral or septicemic infections often occur. Intra-uterine infection of the fetus via the placenta frequently results in abortion in sheep and cattle (Doyle and Schoeni, 1986).

The true incidence of listeriosis in humans is not known, because in the average healthy adult, infections are usually asymptomatic, or at most produce a mild influenza-like disease. Clinical features range from mild influenza-like symptoms to meningitis and/or meningoencephalitis. Illness is most likely to occur in pregnant women, neonates, the elderly and immunocompromised individuals, but apparently healthy individuals may also be affected. In the serious (overt) form of the disease, meningitis, frequently accompanied by septicemia, is the most commonly encountered disease manifestation. In pregnant women, however, even though the most usual symptom is a mild influenza-like illness without meningitis, infection of the fetus is extremely common and can lead to abortion, stillbirth, or delivery of an acutely ill infant (David et al., 1994).

In humans, overt listeriosis following infection with *L. monocytogenes is* usually sporadic, but outbreaks of epidemic proportions have occurred. In 1981, there was an outbreak that involved over 100 people in Canada. Thirty-four of the infections occurred in pregnant women, among whom there were nine stillbirths, 23 infants born infected, and two live healthy births. Among 77 non pregnant adults who developed overt disease, there was nearly 30% mortality. The source of the outbreak was coleslaw produced by a local manufacturer (David et al., 1994.)

In 1985, in California, 142 people developed overt listeriosis. Of these, 93 cases were perinatal, and among the 49 cases that were in non pregnant individuals, 48 were immunocompromised. Thirty fetuses or newborn infants died and 18 adults died. The source of the bacteria was a certain brand of "pasteurized" soft cheese that apparently got contaminated with non pasteurized (raw) milk during the manufacturing process (Kenneth, 2004)..

In 2002, a multistate outbreak of *Listeria monocytogenes* infections with 46 culture-confirmed cases, seven deaths, and three stillbirths or miscarriages in eight states was linked to eating sliced turkey deli meat. One intact food product and 25 environmental samples from a poultry processing plant yielded *L. monocytogenes*. Two environmental isolates from floor drains were indistinguishable from that of outbreak patient isolates, suggesting that the plant might be the source of the outbreak (Kenneth, 2004).

Listeria monocytogenes, commonly referred to as *Listeria*, is a pathogen that causes listeriosis, a serious human illness. It is unlike most other foodborne pathogens because it can grow at proper refrigeration temperatures. In addition, *Listeria* is widely distributed in nature, and the organism has been recovered from farm fields, vegetables, animals and other environments such as food processing facilities, retail stores and home kitchens and ready-to-eat foods (Kenneth, 2004).

3. Symptoms and disease process

L. monocytogenes causes listeriosis, a serious infection with high hospitalization rates for those who become ill. People at highest risk for a severe case include the elderly, the fetuses of pregnant women, and the immunosuppressed. It is unique among foodborne pathogens since its incubation time (time from ingestion of cells to illness) is at least seven days. Listeriosis is a rare disease with a high mortality rate, causing about 43 percent of the food poisoning deaths in the United States.

L. monocytogenes can also cause mild, flu-like symptoms in healthy individuals when consumed at very high levels. A person with listeriosis has fever, muscle aches and occasional gastrointestinal symptoms such as nausea or diarrhea. If infection spreads to the nervous system, symptoms such as headache, stiff neck, confusion, loss of balance, or convulsions can occur. Infected pregnant women may experience only a mild, flu-like illness; however, infections during pregnancy can lead to miscarriage or stillbirth, premature delivery or infection of the newborn (Vishal, 2004).

Primary routes of transmission

Foods can become contaminated with *L. monocytogenes* along the continuum from farm to fork, in the produce growing environment, during processing, or during handling and preparation in retail establishments and consumers' kitchens (ILSI, 2005).

The primary route of transmission is through the ingestion of contaminated food. The International Life Sciences Institute in 2005 described high-risk foods for causing listeriosis as those with the following properties:

1. have the potential for contamination with *L. monocytogenes*;
2. support the growth of *L. monocytogenes* to high numbers;
3. are ready-to-eat;
4. require refrigeration; and
5. are stored for an extended period of time(ILSI, 2005).

Because *Listeria* is abundant in nature and can be found almost anywhere, there can be a constant re-introduction of the organism into the food plant, retail setting, foodservice establishment and home. It is difficult to totally eliminate this contaminant from the food-handling environment, but the goal is to control it as effectively as possible, especially where it can contaminate ready-to-eat, refrigerated foods.

Although *L. monocytogenes* is the only member of the *Listeria* family that causes human illness, the presence of any member of the *Listeria* family in a food processing environment may indicate that conditions are favorable for *L.monocytogenes* proliferation(ILSI,2005)..

4. Control

Effective control of *L. monocytogenes* requires prevention of contamination (to the extent possible) and prevention of growth through time/temperature or formulation control. Knowledge of potential harborage sites is important, as contamination is more likely to occur when the organism has become established in a niche. Food processing plant surveys have found *Listeria* in the following locations (listed approximately in the order of prevalence):

- floors
- drains
- coolers
- cleaning aids such as brushes, sponges, etc.
- product and/or equipment wash areas
- food contact surfaces
- condensate
- walls and ceilings

4.1 Compressed air (ILSI, 2005)

Control of *Listeria* relies on detecting and managing harborage sites with thorough and frequent cleaning. This includes daily cleaning of floors and drains, and adequate attention to less frequently cleaned areas such as HVAC systems, walls, coolers and freezers. Also, damaged equipment, cracks, crevices and hollow areas must be part of sanitation and inspection schedules. It is essential to avoid creation of aerosols during cleaning, especially of floors and drains, to avoid spread of contaminants.

The organism is killed by normal food pasteurization and cooking processes, and is typically sensitive to most sanitizers at recommended rates. Contamination may occur after the cooking process in the processing environment, at retail locations and in the home. For example, post pasteurization contamination of food products can occur when the organism is dispersed via an aerosol. Prevention of growth is essential to avoid the potential for illness, because *L. monocytogenes* can grow at refrigerated temperatures, defeating one of the traditional food safety measures.

L. monocytogenes can survive on cold surfaces and can also multiply *slowly* at 34° F. It has also been shown to grow to a water activity as low as 0.92 and over a pH range of 4.4-9.4(ICMSF, 2004). Because the organism can grow under refrigeration, effective labeling to ensure product rotation in retail settings is an important control measure for ready-to-eat products.

Since this organism continues to elicit concern among consumers, regulators, processors and retailers, studies need to be carefully designed to ensure validity (ILSI, 2005).

5. Background on challenges to the zero tolerance initiative

The FDA/Food Safety and Inspection Service risk assessment reinforces epidemiological conclusions that food borne Listeriosis is a moderately rare, although severe, disease. A study by the Food Products Association showed it is likely that low levels of *L. monocytogenes* are consumed routinely with limited effect. It is believed that 5 percent of the general population may be asymptomatic carriers of *Listeria*, but the percentage may be higher in particular groups, such as slaughterhouse workers.

Extensive risk assessments and analyses have been conducted by the Food Safety and Inspection Service (FSIS, 2005), U.S. Food and Drug Administration/FSIS , World Health Organization/Food and Agriculture Organization and International Life Sciences Institute to identify factors that contribute to risk of illness (Gombas *et al.*, 2003). This research is important because the prevalence in the food supply does not match the rate of illness in the population, and because the outcome of illness in susceptible individuals is very severe. These assessments have generally concluded that the ability of a food to support growth of *Listeria* enhances risk. Because of this, US FDA issued draft Compliance Policy Guidelines in February, 2008 based on the ability of a product to support growth of *L. monocytogenes (ILSI, 2005).* The USDA retains a zero tolerance policy for RTE foods with respect to *L. monocytogenes*, while other countries allow up to 100 Cfu/g in certain foods *(ILSI, 2005).*

6. *Listeria monocytogenes* in the human and animal environment

Listeriosis is essentially a food borne disease caused by *Listeria monocytogenes* and to some extent *L. ivanovii.* The disease conditions vary from severe invasive forms that affect immunocompromised patients to febrile gastroenteritis and perinatal infections associated with fetal loss or abortion in humans and animals (Siegman-Igra *et al.*, 2002). Although rare, the disease is reported (Lyautey *et al.*, 2007) to have a very high mortality rate (20-50%), thus making it of serious public health concern. Despite the general consensus that food is the primary route of transmission of this disease, wastewater has long been reported to be a potential reservoir for *Listeria* species and possible source of transmission (Paillard *et al.*, 2005; Arslan and Ozdemir, 2008). Watkins and Sleath (1981) reported the prevalence of *Listeria* species in sewage at numbers far higher than those of *Salmonella* species. And recent studies suggest that *Listeria* species readily survive conventional wastewater treatment processes even after tertiary treatment (Paillard *et al.*, 2005).

With reports of inadequate removal of *Listeria* pathogens from wastewater coming from the developed world (Paillard *et al.*, 2005), one can safely presume that wastewater treatment plants in developing countries such as South Africa are inefficient at removing these pathogens from wastewater influents prior to discharge of the final effluents into the receiving waters for obvious reasons. Most studies (Mackintosh and Colvin, 2003; Obi *et al.*, 2007; Obi *et al.*, 2008) in the area of water quality in South Africa had focused almost exclusively on drinking or potable water supply with scanty reports in the literature on treated wastewater effluent as a source of pathogens for receiving waters. This may have serious public health implications as about 80 % of South Africans are reported to depend on surface water bodies for drinking, domestic and agricultural purposes (Mackintosh and Colvin, 2003). It is little surprise therefore that about 43, 000 deaths (mostly children) are reported annually in South Africa due to diarrhea diseases (Mara, 2001). The situation is amongst the worst in the Eastern Cape Province due to high level of poverty, low level of sanitation, and lack of appropriate infrastructure (Mackintosh and Colvin, 2003). While reports in the media suggests that cholera may be responsible for the majority of these infections, actual diagnosis suggests that these diseases could have been caused by any other waterborne pathogen apart from *Vibrio* species. A case in point was seen in the report of the Daily Dispatch of Thursday, 30th of January 2003, where out of 446 cases of water related diseases reported to the Eastern Cape health authorities, only 25 (5.6 %) were confirmed to be cholera and yet the disease was termed a "cholera outbreak" without ascertaining the true identities of the pathogens responsible for over 84% of reported cases.

There is a general belief that the larger population of bacteria species grow as adherent to surfaces in all nutrient-sufficient aquatic ecosystems and that these sessile bacterial cells differ profoundly from their planktonic (free-living) counterpart (Costerton *et al.*, 1978). It has also been reported that the existence of pathogens as free-living or plankton-associated cells, is critical to their survival in the environment as well as their transmission from one host to another (Donlan and Costerton, 2002). Several studies have revealed the preponderance of *Listeria* species to exist as biofilms attached to surfaces such as stainless steel, glass and propylene (Mafu et al., 1990), and food and food processing environments (Lunden et al., 2000). There is however little or no report in the literature on Listerio-plankton association in the natural environment. Understanding the distribution of Listeria cells as free-living or plankton-associated niches may provide clues on how best to reduce the survival potentials of these pathogens in the environment and during wastewater treatment, and consequently reduce their ability to interact with human and animal populations.

Nwachukwu et al., 2010 reported the isolation of *Listeria monocytogenes* from two anthropogenic lakes from Lokpa Ukwu, Abia State (Nigeria). The identification of isolates was based on cultural and morphological appearances. The identity of isolates was confirmed by biochemical tests. The results of this study revealed that the pathogen was present in 22 out of 24 samples of water from Lake A, giving a prevalence rate of 91.67% while in lake B, the prevalence rate observed was 79.17%. This high prevalence rate is not surprising as the organism is quite ubiquitous in soil, water, and animal dung samples. *Listeria monocytogenes* is water and food borne bacterial pathogen that is ubiquitous in nature and shows ability to persist in its environment for prolong time (Yutaka *et al.*, 2004).

7. *Listeria monocytogenes* in food and food industries

L. monocytogenes is a bacterium that can contaminate foods and cause a mild non-invasive illness (called listerial gastroenteritis) or a severe, sometimes life-threatening, illness (called invasive listeriosis). Persons who have the greatest risk of experiencing listeriosis after consuming foods contaminated with *L. monocytogenes* are fetuses and neonates who are infected after the mother is exposed to *L. monocytogenes* during pregnancy, the elderly, and persons with weakened immune systems. Invasive listeriosis is characterized by a high case-fatality rate, ranging from 20 percent to 30 percent (USFDA, 2003).

L. monocytogenes is widespread in the environment. It is found in soil, water, sewage, and decaying vegetation. It can be readily isolated from humans, domestic animals, raw

Category	Potential Sources of *L. monocytogenes*
A. Ingredients	Raw foods, such as: Raw meat, poultry, and seafood Raw milk Raw produce
B. Processing aids	Compressed air Ice Brine solutions used in chilling refrigerated RTE foods
C. Contact surfaces for RF-RTE foods	Fibrous and porous-type conveyor belts Filling and packaging equipment Belts, peelers, and collators Containers, bins, tubs and baskets Slicers, dicers, shredders and blenders Utensils Gloves
D. Surfaces that do not contact RF-RTE foods	In-floor weighing equipment Cracked hoses Hollow rollers for conveyances Equipment framework Wet, rusting, or hollow framework Open bearings within equipment Poorly maintained compressed air filters Condensate drip pans Motor housings Maintenance tools (*e.g.*, wrenches and screw drivers) Forklifts, hand trucks, trolleys, and racks On/off switches Vacuum cleaners and floor scrubbers Trash cans and other such ancillary items Tools for cleaning equipment (*e.g.*, brushes and scouring pads) Spiral freezers/blast freezers Ice makers Aprons
E. Plant environment	Floors, walls and drains Ceilings, overhead structures, and catwalks Wash areas (*e.g.*, sinks), condensate, and standing water Wet insulation in walls or around pipes and cooling units Rubber seals around doors, especially in coolers Contents of vacuum cleaners

(SOURCE: Quin et al., 1999; Slustsker and Schuchat, 1999 ; Afnor, 2000 ; EUAHS,2007).

Table 1. Potential Sources of *L. monocytogenes*Scenarios That Could Lead to Contamination with *L. monocytogenes*

agricultural commodities, and food processing environments (particularly cool damp areas) (NACMCF, 1991). Control of *L. monocytogenes* in the food processing environment has been the subject of a number of scientific publications (Fenlon *et al.*, 1996). *L. monocytogenes* can multiply slowly at refrigeration temperatures, thereby challenging an important defense against food-borne pathogens. (Doyle et al, 2001).

Most cases of human listeriosis occur sporadically - that is, in an isolated manner without any apparent pattern. However, much of what is known about the epidemiology of the disease has been derived from outbreak-associated cases, in which there is an abrupt increase in reports of the disease. With rare exceptions, foods that have been reported to be associated with outbreaks or sporadic cases of listeriosis have been foods that can support the growth of *L. monocytogenes* and that are ready-to-eat (including coleslaw, fresh soft cheese made with unpasteurized milk, frankfurters, deli meats, and butter) USFDA, 2003. Outbreaks of listeriosis are often associated with a processing or production failure (Slutsker and Schuchat 1999); this association has been less evident among sporadic cases (Slutsker and Schuchat 1999).

In addition to this information obtained from reported cases of listeriosis, contamination data (largely obtained from samples of foods collected at retail or during storage before sale) are available in published scientific literature, government documents and industry documents, or were made available to us from unpublished government and industry documents (Doyle et al, 2001). These contamination data show that *L. monocytogenes* has been detected to varying degrees in unpasteurized and pasteurized milk, high fat dairy products, soft unripened cheese (cottage cheese, cream cheese, ricotta), cooked ready-to-eat crustaceans, smoked seafood, fresh soft cheese (queso fresco), semi-soft cheese (blue, brick, monterey), soft-ripened cheese (brie, camembert, feta), deli-type salads, sandwiches, fresh-cut fruits and vegetables, and raw molluscan shellfish (Doyle et al, 2001). However, these data also show that most RTE foods do not contain detectable numbers of *L. monocytogenes*. For many RTE foods, contamination of foods with *L. monocytogenes* can be avoided - *e.g.*, through the application of current good manufacturing practices that establish controls on ingredients, listericidal and listeristatic processes, segregation of foods that have been cooked from those that have not, and sanitation. Sanitation controls include effective environmental monitoring programs designed to identify and eliminate *L. monocytogenes* in and on surfaces and areas in the plant (Doyle et al, 2001). The critical control points for food manufacturing industries will include one or more of the following:

- A packaging line is moved or modified significantly.
- Used equipment is brought from storage or another plant and installed into the process flow.
- An equipment breakdown occurs.
- Construction or major modifications are made to an area where RTE foods are processed or exposed (e.g., replacing refrigeration units or floors, replacing or building walls, modifications to sewer lines).
- A new employee, unfamiliar with the operation and *L. monocytogenes* controls, has been hired to work in, or to clean equipment in, the area where RTE foods are processed or exposed.
- Personnel who handle RTE foods touch surfaces or equipment likely to be contaminated (*e.g.*, floor, trash cans) and do not change gloves or follow other required procedures before handling the food.

- Periods of heavy production make it difficult to clean the floors of holding coolers as scheduled.
- A drain backs up.
- Product is caught or hung-up on equipment. (Stagnant product in a system can be a major site of microbial growth during production.)
- Raw or under-processed foods are placed in an area designated for cooked foods.
- Frequent product changes on a packaging line cause you to change packaging film, labels, forming pockets or molds, line speeds, etc.
- Personnel are used interchangeably for packaging raw and cooked foods.
- Increased production causes you to perform wet cleaning of lines that have been taken down from production in the same room as lines that are running product.
- Heat exchangers have become compromised (*e.g.*, with pinholes).
- Equipment parts, tubs, screens, etc. are cleaned on the floor.
- Waste bins in the RTE area are not properly maintained, cleaned and sanitized.
- Personnel handling RTE foods may come into contact with these items and then contaminate the foods and/or food contact surfaces.
- Re-circulating pumps and lines are not cleaned and sanitized.
- Indiscriminate use of high-pressure hoses in cleaning.
- Inappropriate use of footbaths in dry processing areas.

7.1 Laboratory identification of *Listeria monocytogenes*

7.1.1 Traditional method

Current methods for identification of *L. monocytogenes* rely on physiological and biochemical methods. These include Gram stain morphology, catalase, motility, beta haemolysis on blood agar and oblique illumination of colonies on blood free agar.

a. Isolation methods

Conventional methods for the isolation of *L. monocytogenes* from food, water, and soil immediately that have gained acceptance for international regulatory purposes include the United States Food and Drug Administration (FDA) method (Hitchins, 1998), the Association of Official Analytical Chemists (AOAC) official method , the ISO 11290 Standards , the United States Department of Agriculture (USDA)-Food Safety and Inspection Service (FSIS) method (FSIS, 2002).) and the French Standards (AFNOR, 2000; AFNOR, 2004). Depending on the nature of the sample, a particular method might be more suitable than others. The selective Media for the isolation of *Listeria* species include Oxford Agar, Palcam Agar, Listeria Selective Agar (Oxoid, Basingstoke, England), and Nutrient Agar Supplemented with esculine bile salt.

b. Conventional biochemical identification methods

Typical *Listeria* spp. colonies, on the above selective/differential agar plates, are then selected for further identification to the species level, using a battery of tests. The tests include the Gram-staining reaction, catalase, motility (both in a wet mount observed under phase-contrast microscopy and by inoculation into motility test media), haemolysis and carbohydrate use. The Christie–Atkins–Munch–Peterson (CAMP) test is a very useful tool to help identify the species of a *Listeria* spp. isolates. It is used in the ISO and AOAC protocols and it is considered to be optional in the FDA and USDA-FSIS methods. The test is simple to perform and easy to read. It consists of streaking a ß-haemolytic *Staphylococcus aureus* (ATCC strain 49444 or 25923, NCTC strain 7428 or 1803) and *Rhodococcus equi* (ATCC strain 6939, NCTC strain 1621) in single straight lines in parallel, on a sheep blood agar plate or a double-layered agar plate with a very thin blood agar overlay. The streaks should have enough separation to allow test and control *Listeria* strains to be streaked perpendicularly, in between the two indicator organisms, without quite touching them (separated by 1–2 mm). After incubation for 24–48 hours at 35–37°C (12–18 hours if using the thin blood agar overlay),a positive reaction consists of an enhanced zone of ß-haemolysis, at the intersection of the test/control and indicator strains. *Listeria monocytogenes* is positive with the *S. aureus* streak and negative with *R. equi*, whereas the test with *L. ivanovii* gives the reverse reactions (Quinn, 1999).

7.1.2 Molecular approach for identification of *Listeria monocytogenes*

7.1.2.1 Polymerase Chain Reaction (PCR)

Enrichment and DNA extraction

A total of 25 g or 25 ml of food sample, soil, water, animal droppings, is incubated in 225 ml of *Listeria* enrichment broth (Oxoid, England) at 30 ± 1 °C for 24 and 48 h. For DNA isolation, 1 ml of suspension after 24 h and after 48 h is necessary.

Homogenate is centrifuged at 1800 × *g* for 5 min and the supernatant is discarded. The pellet is re-suspended in 100 µl of 0.5 % TRITON X-100 (Sigma, Germany) and the whole process is repeated. Homogenate is incubated at 95 °C for 5-10 min. 2 µl of Proteinase K [20 mg/ml] (Promega, USA) are added to the homogenate after cooling and it is incubated at 55 °C for 2 h. Proteins are removed with a phenol-chloroform-isoamylalcohol [25:24:1] solution (Sigma, Germany). DNA is precipitated with ice-cold absolute ethanol at -70 °C for 2h, Centrifuged at 3500 × *g* for 10 min. Pellet is dried and DNA is re-suspended in 30 µl of sterile distilled water.

PCR amplifications

The first round used primers PRFA1 and PRFA2 (Simon et al. 1996) are directed against nucleotides 181-207 and 1462-1482 of the sequence. Each 50 µl of the reaction mixture contains: 5 µl target DNA, 5 µl 10 x PCR buffer (Gibco BRL, USA), 2mM dNTPs (Promega, USA), 50mM MgCl2 (Gibco BRL, USA), 0.5 µmol/l primer (Generi Biotech, Czech Republic) and 1U Taq DNA polymerase (Gibco BRL, USA), sterile distilled water added to the volume 50 µl.

Hot start is at 94 °C for 2 min. The reaction mixtures are subjected to 35 cycles consisting of heat denaturation at 94 °C for 30 s, primer annealing at 60 °C for 30 s and DNA extension at 74 °C for 1 min. Finally, the samples are maintained at 74 °C for 5 min for the final extension of DNA. These incubation conditions are the same for second round-nested PCR, except those LIP1 and LIP2, since these primers require 45 cycles.

The second round employed primers LIP1 and LIP2 (Simon et al. 1996) directed against nucleotides 634-654 and 886-907 of first product amplified by PRFA1 and PRFA2. 2 µl of completed first round reaction mixture are added to each reaction as target DNA. Remaining components are the same as in the first round.

Visualization of the PCR product

For detection, 10 µl of PCR reaction mixture is electrophoresed on a 2% w/v agarose gel (Gibco BRL, USA), diluted in 1 × TAE buffer (Kaufman et al. 1995), stained with ethidium bromide (Amresco, USA) in concentration 0.1 µg/ml and viewed under the ultraviolet light.

Target gene	Primer sequence (5'-3')	Amplified fragment length	Reference
prfA gene	-TCATCGACGGCAACCTCGG- -TGAGCAACGTATCCTCCAGAGT-	217 bp	Germini et al. 2009
inlA gene	-AGCCACTTAAGGCAAT- -AGTTGATGTTGTGTTAGA-	760 bp	Poyart et al., 1996.
hlyA gene	-CCTAAGACGCCAATCGAA - -AAGCGCTTGCAACTGCTC -	-	Lakićević et. al., 2010
16S rRNA Gene	- CTCCATAAAGGTGACCCT - - CAGCMGCCGCGGTAATWC -	-	Lakićević et. al., 2010
iap gene	-GCCAGCGGCCCGGCGCGGGCCCGGCGGGG GCCGCGGCATGTCATGGAATAA- -GCTTTTCCAAGGTGTTTTT -	-	Lakićević et. al., 2010

Table 2. List of primers for detection of *Listeria monocytogenes* using polymerase chain Reaction

7.2 Practical case report: Studies on isolation of *Listeria monocytogenes* from poultry droppings in some selected farms in Okigwe, Imo State, Federal Republic of Nigeria

7.2.1 Aim and objectives of the study

The aims of this work are to:

i. Investigate the occurrence of *Listeria monocytogenes* in poultry droppings from farms in the study area.
ii. Study the pattern of antibiotic susceptibility of isolates of *L. monocytogenes* from the environment.

7.2.3 Study area

Poultry droppings were collected from three different farms. These farms include: David's Poultry Farm, Harrison's Farm, and Paul's Poultry Farm, all in the Okigwe Local Government Area of Imo State, Nigeria.

7.2.4 Sample collection

The poultry droppings were collected using sterile universal bottles, the screw caps were carefully removed using sterile hand gloves and with the help of an applicator stick, a large quantity of faecal droppings of poultry were collected. The samples were labeled and transported the Microbiology Laboratory, Abia State University, Uturu, Nigeria for laboratory studies.

Pre-enrichment and culture: 1 gram of faecal droppings from each sample was transferred into a test tube containing sterile and freshly prepared peptone water. This was inoculated at room temperature for 18 hours. This was to revive viable but non-culturable cells. Thereafter, a loopfull of the peptone water culture was transferred to a freshly prepared listeria Agar (Oxoid), and streaked on the surface of the solid medium. Incubation was done at 37°C for 48 hours. The pure cultures were subjected to morphologically and biochemically studies. (Nwachukwu *et.al,* 2009).

Antibiotic susceptibility testing

Antibiotic susceptibility testing was performed using the Kirby-Bauer method (Disc diffusion Technique). The discs used were manufactured by optun laboratories, Nigeria. The sensitivity discs were specifically designed and contained appropriate concentrations of different Gram positive antibiotics which include: ciprofoxacin (10μg/disc), norflaxacin (10μg/disc), gentamycin (10μg/disc), streptomycin (30μg/disc). Both cultures of different isolates of the test organism were carefully poured onto the surface of Muellar-Hinton Agar (Previously prepared according to manufacturer's instructions). The plates were incubated at 37°C for 48 hours. The different inhibition zone sizes were measured and recorded in millimeters (mm), and then the zone and size interpretive criteria of the National committees for Clinical Laboratory Standards (NCCLS) were used to interpret the zone sizes.

8. Results and discussions

Microbiological studies in Farm A, showed 100% frequency of occurrence of *L. Monocytogenes* from poultry droppings. In three sampling points in Farm, B, *Listeria monocytogenes* showed a frequency of 75%, 83%, and 66.6% respectively.

Farms	Numbers of Samples examined	No. of times *L. monocytogenes* was isolated (%)
Farm A	12	12 (100)
Farm A	12	12 (100)
Farm A	12	12 (100)
Farm B	12	9 (75)
Farm B	12	10 (83)
Farm B	12	8 (66.60)
Farm C	12	4 (33.3)
Farm C	12	4 (33.3)
Farm C	12	6 (66.60)

Table 3. Isolation of *L. monocytogenes* from Poultry droppings

In Farm C, *listeria monocytogenes* was isolated as frequencies of 33.3%, 33.3%, and 66% from three different locations of poultry droppings. The bacterial organism in Farm A, from poultry droppings showed a 25%, 33%, 50%, 41.7% resistance to ciprofloxacin, norfloxacin, gentamycin, lincocin respectively. *L. monocytogenes* strains from Farm A showed 75% resistance to floxapen and Ampicillin. *L. monocytogenes* showed 83% susceptibility to tarivid (Quinolone).

In Farm 2, the highest resistance was observed against chloramphenicol (77.8%). Ampicillin (75%). The highest susceptibility rate of 77.8% was observed on Tarivid and *L. monocytogenes* isolates from Farm 2

antibiotics		Farm 1		Farm 2		Farm 3	
		(N=9)		(N=12)		(N=9)	
	μg/disc	Ns (%)	NR(%)	Ns (%)	NR(%)	Ns (%)	NR(%)
Ciprnofloxacin	10	9(75)	3(25)	6(66.7)	3(33.3)	4(66.7)	2(33.3)
Norfloxacin	10	8(66.7)	4(33.3)	5(55.6)	4(44.4)	350.0)	2(33.3)
Gentamycin	10	6(50.0)	6(50)	3(33.3)	6(66.7)	2(33.3)	4(66.7)
Lincocin	20	7(58.3)	5(41.7)	4(44.4)	5(55.6)	5(83.3)	1(16.7)
Streptomycin	30	8(66.7)	4(33.3)	5(55.6)	4(44.4)	3(50)	3(50)
Rifampicin	20	6(50)	6(50)	3(33.3)	6(66.7)	5(83.3)	1(16.7)
Erythromycin	30	8(66.7)	4(50)	6(66.7)	3(33.3)	3(50)	3(50)
Chloram-phenicol	30	6(50)	6(50)	2(22.2)	7(77.8)	2(33.3)	4(66.7)
Ampiclox	20	6(50)	6(50)	3(33.3)	6(66.7)	2(33.3)	4(66.7)
Floxapen	20	9(75)	9(75)	6(66.7)	3(33.3)	4(6617)	2(33.3)
Ampicillin	10	3(25)	9(75)	2(22.2)	7(77.8)	1(16.7)	5(83.3)
Tarivid	10	10(83.3)	2(16.7)	7(77.8)	2(22.2)	5(83.3)	1(16.7)

Ns; Number that remained susceptible to the antibiotic, NR; Number that was resistant to the given antibiotics

Table 4. Antibiotic Susceptibility patterns of *L. monocytogenes* isolated from different poultry droppings.

In Farm, resistance was highest in Gentamycin (66.70%), Chloramphenicol (66.70%), Ampiclox (66.70%) and Ampicillin (83.3%).

The *L. monocytogenes* strains from Farm A showed a susceptibility of 83.3%, 83.3% in Lincocin and Tarivid respectively. This observation is in accordance with the report of Walsh et.al, (2001) where *L. monocytogenes* isolates were more susceptible to Drovid than floxapen.

Walsh *et.al,* 2004 also reported high resistance of *L. monocytogenes* to Penicillin. This drug rate of resistance to β-lactains and few quinolones could be as a result of drug abuse, and consequent acquisition of R-plasmid by these strains of *L. monocytogenes*. From this study on poultry droppings, it is now known that drug resistant *L. monocytogenes* are available on poultry droppings. However, Poultry industries are advised to understand that poultry droppings in the farm yard remain a critical control point for the production of chickens for human consumption. In addition, the use of poultry droppings as biofertilizers should be discouraged because of the hazard of transferring *L. monocytogenes* to edible plants and finally humans.

Veterinary Surveillance, especially in the droppings of poultry must be undertaken by Public health agencies in Nigeria, Africa and the entire world.

9. References

Afnor (1997). Norme Française NF V 08-055. Microbiologie des aliments. Recherche de *Listeria monocytogenes.* Méthode de Routine. Paris, France.

Afnor (2000). Normalisation Française XP V 08-062. Microbiologie des aliments. Méthode de dénombrement de *Listeria monocytogenes.* Méthode de Routine. Paris, France.

Arslan S, Ozdemir F (2008) Prevalence and antimicrobial resistance of *Listeria* species in homemade white cheese. Food Control 19: 360-363

Aureli, P. Ferrini, A.M, Hodzie, S., Wedell-Weergard, C., and Oli, B (2006). *Listeria monocytogenes* Isolated from food. International Journal of Food Microbiology, 55: 599-603.

Bailey J., Fletcher, D., and Swaminanthan B (2002). *Listeria, Erysipelothrix* and *Kurthia.* pp.295-314. In: manuel of Clinical Microbiology. 7th Edition Murray, R.P-(ed). American Society for Microbiology, Washington DC.

CDC(2006). Surveillance for Foodborne-Disease Outbreaks, United States, 1998– 2002. MMWR

Centers for Disease Control. (1988). United States Morbidity and Mortality. Weekly Rep. **37**: 377-382, 387-388.

Dijkstra, R.G. (1978). Incidence of *L. monocytogenes* in the intestinal contents of different farm. Tijd schr. Diergeneeskd, 15: 229-231.

Doyle ME, Mazzotta AS, Wang T, Wiseman DW, and Scott VN. (2001). Heat resistance of *Listeria monocytogenes. Journal of Food Protection* 64 (3): 410-429.

EUAHS (2007) European Union Animal Health Strategy. Avialable online at http://one-health.eu/ee/index.php/en/homepage/(Accesed 12th July, 2011)

Fatoki SO, Gogwana P, Ogunfowokan AO (2003) Pollution assessment in the Keiskamma River and in the impoundment downstream. Water SA 29 (3): 183-187

Fenlon DR, Wilson J, and Donachie W. (1996). The incidence and level of *Listeria monocytogenes* contamination of food sources at primary production and initial processing. *Journal of Applied Bacteriology* 81 (6): 641-650. Available in Docket No. 1999N-1168, Volume 0011 bkg1 (08 of 17), Tab 134

FSIS Risk Assessment for *Listeria monocytogenes* in Deli Meats, FDA/FSIS Risk Assessment

Gahan, C.G.M., Hill C. (2005). Gastrointestinal phase of *Listeria monocytogenes* infection. *Journal of Applied Microbiology 98,* 1345-1353.

Germini, A.; Masola, A.; Carnevali, P. and Marchelli, R. (2009). Simultaneous detection of *Escherichia coli* O175:H7, *Salmonella* spp., and *Listeria monocytogenes* by multiplex PCR. *Food Control,* 20:733-738.

Gombas DE, Chen Y, Clavero RS, Scott VN. (2003). Survey of *Listeria monocytogenes* in ready-to-eat foods. J Food Prot., 66(4):559-69

Hitchins A.D. (1998). *Listeria monocytogenes. In:* Bacteriological Analytical Manual, US Food and Drug Administration, AOAC INTERNATIONAL, Gaithersburg, MD, USA, 10.01–10.11

ILSI. 2005. Achieving Continuous Improvement in Reductions in Foodborne Listeriosis - A Risk Based Approach. Journal of Food Protection 68(9):1932-1994.

International Commission on Microbiological Specifications for Foods (ICMSF, 2004). Microorganisms in Foods

Kohne, D. E., A. G. Steigerewalt, and D. J. Brenner. (1984). Nucleic acid probe specific for members of the genus Legionella, p. 107-108. In: C. Thornsberry, et al. (ed.) (Legionella): proceedings of the 2nd international symposium. American Society for Microbiology, Washington, D.C.

Lakićević, B. Stjepanović , A. , Milijašević, M., Terzić- Vidojević, A , Golić, N. and Topisirović, L. (2010.) The Presence of *Listeria* spp. and *Listeria monocytogenes* in A Chosen Food Processing Establishment in Serbia. *Arch. Biol. Sci., Belgrade,* 62 (4), 881-887.

Linnan, M.J., Mascola, L., Lou, X.D., Goulet, V., May, S., Salminen, C., Hird, D.W.,Yonekura, M.L., Hayes, P., Weaver, R., (1988). Epidemic listeriosis associated with Mexican-style cheese. N Engl J Med 319, 823-828.

Lunden JM, Miettinen MK, Autio TJ, Korkeala H (2000) Persistent *Listeria monocytogenes* strains show enhanced adherence to food contact surface after short contact times. J Food Prot 63:1204-1207.

Mackintosh G, Colvin C (2003). Failure of rural schemes in South Africa to provide potable water. Environ Geol 44:101- 105

Mafu A, Roy D, Goulet J, Magny P (1990) Attachment of *Listeria monocytogenes* to stainless steel, glass, polypropylene and rubber surfaces after short contact times. J Food Prot 53: 742-746

Mara I. (2001). Between diarrhea disease and HIV/AIDS: debates in South Africa. Newsletter 20011021, *Health Systems Trust,* Durban, South Africa. Available via DIALOG. http://new.hst.org.za/news/index.php/20011021/ Accessed 13 April 2009

Maugeri TL, Carbon M, Fera MT, Irrrera GP, Gugliandolo C (2004) Distribution of 132

Mead, P.S., Slutsker, L., Dietz, V., McCaig, L.F., Bresee, J.S., Shapiro, C., Griffin, P.M., Tauxe, R.V. (1999). Food-related illness and death in the United States. Emerg Infect Dis., 5, 607-625.

Microbiological Specifications of Food Pathogens. Blackie Academic and Professional, New York. (1996).

Mohammed HO, Stipetic K, McDonough PL, Gonzalez RN, Nydam DV, Atwill ER. Identification of potential on-farm sources of *Listeria monocytogenes* in herds of dairy cattle. Am J Vet Res., 70(3):383-8.

National Advisory Committee on Microbiological Criteria for Foods. (1991). *Listeria monocytogenes*. Recommendations by The National Advisory Committee on Microbiological Criteria for Foods. *International Journal of Food Microbiology* 14 (3-4): 185-246.

Nwachukwu, N.C., Orji, F.A., and Amaike, J.I. (2009). Isolation and Characterisation of *Listeria monocytogenes* from Kunu, a locally produced beaverage marketed in different markets in Abia State of Nigeria. Austraian Journal of Basic and Applied sciences, 3,(4): 4432 - 4436.

Nwachukwu, N.C., Orji, F.A., Iheukwumere, and Ekeleme, U.G. (2010). Antibiotic resistant environmental isolates of *Listeria monocytogenes* from anthropogenic lakes in Lokpa-Ukwu, Abia State of Nigeria. *Australian Journal of Basic and Applied Sciences*, 4(7): 1571-1576.

Obi CL, Igumbor JO, Momba MNB, Samie A (2008). Interplay of factors involving chlorine dose, turbidity flow capacity and pH on microbial quality of drinking water in small treatment plants. Water SA 34: 565-572.

Obi CL, Momba MNB, Samie A et al (2007) Microbiological, physico-chemical and management parameters on the efficiency of small water treatment plants in the Limpopo and Mpumalanga Provinces of South Africa. Water SA 33: 229-237

Paillard D, Dubois V, Thiebaut R et al (2005) Occurrence of *Listeria* spp. in effluents of French urban wastewater treatment plants. Appl Environ Microbiol 71: 7562-7566

Poyart, C., Trieu-Cuott, P., and Berche, P. (1996). The inlA gene required for cell invasion is conserved and specic to *L. monocytogenes*. Microbiology, 142, 173-180.

Quinn P.J., Carter M.E., Markey B. & Carter G.R. (1999). Clinical Veterinary Microbiology. Mosby International, Edinburgh, Scotland, UK.

Quinn P.J., Carter M.E., Markey B.K., Carter G.R. (1999). *Listeria* species. In: Quinn P.J., Carter M.E., MarkeyB.K, Carter G.R. (editors). *Clinical Veterinary Microbiology*. Mosby, Edinburgh, p. 170-174.

Ryser, E.T. & Marth, E.H. (1991). *Listeria*, Listeriosis & Food Safety. New York, Marcel Dekker.

Simon, C. M., Gray, D. I., Cook, N. (1996): DNA Extraction and PCR Methods for the Detection of *Listeria monocytogenes* in Cold-smoked Salmon. Appl. Env. Microbiol. **62**: 822-824

Slutsker L, and Schuchat A. (1999). Listeriosis in humans. In *Listeria, Listeriosis and Food Safety*, eds ET Ryser and EH Marth, 75-95. New York: Marcel Dekker, Inc. Available in Docket No. 1999N-1168, Volume 0018 bkg1 (15 of 17), Tab 389

Swanson, K.M.J. 2005. *L. monocytogenes* Challenge Study "How To" Guidelines. Food Safety Magazine. June/July 2005.

U.S. Food and Drug Administration, and U.S. Food Safety and Inspection Service. (2003). Quantitative Assessment of the Relative Risk to Public Health from Foodborne *Listeria monocytogenes* Among Selected Categories of Ready-to-Eat Foods.

U.S. Food and Drug Administration. 2003. Chapter 10. *Listeria monocytogenes*. Detection and Enumeration of *Listeria monocytogenes* in Foods. In *Bacteriological Analytical Manual Online*.

Vishal, S.P. (2004). Zoonotoc aspects of *Listeria monocytogenes. M.Sc. thesis submitted to Department of food Hygiene. Swedish University of Agricultural Sciences.*

Walsh, D., Duffy, G., Sheridan, J.J., Blair S.I. and McDowell D.A. (2001). Antibiotic, *Listeria* including *Listeria monocytogenes* in: Retail foods, Journal of Applied and Environmental Microbiology, 90: 517 - 520.

Yutaka, S., S. Naohira, D. Yohei and A. Yoshichika, 2004. *Escherichia coli* Producing CT X-m-z-betalactamase in cattle in Japan. Emerg. Infect. Dis., 10(1): 69-75.

Part 4

New Technologies

9

Linkages Between Clean Technology Development and Environmental Health Outcomes in Regional Australia

Susan Kinnear[1] and Lisa K. Bricknell[2]
[1]*Sustainable Regional Development Programme, Centre for Environmental Management, CQUniversity,*
[2]*School of Health and Human Services, Faculty of Sciences, Engineering and Health; CQUniversity, Australia*

1. Introduction

1.1 What is 'cleantech'?

By technical definition, clean technology (also referred to as 'cleantech' or 'eco-innovation') reflects 'a diverse range of technologies, products, services and processes that measure, reduce, eliminate or remediate negative environmental impact, and/or improve the productive and responsible use of natural resources while returning a profit to the provider' (DEEDI 2010). However, more simply defined, a clean technology practice, product or industry is typically one that combines the three essential components of efficiency, environmental outcomes, and profitability. Consequently, the focus for clean technology development is usually about the simultaneous pursuit of increased profitability as well as environmental benefit.

1.2 Current status of the cleantech industry

At the global level, clean technology is being embraced across all business and industry sectors. Indeed, 'cleantech' is now often considered as an industry in its own right. In 2010, the Australian cleantech review identified a number of national cleantech industry sub-sectors, including renewable energy, water, waste and recycling, energy efficiency, carbon trading and environmental services (ACT, 2010). At the global scale, significant investment in cleantech is already occurring in both developing and developed economies; with the Americas, Asia and – to a lesser extent – Europe dominating the market in terms of venture capital expenditure (ACT, 2010; 2011; Cleantech Group 2011). The Australian clean technology industry is still emerging, but it is a rapidly growing sector: in 2011, Australian cleantech companies had combined revenue of $22 billion, and employed over 25,000 people (ACT, 2010). This represents more than doubling in the value of the sector as well as an increase of some 12,000 jobs since 2010 (ACT 2010). Recent data show that the national emphasis in cleantech is currently centred on solar, energy efficiency and transport technologies (ACT, 2011). These trends largely mirror those at the global level, where energy efficiency, solar, biofuels and recycling are capturing large investment and interest (Cleantech Group 2011). It is more than coincidental that it is these same industries who are leading the way in terms of transiting countries to a lower-carbon and more environmentally sustainable future: the ongoing policy and economic focus on this area means that 'cleantech' is likely to continue to experience strong growth. Consequently, it will be important that the risks and benefits of this sector be well understood and managed.

1.2.1 The role and importance of 'cleantech' to regional Australia

Australia's regional areas are vital in helping to deliver national goals in social, economic and environmental issues, and they have strong drivers to be sustainable: regional communities represent an important and complex nexus between climate change, population growth, regionalisation, business and industry growth, natural resource management, liveability and land use conflicts. However, many of Australia's regions are facing an important challenge: where economic growth relies solely on industries that consume finite natural resources, a region's economic position can only decline as those resources are extracted (Clement, 2000). Ecological concerns and issues of resource depletion have been largely absent from the management of regional economic development in Australia (Courvisanos, 2009, p. 256). There is now a need to change this trajectory, and establish new regional economies around ecosystem services which enable regional areas to recapture value and create market and consumption niches (Marsden, 2010). Clearly, 'cleantech' is one way of exploring this.

The value of clean technology to regional development has already been demonstrated with clean technology 'hubs' being established in a number of locations worldwide. These areas are characterised by a concentration of industry in one or more clean technology applications. For example, globally significant sites include Denmark (wind power), Jiangsu Province and Baoding in China (solar and biomass energy facilities), India and North Africa (solar power), and Abu Dhabi (a green/renewable energy consortium).

Australia is a developed and technological nation of strong economic standing and one which has the ability to offer a stable operating environment. It is richly endowed with natural resources; it also faces a number of key environmental challenges including those related to energy, water, waste and climate. There are many locations that could host significant developments in the cleantech arena, thus exploiting the natural advantages that Australian regions have for innovation and solving environmental challenges. There are also many factors to support the use of a regional approach to establish and grow Australian cleantech: these include the strong regional drivers for sustainability and the importance of regions in the national innovation agenda. Using a regional-level approach also brings cleaner production and environmental gains almost by default: for example, the recovery, reuse and/or substitution of raw input materials with locally sourced alternatives reduces transport emissions and encourages recycling (van Berkel, 2007). Furthermore, 'green' businesses and industries tend to be established in response to local markets for sustainable goods and services (Chapple and Hutson, 2010). Despite these features and benefits, remarkably few cleantech hubs (or clusters) are yet to exist in Australia. This is likely to change as the economic and environmental drivers for cleantech in regional Australia are increasingly recognised, and as policy imperatives in the areas of carbon, renewable energy targets and other sustainability goals are pursued. However, cleantech hubs are now beginning to be viewed not only for their commercial potential and their ability to respond to environmental challenges, but also for their ability to blend social challenges and issues into existing decision-making by industry (Horwitch and Mulloth, 2010). Perhaps one of the most important social elements of cleantech that is yet to be properly investigated and exploited is the possible effects on public and occupational environmental health outcomes.

2. Environmental health and industry in regional Australia

In 2006, the World Health Organisation (WHO) published estimates on the environmental burden of disease. Here, the WHO researchers attempted to determine the proportion of global disease that could be prevented through environmental modification, specifically with respect to the following:

- air, soil and water pollution with chemicals or biological agents;
- ultraviolet and ionising radiation;
- built environment;
- noise and electromagnetic fields;
- occupational risks;
- agricultural methods, including irrigation schemes;
- anthropogenic climate change and ecosystem degradation; and
- individual behaviours related to the environment, such as hand washing, food contamination with unsafe water or dirty hands.

According to the report, "an estimated 24% of the global disease burden and 23% of all deaths can be attributed to environmental factors". As part of this research, the WHO has also published profiles for each of its member states, detailing the impact that environmental factors have on health in terms of deaths and disability adjusted life years (DALYs) lost. The figures for Australia indicate that outdoor air pollution is the most significant risk factor for environmentally related morbidity and mortality, with an estimated 700 deaths per annum and 0.2 DALYs /1,000 people/ year attributable to these exposures (WHO 2009).

Industry has long been known to adversely affect the health of communities living in surrounding regions. While it is clear that the entirety of the environmental burden of disease identified by the WHO cannot be attributed solely to industry, there is ample evidence to illustrate the significant effects that industrial activity can have upon human health. Perhaps the best known example of this is the fishing village of Minamata in Japan, where a chemical manufacturing plant released methylmercury-contaminated waste into the bay. The impacts were wide ranging, including severe neurological effects and birth defects as well as the effective destruction of the local fishing industry, the traditional basis of the town's economy (Tsuda et al., 2009).

Australian examples of industry-linked health impacts include the excessive blood lead levels identified in children and adults residing in Australian smelter towns such as Mt Isa (Queensland Health 2008), Port Pirie (Wilson et al. 1986) and Broken Hill (Boreland & Lyle

2009). In these towns, the smelting process has released airborne lead for decades, resulting in significant levels of soil contamination. This has consequently led to a significant increase in blood lead level, particularly in children (Boreland & Lyle 2009; Queensland Health 2008; Wilson et al., 1986).

These examples are consistent with the results published by the WHO, indicating that industrial air pollution and the related deposition of contaminants is of concern with respect to the health of communities located in some industrialised regions of Australia. A report by the Bureau of Transport and Regional Economics (BTRE, 2005) also noted that rural and regional Australia is particularly challenged by managing windblown dust from mining and agriculture, including smoke and agricultural sprays. There are also a number of other environmental health outcomes in Australia that are impacted upon by industry, including:

- water quality, particularly natural aquifers: for example, recent growth in the development of the coal seam gas industry in central and south-eastern Queensland has been associated with groundwater contamination (Moran & daCosta 2011)
- noise and odour problems: complaints to environmental heath regulatory agencies often arise as a consequence of population growth into declining industrial areas. Unfortunately, the pre-existing industries tend to be older facilities with less investment in environmental controls, thus resulting in residents' exposure to odour, noise and pollutants.
- vapour intrusions: contamination of soil and groundwater by volatile organic compounds can be the result of spills, leaks and past disposal practices from previous industrial activity. These compounds can leak into dwellings built on past industrial sites through pores and cracks in soil and foundations and present a risk to the health of residents (Evans et al., 2010)

In addition to these, in the long term, anthropogenic climate change (i.e., that resulting from high levels of greenhouse gas emissions from industry) has been predicted to impact upon health in a variety of ways. Some examples include heat-related mortality and morbidity (e.g., heatstroke in the elderly); waterborne diseases relating to a reduction in water quality associated with reduced riverine flows; flood- related deaths, injuries and economic impacts relating to rainfall events of greater intensity; increased food-borne disease related to temperature increases and the spread of vector-borne disease, particularly dengue fever, Ross River virus infection and potentially malaria (McMichael et al., 2002).

3. Establishing cleantech hubs to help drive healthy regions

The basic relationship between emerging 'cleantech' industries and environmental health outcomes has been recognised for over a decade: it was succinctly described in 1998 by the World Resources Institute:

"A long-term strategy for preventing exposure to hazardous industrial pollutants is to reduce their use in the first place through cleaner production… industry must reduce raw material inputs - chemicals, natural resources, energy, water - and at the same time reduce air, water, and solid pollutants for each unit of production. This push toward cleaner production is typically driven by environmental and economic concerns rather than by health concerns, although it seems certain that cleaner production would benefit public health as well' (WRI et al., 1998, online source).

However, according to Briggs (2003), the actual associations between environmental pollution and health outcomes are complex and often poorly characterized. Partly, this may be due to the emerging nature of the 'cleantech' industry, but it is also likely to reflect the particularly complex nature of relationships between industry and environmental health. As Briggs noted, this is a difficult field of study with 'long latency times, the effects of cumulative exposures, and multiple exposures to different pollutants which might act synergistically' (Briggs, 2003, p. 1). For example, even the public health outcomes of a particular industry sub-sector may be contrasted by the different scales in developed compared with developing nations. A case in point is the clean technology that is being rapidly adopted by advanced nations (e.g., US, Japan), as well as in developing economies (China, India, Africa). The latter nations are likely to experience particularly strong environmental health benefits from this growth, since developing nations often experience high 'baseline' health risks from industrial pollution: this results from a lack of investment in modern technology, combined with less-stringent environmental regulations that allow high pollutant loads (Briggs, 2003).

Another difficulty in measuring the health impacts of clean technology are temporal and spatial influences. There are large differences in the nature and extent of the short-term health impacts (0-5 years) that might result from clean technology adoption, compared with those in the long-term (20+ years). For example, in the short-term, benefits may flow from reduced noise, water and air pollution burdens and the direct impacts of these would be relatively easy to measure. In one recent case, Hixson et al. (2010) performed modelling of emissions to 2030 in order to examine the likely public exposures to air pollution under different regional planning, land use and transportation scenarios. On the other hand, in the long-term, clean technology may contribute to climate change mitigation, thus driving vastly improved health outcomes. However, isolating and quantifying the specific role of 'clean' industries in achieving this would prove extremely difficult. Similarly, pinpointing the health benefits of large-scale industrial changes in (for example) air pollution will require a strong understanding of airshed issues and an appreciation of how a local area may be impacted by weather and other influences: pollutants (especially airborne materials) dissipate with distance, so human populations that are located more closely to the source will naturally experience greater impacts (US EPA, 2010).

These kinds of experimental and analytical difficulties means that the relationship(s) between clean technology development (clean, green business technologies and behaviours) and public health outcomes are poorly articulated, and are likely to remain so for some time. Nevertheless, the discussion below attempts to begin identifying some of keyways in which clean technology can impact upon environmental health outcomes, with respect to both the general population as well as the cleantech workforce.

3.1 Direct and indirect health benefits

There are a number of ways that development and/or adoption of cleantech technologies and practices can assist with improving environmental health outcomes, and these can be both direct and indirect. At its ultimate level, the development of clean technology industries may displace entire sectors (e.g., coal-fired power generation), thus removing the impacts associated with them either in the workplace, or in surrounding communities. For example, a study is already underway to examine the excess burden of respiratory disease, mental health disorders, cancer, injury and death that is associated with coal mining in the Hunter Valley and Liverpool Plains regions in Australia, including impacts on social health and sense of community. This work will help to identify the environmental health risks of the conventional resource industries, thereby helping to quantify the nature and extent of health benefits that could be expected when those operations are replaced with industries of a different 'cleantech' kind.

At a more modest level, introducing 'cleantech' into existing industries through retrofitting or changed operational and behavioural practices can also introduce employee and public health benefits. Where safer, less toxic, or non-toxic chemical alternatives can be identified and used in place of environmentally hazardous substances, a reduction in chemical waste and public exposures should follow (LCSP, 2010). A good example of this is the use of biofuels: Traviss et al. (2010) reported that employee health risks related to exhaust exposures were much lower when biodiesel blends were used to power heavy-duty equipment, compared with regular petroleum diesel. Industries that adopt cleantech principles may also be able to use existing industrial, commercial or domestic waste as process inputs (e.g., feedstock for bio-energy): this further reduces the public health burden associated with waste management from neighbouring sectors. As cleaner production technologies lead to greater efficiency in natural resource and energy use, they are also usually linked with decreases in the amounts and toxicity of generated waste products (Kohler, 1998). A key example of the reduction of air pollutants with clean energy generation, especially fine particulate matter (PM_{25}), volatile organic compounds and ozone, which have each been linked with both respiratory and cardiovascular illnesses and death (US EPA, 2010). Other benefits that may result from reduced pollution, disease and injury burdens as a result of new, clean industries are summarised in Table .

One of the most specific studies into the public health benefits of developing a 'cleantech' culture focussed not on the industrial sector, but instead on the advantages of energy efficiency initiatives in residential buildings. Wilksinson et al. (2009) reported that a mix of actions designed to improve the energy efficiency of UK housing stock would be associated with 850 fewer DALYs per million head of population in one year. The study concluded that there are therefore 'important co-benefits in pursuing health and climate goals' (Wilkinson et al., 2009, p. 1917).

In a more indirect sense, clean technology - through its focus on environmental efficiency - may lead to new techniques in impact assessment, life-cycle analysis, auditing and risk assessment: this helps to culture of awareness and understanding that can lead to reduced exposures in the workplace as well as the general community (Kohler, 1998). Moreover, even in the absence of process or technological changes, existing industries may be able to embrace cleantech by committing to greater environmental monitoring and reporting. This in itself may contribute to improved public health benefits in the long-term, through development of an evidence base that will allow a better understanding of the linkages between 'conventional' versus cleantech-based resource use or development and public

'Clean tech' practice (behaviour or technology adoption)	Possible environmental health benefits
Use of integrated pest management in place of synthetic agrichemicals	Reduced risk of non-target pesticide drift and related respiratory complaints
Agricultural best practice in land management	Reduced runoff and eutrophication, leading to reduced public health risk from toxic algal blooms
Better agricultural efficiencies and productivity	Improved food quality (higher nutritional content, decreased antibiotic use and reduced hormone loads).
Improved water efficiencies at the regional level	Reduced need for river regulation (dams and weirs), thus avoiding climbing salinity levels that are harmful to residents with high blood pressure or are on dialysis treatment.
Introduction of solar technology	Avoidance of cooling towers associated with conventional coal-fired technologies, thus decreasing the risk of harboured Legionnaire's disease.
Improved waste and wastewater management practices	Reduced the load of disease-carrying vectors and pollutants
Improved transport networks, use of regional supply chains	Decrease in regional nitrous oxide emissions

Table 1. Examples of direct human health benefits from adoption of clean technology practices

health. It may also assist in better preparedness and rapid response to environmental hazards on industrial sites. For example, combining wireless sensor networks with web-based real-time data reporting provides an efficient and powerful way to detect health hazards and respond accordingly (Morreale et al., 2010).

Investing in cleantech research and development can also have wider benefits. For example, in agriculture, it has recently been acknowledged that a greater understanding of microbial ecology within livestock will help with reducing greenhouse gas emissions from ruminants; and that these studies may also assist in a better understanding of human health complaints linked with microbial dysfunction (such as inflammatory bowel disease and obesity) (Frank, 2011). Furthermore, technological advances that are engineered for 'cleantech' purposes may also have spillover into health care and treatment: for example, installing high-reliability renewable energy systems in rural, regional and remote areas may enable the operation of advanced health infrastructure (e.g., sensitive health monitoring equipment). One final example of an indirect public health effect of clean technology innovation is the potential for new industries to drive regional job creation and economic growth. In turn, this can lift the unemployment rate and thus cause flow-on advantages in terms of overcoming the socio-economic disadvantage that is typically linked with poor health outcomes. Since it has been shown that that work can be beneficial for people's physical and emotional wellbeing (ABS, 2011), this is a positive public health result.

3.2 Environmental health risks of cleantech

Unfortunately, there may also be some disadvantages associated with cleantech in terms of public health risks. In Australia, the potentially negative health impacts of wind farms has attracted significant interest; with a recent Senate report being published on the potential social and economic impacts of these facilities (CARC, 2011). This document noted the potential for noise and vibration associated with individual wind turbines and/or wind-based generation facilities to be linked with ill health and poor quality of life. The reported health complaints have predominantly included sleep disturbance and fatigue, headaches, dizziness/vertigo, tinnitus, and ear pressure/pain (CARC, 2011). There has also been discussion on the potential for 'shadow flicker' (caused when sunlight is interrupted by the turbine blades) to be associated with seizures; and for turbines to cause unhealthy exposures to electromagnetic radiation (NHMRC, 2010). However, there continues to be questions over the scientific rigour of each of these claims, with a number of international studies opposing the view that noise, vibration or other aspects of wind farms are linked with health effects (be it either audible or inaudible) (NHRMC, 2010). The Australian senate report thus called for 'adequately resourced epidemiological and laboratory studies of the possible effects of wind farms on human health' to close this knowledge gap (CARC, 2011, p. 9).

There are also some technical (operational) aspects of 'cleantech' where environmentally friendly practices must be carefully deployed so that public health risks are minimized: here, wastewater reuse and recycling and of various solids wastes are two good examples. For example, alternative waste technology (AWT), which involves a range of waste treatment (e.g., incineration) and resource-recovery (e.g. recycling) activities, is an increasingly important part of clean technology systems. Within these, there are a range of complex materials handling and occupational health issues, such as concerns over odour, hazardous emissions, vermin and disease (Hamer, 2003). The re-use of purified wastewater to augment drinking water supplies carries with it a potential increase - albeit a slight one - in the incidence of some human diseases; it also requires additional electricity demand to operate reverse osmosis and ultraviolet disinfection systems as well as the use of chemicals for disinfection (Gardner et al., 2008). However, as many of these issues are also shared by traditional technologies, the use of clean technology in this sense does not necessarily introduce new environmental health risks, excepting facilities that bring new types of wastes (e.g., heavy metals) into the region for processing. This latter may be particularly important in the context of establishing e-waste recycling centres that may deal in regulated waste (e.g., mercury, lead).

4. A regional cleantech case study from Central Queensland

4.1 The Central Queensland region

Building comprehensive business cases for clean technology hubs in regional Australia will require data on not only the economic and environmental benefits that these initiatives can bring, but also the social wellbeing and human health advantages. The following case study therefore attempts to provide an evidence base for the latter, by identifying the likely environmental health implications of establishing a cleantech hub in the central Queensland region. For the purposes of this study, Central Queensland (CQ) will be taken to mean the Fitzroy statistical division, which is located on Queensland's central coast and extends for some way inland. Rockhampton is the major city in the region and other major localities include the industrial and mining areas of Gladstone and Emerald (Figure).

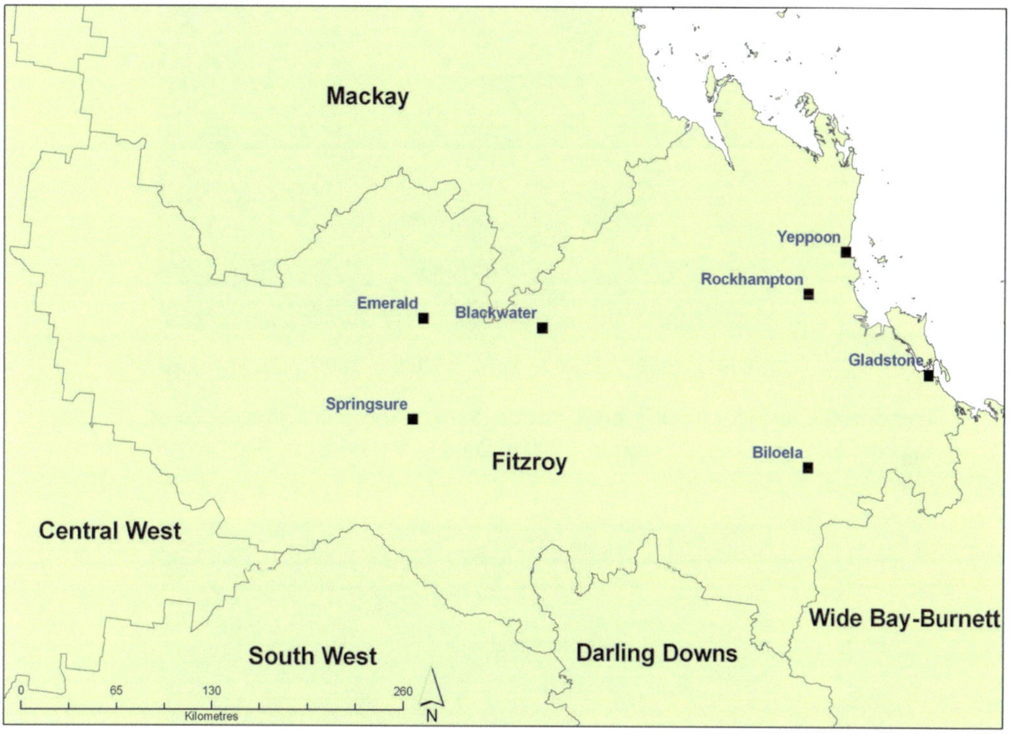

Fig. 1. The Fitzroy Statistical Division (Australian Standard Geographical Classification 2006). Source: provided on request from the Queensland Office of Economic and Statistical Research, Brisbane.

4.2 Climate conditions and climate change

Specific data on climate and climate projections can be difficult to source at the regional level in Queensland. However, with the threat of climate change, this is gradually improving. In 2009, a study by Kinnear et al. (2010) examined the available data for Central Queensland, with the objective of exploring climate change risk for local businesses. This study indicated that historically, CQ has experienced a subtropical climate with wet summers accompanied by low winter rainfall, and coastal areas experiencing a slightly milder climate compared with inland locations. However, the region is showing a warming trend, with hotter seasons (particularly spring and autumn), an increase in the number of days exceeding 35°C, and a decline in periods where temperatures are below 4°C (Fig. 2; Fig. 3). The region has also experienced a steady annual decline in total annual rainfall over the past two decades, but an increase in rainfall intensity (Kinnear et al., 2010).

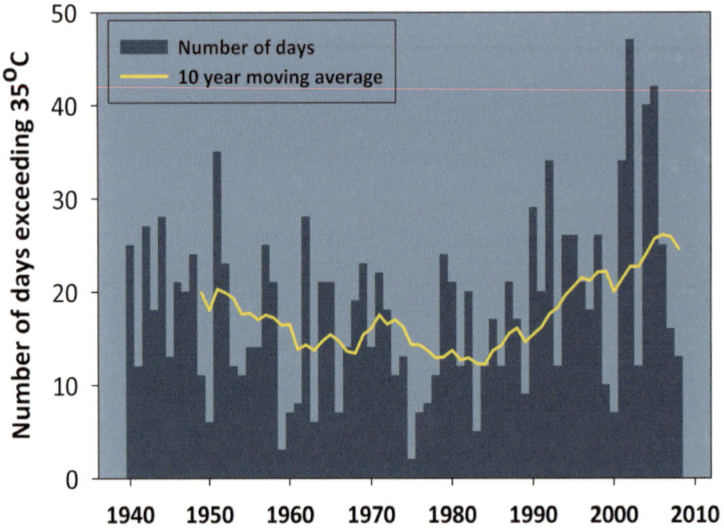

Fig. 2. Trend in the number of extremely hot days (exceeding 35°C) recorded at Rockhampton Aero monitoring station, 1940 to 2008 (adapted from BoM weather data).

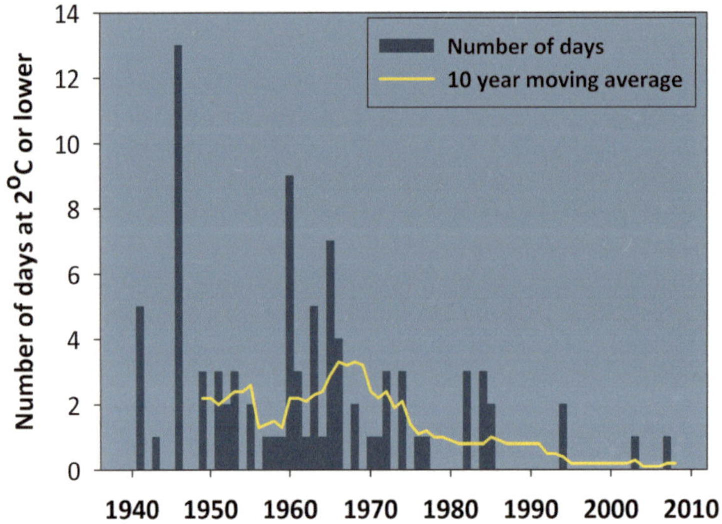

Fig. 3. Trend in the number of extremely cold days (2°C or lower) recorded at Rockhampton Aero monitoring station, 1940 to 2008 (adapted from BoM weather data).

Kinnear et al. (2010) also reported that current climate change modelling, specific for the Rockhampton region, shows that by 2030:

- the average annual temperature in the region is expected to rise by 1°C; and
- there will be a further decline of 50-100mm in annual rainfall (comprised of moderately increased late-summer rainfall and substantial decreases in the remaining three seasons).

A seasonal shift of approximately six weeks is also expected (e.g., 'summer' will be from January-March, rather than December-February); together with a sea-level rise of 18 - 59 cm along the Queensland coast (Kinnear et al., 2010).

4.3 Economic profile and key industry sectors

In economic terms, the key sectors in the Central Queensland regional economy are the mining, construction and manufacturing sectors, which together comprise some 63% of the economic output for the region (Fig.). However, retail trade, manufacturing, and health and community services are also key industries in terms of employment creation; whilst mining, manufacturing and property and business services contribute most significantly to the regional value-add (Fig.). Thus, Central Queensland has a diverse economy built on an array of different industries, each playing different, but important roles.

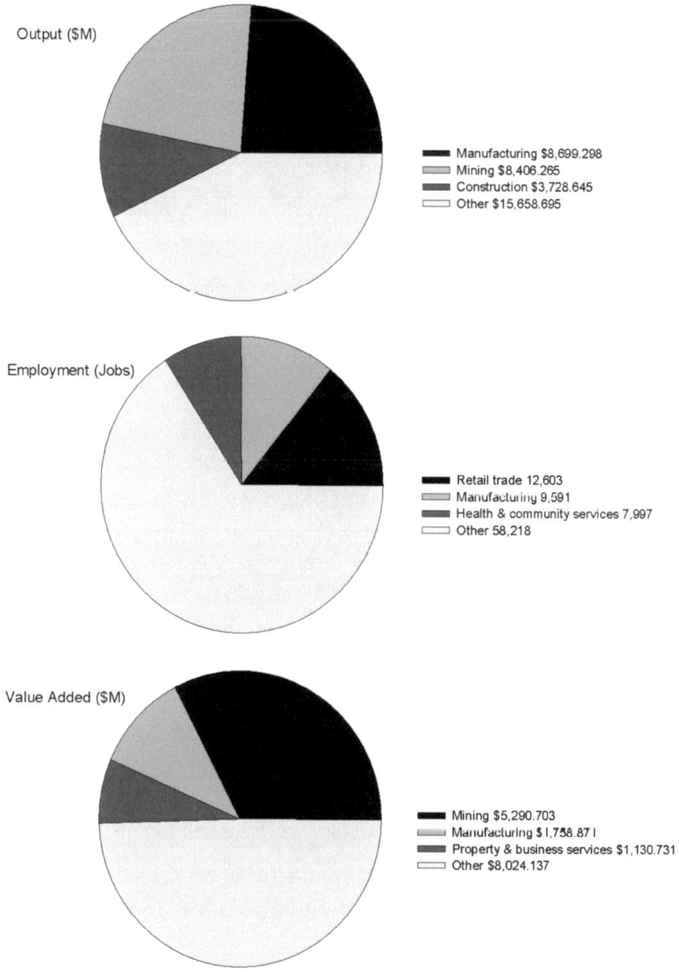

Fig. 4. Analysis of key contributing industries in the Central Queensland region (Fitzroy and Central West Statistical divisions) - economic output, employment, and value-added totals (as at June 2010). Source: REMPLAN Economic Modelling Tool.

4.4 Current and projected socio-demographic statistics

In addition to being an 'economic powerhouse' the CQ region houses a significant percentage of the state's population. The region will grow to 344,938 people by 2031, from a 2006 base population of 206,166 (Table). The region is currently experiencing a loss of young adults, but an increase in the aged population, and both these trends are set to continue (Table). Socio-demographic trends in the CQ population are heavily influenced by the presence of mining and other industrial activity in the Bowen Basin coal and energy reserves. The 2009 reported unemployment rate for Fitzroy statistical division was 5.0% (OESR, 2010). However, based on 2006 Census data[1], over 40% of employed males in the Bowen Basin (more than 38,000 people) work in the mining, construction and/or manufacturing industries, and 80% of these work full time. This is much higher than the Queensland average of only 74% full time. Around one in seven workers (15%) in the Bowen Basin are fly in/ fly out (FIFO) and/or drive in/drive out (DIDO) workers, and this trend for non-resident workers is expected to increase (OESR, 2011).

Age group	As at 30 June					
	2006 ERP	2011	2016	2021	2026	2031
0–4	14,733	17,075	18,696	20,432	21,960	23,531
5–9	15,630	16,254	18,845	20,297	22,149	23,845
10–14	16,504	16,764	17,494	20,108	21,615	23,573
15–19	14,871	16,314	16,458	17,125	19,678	21,192
20–24	14,080	15,895	17,530	17,704	18,630	21,369
25–29	13,221	16,747	18,601	19,906	20,478	21,792
30–34	14,305	15,423	19,140	20,772	22,186	23,088
35–39	14,827	16,305	17,508	21,088	22,848	24,380
40–44	15,817	16,299	17,946	19,131	22,803	24,682
45–49	15,550	16,409	17,268	18,813	20,115	23,805
50–54	13,623	15,302	16,494	17,412	18,936	20,304
55–59	11,894	13,018	14,920	16,093	17,118	18,622
60–64	9,184	11,078	12,605	14,421	15,661	16,766
65–69	7,090	8,464	10,781	12,221	14,049	15,356
70–74	5,428	6,443	8,119	10,393	11,834	13,683
75–79	4,330	4,717	5,916	7,545	9,766	11,205
80–84	2,807	3,507	4,007	5,109	6,632	8,696
85+	2,271	3,161	4,318	5,361	6,859	9,051
Total	206,166	229,173	256,644	283,931	313,314	344,938

Table 2. Projected population by age group, medium series projections, Fitzroy Statistical Division, 2006 to 2031. ERP = Estimated resident population. (Source: Queensland Treasury, Office of Economic and Statistical Research[2])

[1] These are the most recently available data; 2011 Census datacubes are not yet published.

[2] Available online at http://www.oesr.qld.gov.au/regions/fitzroy/tables/proj-pop-series-age-group-sd-qld/proj-pop-series-age-group-fitz-sd.php.

Also based on 2006 Census data, over 15% of employed Indigenous males in the Bowen Basin work in the construction sector, with a similar number working in manufacturing; mining accounts for another 11% of the workforce. Most of the Indigenous workforce of the Bowen Basin receives lower weekly gross incomes than do the remainder of the population.

In 2009, tradespeople and labourers together represented 29.1% of the wage and salary earners by occupation, with production and transport workers representing a further 11.4% (ABS, 2010). This is relevant in an environmental health sense because data from the ABS has shown that the 'the types of risks to which people are exposed in the workplace vary considerably according to the type of job they do and the industry in which they work' (ABS, 2011, p. 3). For example, in 2009-10, the National Health Survey reported that the highest rates of injuries were found among labourers (88 per 1,000), machinery operators and drivers (86 per 1,000), and Technicians and Trades Workers (78 per 1,000); meanwhile, much lower injury rates are found in professionals and managers (42 and 45 per 1,000, respectively) (ABS, 2011). For this reason, encouraging the development of a cleantech workforce - one that is strongly centred on new knowledge creation through sophisticated research and trialling, may suggest that the region could experience a lower overall rate of work-related injuries. Similar trends are also evident for workplace fatalities. Furthermore, a move away from resource-based enterprises may also assist in reducing injuries: national data indicate that the agriculture, forestry and fishing sector had amongst the highest rates of workplace injuries (some 77 injuries per 1,000)(ABS, 2011). The agricultural, fisheries and forestries sectors also suffered the highest fatality rate in 2009-10, followed by mining and construction.

4.5 Key health issues

4.5.1 Population health statistics

Data from the Social Health Atlas of Australia indicate that Fitzroy statistical division generally has poor population health statistics when values are compared with the state and national averages (Table 3). In particular, residents of Fitzroy statistical division suffer higher risk of respiratory system disease, and report high levels of physical inactivity.

4.5.2 Community health concerns

Within the area managed by the Central Queensland Rural Division of General Practice[3], the three major causes of premature mortality are lung cancer, circulatory system diseases, and injuries and poisonings, despite rates of both these being lower than the averages for country Queensland and Australia (PHIDU, 2005a). However, rates of physical inactivity (15+ years) are much higher in the Division (377.4 per 1,000 people) than the State and national averages, as are people with high health risks due to alcohol consumption (64.3 per 1,000 people)(PHIDU, 2005a). Some residents of also have psychological distress levels more than 5% above the Australian average (PHIDU, 2005a).

---

[3] The CQRDGP services nearly 66,000 people living in the region bounded by Moranbah in the north, Theodore in the south and west to the Gemfields, a total of 163,919 km^2.

Average rate per 1,000			
2007-08/synthetic predictions			
Type 2 diabetes	3.6	3.5	3.4
High cholesterol	5.6	5.5	5.6
Males with mental/behavioural problems	10.0	10.4	10.1
Females with mental/behavioural problems	11.9	12.0	11.8
Circulatory system diseases	16.5	16.0	16.0
Respiratory system diseases	24.9	26.0	26.6
Asthma	11.7	11.4	9.7
Chronic obstructive pulmonary disease	2.5	2.4	2.3
Physical inactivity (persons 15 years and over)	38.4	36.9	34.3
Overweight males (persons 18 years and over)	36.8	36.2	36.0
Obese males (persons 18 years and over)	21.7	20.9	19.6
Overweight females (persons 18 years and over)	23.4	23.1	22.7
Obese females (persons 18 years and over)	18.3	17.1	16.4
Average annual rate per 100,000			
Population deaths, (15-64 years), 2003 to 2007			
Deaths from cancer	75.4	74.6	74.9
Deaths from circulatory system diseases	35.3	34.4	35.1
Deaths from respiratory system diseases	8.8	7.4	7.4

Table 3. Summary of selected health statistics in Central Queensland (Fitzroy Statistical Division). Source: adapted from PHIDU (2010). Shaded cells indicate where the Central Queensland region performs poorly compared with the state and/or national averages

For the Capricornia Division of General Practice[4], the population is characterized by a slightly higher proportion of children and young people, and of aged adults (65+ years) in the Rockhampton area; the coastal centre of Gladstone is instead populated by a higher proportion of young adults (35-44 years), more males than females, and a lower proportion of aged adults (65+ years) than the Queensland averages (PHCRIS, 2008). In addition, the Indigenous population of Rockhampton (the 'regional capital') is higher than the national average, and that township also has a greater proportion of people with socioeconomic disadvantage. Lung cancer is by far the leading cause of premature death (before age 75) in the CDGP, at 108.8 per 1,000 people, followed by circulatory disease and injuries and poisonings (PHIDU, 2005c).

Within the broader Bowen Basin area, many subregional areas have a higher proportion of middle aged adults, and sometimes of aged adults. According to Harper *et al.* (2004), the major causes of death and illness in these groups are chronic obstructive pulmonary disease, coronary heart disease, stroke, depression, suicide and self-inflicted injury, diabetes and lung cancer (as reported in Harper *et al.*'s Health Determinants Queensland 2004). The key pressures impacting on the health of the general population in both Central Queensland and Capricornia general practice divisions include harmful alcohol consumption, illicit drug use (Gladstone only), smoking, obesity, diabetes and mental health (including suicide), along with

[4] The Capricornia Division represents over 144 GPs practising in approximately 43 general practices in the Rockhampton, Capricorn Coast and Gladstone areas.

poor nutrition, physical inactivity, high blood pressure and poor vaccination rates (PHCRIS, 2008). Skin cancer detection and treatment is also a key issue given the geographic location of the region and sun exposure, and, for the Capricornia region particularly, rates of cervical cancer screening and asthma management have been raised as key issues (PHCRIS, 2008).

A recent study by Greer et al. (2010) examined community perceptions of the health effects of large industry operating in the Gladstone region. Industrial emissions, air quality and the possible associated human health risks have been a topic of ongoing concern in Gladstone, despite laboratory testing indicated that industry emissions are below levels that are harmful for human health. The report by Greer et al. noted that residents had the highest levels of concern about dust and air quality impacts, including coal dust from the rail and port facilities and odours and caustic vapours from the alumina refinery. Other high-ranking emissions included chemicals, water pollution, fumes, and land pollution.

4.5.3 Industrial and occupational health

In recent years, Central Queensland has had a number of reported health problems that are linked with existing industries. Firstly, in general terms, the key industry sectors upon which the Central Queensland economy is built tend to be those that have high reported rates of occupational hazards. For example, construction, manufacturing and agriculture each feature prominently in the CQ region, and these have consistently recorded the highest rates of workers' compensation claims at the national level (Fig. 5). Interestingly, the coal sector is an industry that often receives strong focus on safety outcomes. However, at the national level, data for lost time injury rates show that the performance of the sector has been steadily increasing in the past decade (Figure 6).

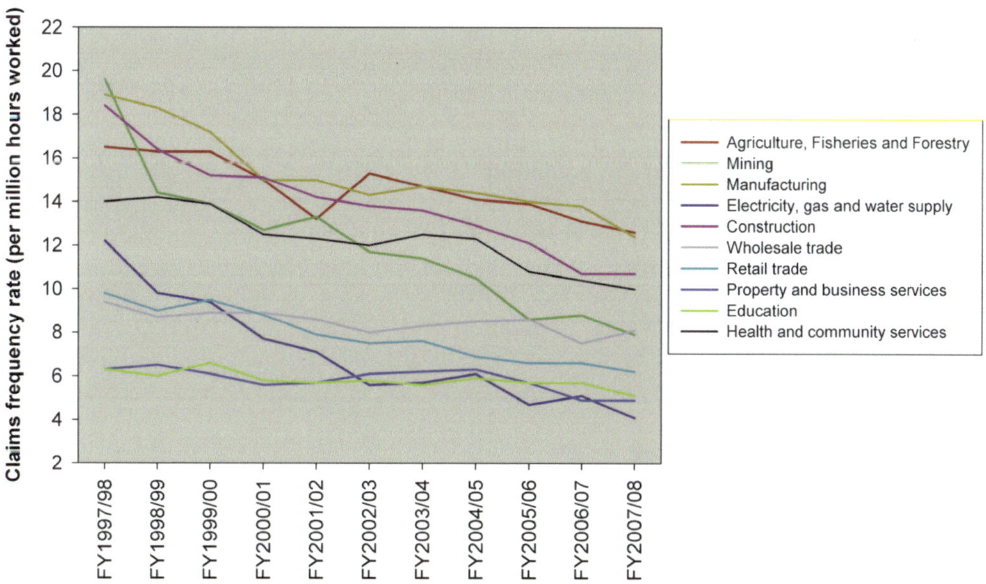

Fig. 5. Frequency Rate (per million hrs worked) of worker's compensation claims for 10 industry sectors relevant to Central Queensland. Data are national values sourced from Safe Work Australia. FY = financial year.

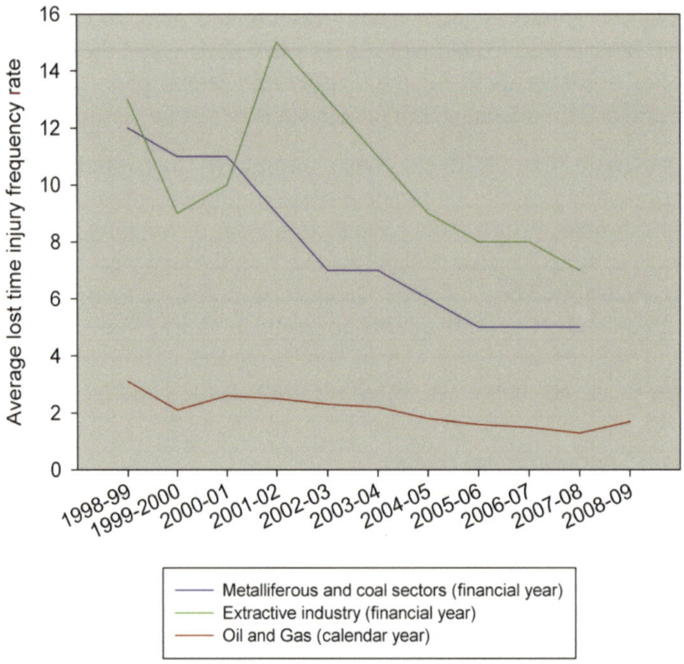

Fig. 6. Average lost time injury frequencies rates for metalliferous, coal, extractive industry and oil and gas sectors. Source: adapted from ABS Category 8417.0 Mining Indicators, Australia, December 2009.

Recent reports have also highlighted some specific problems with key industries. For example, both the mining industry, and the construction, electricity, gas and water industries show a high tendency to have workers that are overweight or obese, with 76% and more than 60% of mining workers in this classification, respectively (ABS 2005).

Secondly, the aluminium industry (both refining and smelting) has been recognised as the most significant contributor to air pollutants in the Gladstone region. According to the National Pollutant Inventory, in 2009-2010 basic non-ferrous metal manufacturing contributed to over 96% of the total 35,365 tonnes of reported carbon monoxide emissions. The industry was also responsible for over 89% of the total 654 tonnes of $PM_{2.5}$, 41% of 42,502t of SO_2 and 22% of a reported 47,815t of oxides of nitrogen (Department of Sustainability, Environment, Water, Population and Communities, 2011). Each of these pollutants is known to cause or contribute to health effects, including respiratory and cardiovascular complaints.

4.6 Establishing a cleantech CQ hub[5]

Simply put, the 'Cleantech CQ' concept refers to a deliberate and strategic effort to attract, develop and/or adopt a concentration of clean technology industries and practices within

[5] This material draws heavily on Susan Kinnear and Ian Ogden, 2010, 'Beyond Carbon: a case study of Cleantech and innovation for sustainable regional development in Central Queensland, *Proceedings of the Social and Economic Growth for Regional Australia (SEGRA) 13th National Conference*, 19-21 October 2010, Townsville, QLD.

the central Queensland region. This might include some or all of retrofitting or redesigning existing industry (including introducing new products and technologies), and/or the establishment of entirely new industries based on better resource efficiencies or resource re-use. Ideally, a culture of environmental awareness and appreciation would develop, and the regional communities would look toward capacity-building in clean technology wherever possible. For example, this might include dedicated cleantech skilling and training programs, as well as new knowledge creation for application in regional industries and/or for export potential. The latter might include the design and creation of novel environmental monitoring devices.

5. The Central Queensland advantage

Central Queensland (CQ) has a number of features that make it particularly attractive and competitive as a region in which clean technology might be developed as a key sector. For example, Central Queensland has exceptionally high demand for clean technology, which results from a combination of pressures including:

- the number of existing and planned heavy industries operating in the region, with all of these under pressure to perform sustainably whilst maintaining profits;
- the high carbon-intensity of the region: one report predicted that Fitzroy Division would bear costs twice as high as any other location in Queensland if carbon trading was introduced[6] (KPMG 2009);
- the location of the region being directly upstream of the Great Barrier Reef, meaning that regional industries are under considerable pressure to improve the water quality flowing through the Fitzroy catchment and onto the GBR lagoon, whilst not sacrificing productivity;
- the pressures of regional climate change (as already described above);
- the need for small businesses to reduce operating costs in order to compete with the mining industry as well as in the global supply chain; and
- since CQ straddles Queensland, cleantech development in the regional transport sector is particularly valuable because of the high costs of transporting goods throughout the region, and into the region from other areas.

Central Queensland also boasts a profile of key physical resources and characteristics that are relevant to developing a Cleantech industry. For example, these include:

- good land availability (including rehabilitated industrial lands and lands accessible to ports and other transport infrastructure);
- a bountiful regional water supply; and
- a number of existing coal-fired power generators, well-developed transmission networks; and a diversity of natural energy resources (including solar, gas fields, and waste products suitable for adaptation into biofuels or other industrial feedstocks).

Central Queensland has a diverse economy built on a wide array of sectors including mining, agriculture, manufacturing and processing (e.g., two significant meat processing

---

[6] Please note that these data were prepared based on the first iteration of the Emissions Trading Scheme, which was later defeated in the Senate.

plants), education, tourism and a regional transport hub: each of these can contribute to the development of a Cleantech industry. Indeed, one of the key strengths of Central Queensland as a Cleantech destination is because the region is not solely linked to the resources sector: CQ also has a range of secondary industries (tourism, transport, SMEs) in which cleantech could be adopted.

A cleantech CQ hub would achieve a natural fit with a number of existing regional planning mechanisms and agendas. For example, the CQ Strategy for Sustainability already has key themes of responding to regional climate change; issues regarding carbon emissions, business resilience and competitiveness; social targets such as community awareness and adoption; and regional coordination. Furthermore, in many respects, establishing such a Hub would not require a huge diversion from existing plans. For example, there are already a number of non-renewable green energy projects planned for Central Queensland, particularly in the area of coal-seam gas generation (Kinnear et al., 2010) (Figure 7).

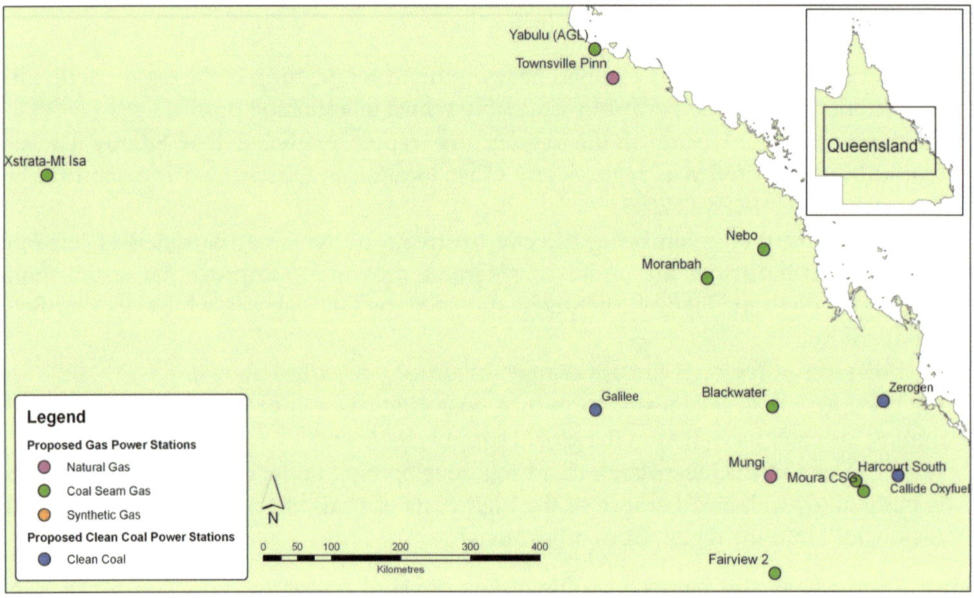

Fig. 7. Planned or proposed clean-coal or natural-gas fired energy generation sites in Central Queensland.

5.1 Potential environmental health benefits from a cleantech CQ hub

Identifying and quantifying the environmental health benefits that may be afforded by a cleantech CQ hub first requires an understanding of the changed regional profile under two future scenarios: one based on a continuation of business as usual (i.e., ongoing expansion of the heavy industry that is already in the region) and the other being the deliberate development of a cleantech CQ hub. This kind of scenario-building can be used in order to conceptualise what environmental health outcomes might be realised across the region, including the comparative health risks and benefits of 'conventional' versus 'cleantech' industry approaches. For CQ, generally speaking, the 'business as usual' scenario is likely to be associated with the continuation of CQ as a resource-based economy (i.e., trading in the mining boom): this would involve strong activity in coal extraction and coal-fired energy production, minerals processing and manufacturing industries, and conventional agriculture. In contrast, a 'cleantech CQ' future would witness the development of the region as an innovative, environmentally-conscious and knowledge-based economy (trading in the "the mind boom"): here, key industries would involve growth in renewable energy, education and skilling, eco-tourism, environmental monitoring and management, new generation agriculture, climate adaptation and mitigation.

Clearly, in the absence of specific data and predictions about the nature and number of new industries, and/or the adaptations that might be embraced by existing industries under a 'cleantech CQ hub', it is very difficult to forecast the specific environmental health benefits that might be associated with this initiative. However, considering the geographic, demographic and socio-economic profile of CQ, there are a number of generic environmental health benefits that could be expected, and some of these are described in further detail below.

5.1.1 Direct regional impacts

Establishing a 'Cleantech CQ' hub could be linked with a number of specific and direct environmental health benefits in the region. For example, the hub may foster a regional culture that incentivizes existing polluting industries to perform more cleanly - thus reducing aerosols such as coal dust, NOx, SOx, and VOCs. For example, the 'Clean and Healthy Air for Gladstone' project was largely initiated due to concerns voiced in the community. Of note here is that the Yarwun alumina refinery in Central Queensland will more than double its production capacity in 2012. While the emissions from this site can be expected to increase accordingly, advances in technology ('cleantech') should ensure that this is not at a proportionate scale. Furthermore, one of the major sources of pollutants in the alumina industry is linked with the intensive electricity demand by the refining process. Traditionally, this electricity has been provided by coal-fired plants. However, the Yarwun 2 refinery is powered by a gas-fired cogeneration plant to produce steam and power for the operation, emitting significantly less CO_2 and particulate matter than a comparable coal-fired plant (Bechtel 2011).

More data are needed on the benefits that might flow from the ability of a cleantech hub to help the regional community mitigate and adapt to climate change. This will be important information given that regional predictions for CQ point to warmer and drier temperatures, both of which pose health issues.

5.1.2 Indirect regional impacts

In terms of indirect impacts, the cleantech hub can be used as a driver for economic prosperity, particularly in the western subregional areas of central Queensland, which are currently underperforming in terms of economic development. Where a regional cleantech hub contributes to overall increase in employment, as well as to better wage conditions, then general improvements in public health could be expected, because lower socio-economic status has been shown to be linked with poor health outcomes. Thus, as fewer regional residents are unemployed and a greater proportion of the region receive higher wages, an improvement in health indicators should follow. This would be especially true if project components could be developed specifically within the Woorabinda Aboriginal Shire Council area, where health and income statistics are extremely poor. The hub would also provide for economic diversity, therefore reducing dependency on the coal mining industry - the latter being associated with poor liveability and poor health outcomes in terms of fatigue, depression, heart disease and domestic violence.

5.1.3 Impacts at other scales

The environmental health benefits of a cleantech hub in CQ will manifest at regional, national and global scales. As an example, changed climatic conditions have been predicted to impact upon agricultural production across Australia- one example being an increased potential for mycotoxin contamination of grains intended for human and animal consumption (Bricknell, 2008). The reduction in greenhouse gas emissions associated with cleantech hubs have the potential to contribute to a reduction or slowing of this effect, depending on the scale and extent of their operations.

A present, the nature of such impacts is speculative, as the ability of practitioners and decision-makers to clearly identify and quantify them is extremely limited. Furthermore, the relative importance of these will decrease in that order: whilst it is possible that the regional health impacts may be specific and (in time) measurable, any contribution to national and international health parameters will always be vague and very limited, given the scale and complexity of natural, industrial and human systems at those levels.

6. Future directions for cleantech and environmental health

6.1 Research and knowledge gaps

Clean technology development has a potentially significant role in optimising both direct and indirect environmental health outcomes. Clearly, at the regional level, the nature of any public health risks or benefits of cleantech will be dependent on:

- the type of clean technologies adopted
- the type of existing industry they replace (if any); and
- the regional profile in terms of
    - climate (including expected climate change);
    - population demographics (especially in terms of proportions of very young, very old, and indigenous subgroups, and how these are expected to change in coming decades); and
    - the pre-existing and/or prevalent health conditions within the region (particularly respiratory complaints).

However, the knowledge and data in this space is very limited and needs to grow: there are a paucity of studies on the health impacts of existing industry, as well as the health benefits of newer or alternative technologies. Consequently, specific figures on the health conditions that are reduced or avoided through the regionally wide adoption of cleaner technologies (such as in a regional 'hub' approach) are extremely difficult to calculate.

The environmental health benefits of cleantechnology development need to be included as part of the overall business case and argument for cleantech hubs, particularly in rural-regional areas of Australia where poorer health outcomes may be evident. However, detailed datasets and modelling will be required in order to gain a clear picture of the risks and benefits of the development of cleantech industries at the regional-level. Fortunately, the increasing focus on carbon and other greenhouse gas emissions is accelerating research in this space. For example, work on the use of geographic information systems (GIS) to collect and analyse data on the health impacts of vehicle emissions, including the role of key parameters such as population, baseline mortality and background air quality, is already underway (ICCT, 2011).

Future research in this space should be centred on answering questions such as:

- what is known about the links between economic development/resource use and environmental health outcomes in the regional areas of Australia?
- what are the key issues that need to be addressed for better regional environmental health outcomes, and how might these be actioned?

Furthermore, a greater focus needs to be dedicated to our understanding of the crossovers between ecological and environmental health, and how these could be better pursued simultaneously. There is also a need to develop (or adapt existing) methodologies to quantify the environmental health benefits of clean technology development and adoption. For example, a simple method might be to compare lost time injury rates of conventional coal-fired power stations with those of renewable energy generators, thus describing the actual value of the occupational health outcomes. The US EPA (2010) has pioneered a staged approach to estimating the environmental and health benefits of clean energy options, comprising a four-step process as detailed below:

1. Develop and project a baseline emissions profile (compiling air pollutants and/or greenhouse gases from available sources into an inventory and develop a forecast);
2. Quantify air and greenhouse gas emission reductions from clean energy measures (noting the operating characteristics of the clean energy resources, and profiling the impacts when they occur);
3. Quantify the air quality impacts by using air pollutant data in an air quality model; and
4. Quantify the human health (and related economic effects) through a combination of air quality changes data, epidemiological and population information; and economic values of avoided health effects (US EPA, 2010, p. 99).

However, this kind of study remains very data-intensive, which is a discouragement to local planning authorities.

6.2 Policy and planning implications

There are a number of international examples that highlight the policy implications of the linkages between regional development, cleantech growth and public environmental health outcomes. For example, Mead (2011) recently commented on the positive health outcomes that would result from the Chinese policy shift towards clean energy technology, renewable energy targets and national fuel efficiency standards; together with more stringent enforcement of existing laws in pollution abatement, resource conservation and ecological management. Mead (2011) noted that one of the key drivers for China's investment in these areas was the high premature death rates linked with outdoor and indoor pollution from energy generation: this is a clear example of environmental health concerns being a key driver for policy, despite the fact that the specific health outcomes (benefits) that may result from a cleaner Chinese energy production system have not yet been described.

In the Australian context, some industries are already required to report annually on various statistics related to employee safety (e.g. lost time injury rates), but not on public health risks associated with their operations. On the other hand, since 2007, many companies have been mandated to participate in the National Greenhouse and Energy Reporting System (NGERS), which reports greenhouse gas emissions. Proposals for significant new projects are required to undertake detailed environmental and social impact assessment processes, including information on the possible health implications (noise, odours, air and water pollution) of their operations. However, this process could be strengthened by asking for an identification of viable fuel and process alternatives, together with a consideration of the differing public health benefits that would be associated with each.

Establishing new planning strategies for the development of cleantech hubs may help to bring forward new ways of scanning the multiple and cumulative impacts of key industries operating in a region, and encourage coordination in the way these risks are measured and managed. Consideration also needs to be given to the planning and environmental health implications of 'cleantech hubs' and how these should be recognised and managed in the pre-developmental phase. For example, in Australia, it has recently been acknowledged that the National Wind Farm Development Guidelines should be redrafted to include provisions for adverse health effects (CARC, 2001). Furthermore, following a study of future air pollution emissions in the San Joaquin Valley region of central California, Hixson et al. (2010, p. 11) recommended that 'regional planning agencies should develop thresholds of population-weighted primary emissions exposure to guide the development of growth plans'. Finally, clean technology industries should also be developed with a consideration of how environmental health (and indeed, other socioeconomic) benefits can be maximised, such as deliberate attraction of an Indigenous workforce, strategic placement of operational sites, and optimal use of regional resource bases (including waste).

7. Conclusions

Developing a 'cleantech' sector is an excellent way to advance the sustainable regional development agenda in Australia. The development of cleantech hubs in regional settings have the potential to solve not only environmental issues, but also environmental health issues, and in turn, regional development issues (e.g., relieving pressure on regional health and services infrastructure in the long-term). In its widest sense, cleantech urges a shift in economic development thinking, from one of growth based on natural resource extraction and/or utilization, to instead the building of knowledge- and skills-based economies that do not require drawdown on, or damage to, natural assets. In this sense, public health gains are achieved by default, as the health complaints linked with conventional mining, energy production or other resource development and transport systems are avoided. Unfortunately, there are few specific examples of the human health outcomes that are linked with clean technology. A review of the existing works suggests that in terms of occupational health, the key benefits of cleantech are likely to be predominantly linked with a decrease in workplace risk factors related to cancers (carcinogenic exposures), respiratory disease (air emissions), and accidents. Meanwhile, in terms of wider public environmental health, the role of cleantech in decreasing air emissions burden is likely to be significant, especially where this reduces hazardous emissions associated with heavy industrial operations and coal-fired electricity generation.

A cleantech CQ hub is one way that Central Queensland can simultaneously address goals of sustainability, productivity, innovation, regional competitiveness and strengthened communities. The CQ region is uniquely placed to resource and support a vibrant cleantech sector, but to date, the value of this development has only ever been considered from an economic and environmental (ecological) perspective. This case study has helped to highlight the linkages between ecological and human health effects, as well as identify examples of the likely environmental health benefits (both employee and public) that might be expected to occur under the development of a regional cleantech hub. However, far more studies are required if a strong case for clean technology is ever to be based on its environmental health advantages.

8. References

ABS (Australian Bureau of Statistics). (2010) *National Regional Profile: Fitzroy (Statistical Division)*, Australian Bureau of Statistics, Canberra, available online at www.abs.gov.au.

ABS (2011) *Australian Social Trends June 2011 Work and Health,* Australian Bureau of Statistics, Canberra, 10 pages, available online at www.abs.gov.au/socialtrends.

ACT (Australian CleanTech). (2011) *Australian Cleantech Review, 2010 Industry Status and Forecast Trends,* Australian Cleantech, Goodwood, South Australia, April 2011.

ACT (Australian CleanTech). (2010) *Australian Cleantech Review, 2010 Industry Status and Forecast Trends,* Australian Cleantech, Goodwood, South Australia, April 2010.

Bricknell, L.K. (2008) Bricknell, LK (2008) Aflatoxins in Australian maize: potential implications of climate change Proceedings of the 10th International Federation of Environmental Health World Congress "*Environmental health: a sustainable future, 20 years on*" Brisbane.

Briggs, D. (2003) Environmental pollution and the global burden of disease. *British Medical Bulletin,* 68, 1-24.

CARC (Australian Senate Community Affairs References Committee). (2011) *The Social and Economic Impact of Rural Wind Farms,* Commonwealth of Australia, ISBN 978-1-74229-462-9.

Boreland, F & Lyle, D (2009) 'Using performance indicators to monitor attendance at the Broken Hill blood lead screening clinic', *Environmental Research,* 109(3), 267-72.

BTRE (Bureau of Transport and Regional Economics), 2005, Health impacts of transport emissions in Australia: economic costs. BTRE Working paper 63, Australian Department of Transport and Regional Services, 169 pages, available online at http://www.bitre.gov.au/publications/94/Files/wp63.pdf

Chapple, K. & Hutson, M. (2010) *Innovating the Green Economy in California Regions,* Centre for Community Innovation, University of California, Berkeley, 180 pages.

Cleantech Group. (2011) *Global Cleantech '10 100 A barometer of the changing face of global cleantech innovation,* San Francisco, 48 pages, available online at http://www.cleantech.com/wp-content/uploads/2010-Global-Cleantech-100-Report.pdf

Chapple, K. & Hutson, M. (2010) Innovating the Green Economy in California Regions. pp. 180 pages. Centre for Community Innovation, University of California, Berkeley.

Clement, K. (2000) *Economic development and environmental gain European Environmental Integration and Regional Competitiveness.* Earthscan Publications Limited, London.

Courvisanos, J. (2009) Innovation Policy and Social Learning: An Economic Framework for Sustainable Development in Regional Australia. *Climate Change in Regional Australia: Social Learning and Adaptation* (eds J. Martin, M. Rogers & C. Winter), pp. 256-281. Victorian Universities Regional Research Network Press, Ballarat, Australia.

DEEDI (Queensland Department of Employment, Economic Development and Innovation), 2010, *Queensland Cleantech Industry Development Strategy, Issues Paper: Growing Queensland's Cleantech Industry*, April 2010.

Department of Sustainability, Environment, Water, Population and Communities (2011) National Pollutant Inventory, Commonwealth of Australia, viewed 4 August 2011, <http:/www.npi.gov.au/>Moran, C.J. & daCosta, J. 2011 *Summary of considerations and recommendations on the Environmental Evaluations of Cougar Energy* Report of the Independent Scientific Panel on Underground Coal Gasification, Queensland Government, Brisbane Available online at , <http://www.derm.qld.gov.au/environmental_management/ucg/documents/cougar-energy-report.pdf>

Frank, D. N. (2011) Growth and Development Symposium: promoting healthier humans through healthier livestock: animal agriculture enters the metagenomics era. *Journal of animal science,* 89, 835-844.

Gardner, T., Yeates, C. and Shaw, R. 2008 *Purified recycled water for drinking: the technical issues* Queensland Water Commission, available online at <http://www.qwc.qld.gov.au/prw/pdf/prw-technical-issues.pdf>

Greer, L., Akbar, D., Rolfe, J. & Mann, J. (2010) *Gladstone industry – community perception study 2010,* CQUniversity Centre for Environmental Management, Rockhampton, 85 pages.

Hamer, G. 2003, Solid waste treatment and disposal: effects on public health and environmental safety, *Biotechnological Advances 22(1-2)*: 71-9.

Hixson, M., Mahmud, A., Hu, J., Bai, S., Niemeier, D. A., Handy, S. L., Gao, S., Lund, J. R., Sullivan, D. C., Kleeman, M. J. (2010). Influence of Regional Development Policies and Clean Technology Adoption on Future Air Pollution Exposure. *Atmospheric Environment* 44 (4), 552 - 562. KPMG (2009) *Carbon Outlook Final Report,* Prepared for Queensland Department of Employment, Economic Development and Innovation, Brisbane, 212 pages.

Horwitch, M. & Mulloth, B. (2010) The interlinking of entrepreneurs, grassroots movements, public policy and hubs of innovation: The rise of Cleantech in New York City. *Journal of High Technology Management Research,* 21, 23-30.

ICCT (International Council on Clean Transportation), 2011, *Estimating Current Global Health Impacts of Vehicle Emissions*, available online at http://www.theicct.org/2011/07/intern-global-health-assessment/

Kinnear, S., Mann, J. & Miles, B. (2010) Uncertainty as an impediment to climate action: a regional analysis of climate change and business preparedness in Rockhampton, Central Queensland. *The International Journal of Climate Change: Impacts and Responses* 2, 209-222.

Kinnear, S., Tucker, G., Mann, J. & Akbar, D. (2010) Profiling Queensland's non-renewable green energy sectors (clean coal and natural gas). Centre for Environmental Management CQUniversity, Rockhampton.

Kohler, L. (1998) Environment and the world of work: an integrated approach to sustainable development, environment and the working environment, *Encyclopaedia of occupational health and safety* (ed J. M. Stellman). International Labour Office, Geneva.

LCSP (Lowell Centre for Sustainable Production), 2010, *Cleantech: An Agenda for a Healthy Economy January 2010,* Lowell Center for Sustainable Production at the University of Massachusetts Lowell, 32 pages.

Marsden, T. (2010) Mobilizing the regional eco-economy: evolving webs of agri-food and rural development in the UK. *Cambridge J Regions Econ Soc,* 3, 225-244.

Mead, M. N. (2011) A Shift in Policy? Learning from China's Environmental Challenges and Successes, *Environmental Health Perspectives 119* (7) July 2011, p. A307.

Morreale, P., Qi. F., Croft, P., Suleski, R., Sinnicke, B., Kendall, F. Real-Time Environmental Monitoring and Notification for Public Safety, *Computing now,* April-June 2010, pp. 4-11.

NHMRC (National Health and Medical Research Council), 2010, *Wind Turbines and Health A Rapid Review of the Evidence July 2010,* 11 pages, available online at http://www.nhmrc.gov.au/_files_nhmrc/publications/attachments/new0048_evidence_review_wind_turbines_and_health.pdf

OESR (Office of Economic and Statistical Research), (2011) *Bowen Basin Population Report, 2010 Full-time equivalent (FTE) population estimates, June 2010,* Queensland Treasury, Office of Economic and Statistical Research, Brisbane, 60 pages.

PHIDU (Public Health Information Development Unit), 2010, *A social health atlas of Australia, 2010* The University of Adelaide, available online at http://www.publichealth.gov.au/data/a-social-health-atlas-of-australia_-2010.html

Queensland Health 2008 *Mount Isa Community Lead Screening Program 2006–2007: A Report into the Results of a Blood-lead Screening Program of 1–4 year Old Children in Mount Isa, Queensland,* viewed 4 August 2011 <http://www.health.qld.gov.au/ph/documents/tphn/mtisa_leadrpt.pdf>

Evans, R., Delaere, I., Babina, K., Simon, D. and Mitschke, M. (2010) Vapour intrusion in suburban dwellings *Public Health Bulletin* 7(1), 48-52

Traviss, N., Thelen, B. A., Ingalls, J. K. & Treadwell, M. D. (2010) Biodiesel versus diesel: A pilot study comparing exhaust exposures for employees at a rural municipal facility. *Journal of the Air and Waste Management Association,* 60, 1026-1033.

Tsuda, T, Yorifuji, T, Takao, S, Miyai, M & Babazono, A 2009, 'Minamata disease: Catastrophic poisoning due to a failed public health response', *Journal of Public Health Policy,* 30(1), 54-67.

US EPA (United States Environmental Protection Agency), (2010). *Assessing the Multiple Benefits of Clean Energy A resource for states,* 168 pages, available online at

http://www.epa.gov/statelocalclimate/documents/pdf/epa_assessing_benefits.pdf

van Berkel, R. (2007) Cleaner production and eco-efficiency in Australian small firms. *International Journal of Environmental Technology and Management*, 7, 672-693.

Wilkinson, P., Smith, K. R., Davies, M., Adair, H., Armstrong, B. G., Barrett, M., Bruce, N., Haines, A., Hamilton, I., Oreszczyn, T., Ridley, I., Tonne, C., Chalabi, Z., (2009), Public health benefits of strategies to reduce greenhouse-gas emissions: household energy, *The Lancet* 374:1917-29.

Wilson, D, Esterman, A, Lewis, M, Roder, D, & Calder, I 1986, 'Children's Blood Lead Levels in the Lead Smelting Town of Port Pirie, South Australia', *Archives of Environmental Health*, 41(4), 245-250

WRI (World Resources Institute), United Nations Economic Programme and The World Bank, (1998) 'Chapter 3. Improving health through environmental action', *World Resources 1998-99: Environmental change and human health.* World Resources Institute, Washington, DC, available online at http://www.wri.org/publication/world-resources-1998-99-environmental-change-and-human-health

Part 5

Health Impacts

10

Heavy Metals and Human Health

Simone Morais[1], Fernando Garcia e Costa[2] and Maria de Lourdes Pereira[3]

[1]REQUIMTE, Instituto Superior de Engenharia do Porto, Porto,
[2]Departamento de Morfologia e Função, CIISA, Faculdade de Medicina Veterinária, Universidade Técnica de Lisboa, Lisboa,
[3]Departamento de Biologia & CICECO, Universidade de Aveiro, Aveiro, Portugal

1. Introduction

Metals occur naturally in the earth's crust, and their contents in the environment can vary between different regions resulting in spatial variations of background concentrations. The distribution of metals in the environment is governed by the properties of the metal and influences of environmental factors (Khlifi & Hamza-Chaffai, 2010). Of the 92 naturally occurring elements, approximately 30 metals and metalloids are potentially toxic to humans, Be, B, Li, Al, Ti, V, Cr, Mn, Co, Ni, Cu, As, Se, Sr, Mo, Pd, Ag, Cd, Sn, Sb, Te, Cs, Ba, W, Pt, Au, Hg, Pb, and Bi. Heavy metals is the generic term for metallic elements having an atomic weight higher than 40.04 (the atomic mass of Ca) (Ming-Ho, 2005). Heavy metals enter the environment by natural and anthropogenic means. Such sources include: natural weathering of the earth's crust, mining, soil erosion, industrial discharge, urban runoff, sewage effluents, pest or disease control agents applied to plants, air pollution fallout, and a number of others (Ming-Ho, 2005). Although some individuals are primarily exposed to these contaminants in the workplace, for most people the main route of exposure to these toxic elements is through the diet (food and water). The contamination chain of heavy metals almost always follows a cyclic order: industry, atmosphere, soil, water, foods and human. Although toxicity and the resulting threat to human health of any contaminant are, of course, a function of concentration, it is well-known that chronic exposure to heavy metals and metalloids at relatively low levels can cause adverse effects (Agency for Toxic Substance and Disease Registry [ATSDR], 2003a, 2003b, 2007, 2008; Castro-González & Méndez-Armenta, 2008). Therefore, there has been increasing concern, mainly in the developed world, about exposures, intakes and absorption of heavy metals by humans. Populations are increasingly demanding a cleaner environment in general, and reductions in the amounts of contaminants reaching people as a result of increasing human activities. A practical implication of this trend, in the developed countries, has been the imposition of new and more restrictive regulations (European Commission, 2006; Figueroa, 2008).

Considering the importance of this subject, this chapter gives an overview of the main features of heavy metals and their health effects. The early part of this chapter is dedicated to the most found and toxic heavy metals, lead, cadmium, mercury, and arsenic. The next piece deals with several approaches for assessment of human exposure, namely the use of biomarkers. The most widely applied separation and detection techniques for quantification of these elements in biological and environmental samples is included, as they provide valuable toxicological data for hazard and risk assessments. Then, finally, the example of the wood preservative chromated copper arsenate (CCA) illustrates the effect of some hazardous substances on the health of humans and the environment.

2. Heavy metals

Lead (Pb), cadmium (Cd), mercury (Hg), and arsenic (As) are widely dispersed in the environment. These elements have no beneficial effects in humans, and there is no known homeostasis mechanism for them (Draghici et al., 2010; Vieira et al., 2011). They are generally considered the most toxic to humans and animals; the adverse human health effects associated with exposure to them, even at low concentrations, are diverse and include, but are not limited to, neurotoxic and carcinogenic actions (ATSDR, 2003a, 2003b, 2007, 2008; Castro-González & Méndez-Armenta, 2008; Jomova & Valko, 2011; Tokar et al., 2011).

2.1 Lead

Lead as a toxicologically relevant element has been brought into the environment by man in extreme amounts, despite its low geochemical mobility and has been distributed worldwide (Oehlenschläger, 2002). Lead amounts in deep ocean waters is about 0.01-0.02 µg/L, but in surface ocean waters is *ca.* 0.3 µg/L (Castro-González & Méndez-Armenta, 2008). Lead still has a number of important uses in the present day; from sheets for roofing to screens for X-rays and radioactive emissions. Like many other contaminants, lead is ubiquitous and can be found occurring as metallic lead, inorganic ions and salts (Harrison, 2001). Lead has no essential function in man.

Food is one of the major sources of lead exposure; the others are air (mainly lead dust originating from petrol) and drinking water. Plant food may be contaminated with lead through its uptake from ambient air and soil; animals may then ingest the lead-contaminated vegetation. In humans, lead ingestion may arise from eating lead-contaminated vegetation or animal foods. Another source of ingestion is through the use of lead-containing vessels or lead-based pottery glazes (Ming-Ho, 2005). In humans, about 20 to 50% of inhaled, and 5 to 15% of ingested inorganic lead is absorbed. In contrast, about 80% of inhaled organic lead is absorbed, and ingested organic Pb is absorbed readily. Once in the bloodstream, lead is primarily distributed among blood, soft tissue, and mineralizing tissue (Ming-Ho, 2005). The bones and teeth of adults contain more than 95% of the total body burden of lead. Children are particularly sensitive to this metal because of their more rapid growth rate and metabolism, with critical effects in the developing nervous system (ATSDR, 2007; Castro-González & Méndez-Armenta, 2008).

The Joint FAO/ World Health Organization Expert Committee on Food Additives (JECFA) established a provisional tolerable weekly intake (PTWI) for lead as 0.025 mg/kg body weight (bw) (JECFA, 2004). The WHO provisional guideline of 0.01 mg/L has been adopted as the standard for drinking water (WHO, 2004a).

2.2 Cadmium

The use of cadmium by man is relatively recent and it is only with its increasing technological use in the last few decades that serious consideration has been given to cadmium as a possible contaminant. Cadmium is naturally present in the environment: in air, soils, sediments and even in unpolluted seawater. Cadmium is emitted to air by mines, metal smelters and industries using cadmium compounds for alloys, batteries, pigments and in plastics, although many countries have stringent controls in place on such emissions (Harrison, 2001).

Tobacco smoke is one of the largest single sources of cadmium exposure in humans. Tobacco in all of its forms contains appreciable amounts of the metal. Because the absorption of cadmium from the lungs is much greater than from the gastrointestinal tract, smoking contributes significantly to the total body burden (Figueroa, 2008; Ming-Ho, 2005).

In general, for non-smokers and non-occupationally exposed workers, food products account for most of the human exposure burden to cadmium (ExtoxNet, 2003). In food, only inorganic cadmium salts are present. Organic cadmium compounds are very unstable. In contrast to lead and mercury ions, cadmium ions are readily absorbed by plants. They are equally distributed over the plant. Cadmium is taken up through the roots of plants to edible leaves, fruits and seeds. During the growth of grains such as wheat and rice, cadmium taken from the soil is concentrated in the core of the kernel. Cadmium also accumulates in animal milk and fatty tissues (Figueroa, 2008). Therefore, people are exposed to cadmium when consuming plant- and animal-based foods. Seafood, such as molluscs and crustaceans, can be also a source of cadmium (Castro-González & Méndez-Armenta, 2008; WHO 2004b; WHO 2006).

Cadmium accumulates in the human body affecting negatively several organs: liver, kidney, lung, bones, placenta, brain and the central nervous system (Castro-González & Méndez-Armenta, 2008). Other damages that have been observed include reproductive, and development toxicity, hepatic, haematological and immunological effects (Apostoli & Catalani, 2011; ATSDR, 2008).

The Joint FAO/WHO has recommended the PTWI as 0.007 mg/kg bw for cadmium (JEFCA, 2004). The EPA maximum contaminant level for cadmium in drinking water is 0.005 mg/L whereas the WHO adopted the provisional guideline of 0.003 mg/L (WHO, 2004a).

2.3 Mercury

Mercury is one of the most toxic heavy metals in the environment (Castro-González & Méndez-Armenta, 2008). Man released mercury into the environment by the actions of the agriculture industry (fungicides, seed preservatives), by pharmaceuticals, as pulp and paper preservatives, catalysts in organic syntheses, in thermometers and batteries, in amalgams and in chlorine and caustic soda production (Oehlenschläger, 2002; Zhang & Wong, 2007). Exposure to high levels of metallic, inorganic, or organic mercury can permanently damage the brain, kidneys, and developing fetus (ATSDR, 2003b).

The toxicity of mercury depends on its chemical form (ionic < metallic <organic) (Clarkson, 2006). Up to 90% of most organic mercury compounds are absorbed from food (Reilly, 2007).

Mercury can be detected in most foods and beverages, at levels of < 1 to 50 μg/kg (Reilly, 2007). Higher levels are often found in marine foods. Organic mercury compounds easily pass across biomembranes and are lipophilic. Therefore elevated mercury concentrations are mainly found in liver of lean species and in fatty fish species. Methyl mercury has a tendency to accumulate with fish age and with increasing trophic level. This leads to higher mercury concentrations in old fatty predatory species like tuna, halibut, redfish, shark, and swordfish (Oehlenschläger, 2002). In the year 2003, the JECFA revised its risk assessment on methylmercury in fish and adopted a lower PTWI of 1.6 μg/kg body weight/week to replace the previous PTWI of 3.3 μg/kg b.w./week of total mercury for the general population (Castro-González & Méndez-Armenta, 2008; JECFA, 2004). This risk assessment was based on two major epidemiology studies which investigated the relationship between maternal exposure to mercury through high consumption of contaminated fish and seafood and impaired neurodevelopment in their children (Castro-González & Méndez-Armenta, 2008; Grandjean et al., 1997; Murata et al., 2007). Because of the extreme health effects associated with mercury exposure, the current standards for drinking water were set by EPA and WHO at the very low levels of 0.002 mg/L and 0.001 mg/L, respectively (WHO, 2004a).

2.4 Arsenic

Arsenic is a metalloid. It is rarely found as a free element in the natural environment, but more commonly as a component of sulphur-containing ores in which it occurs as metal arsenides. Arsenic is quite widely distributed in natural waters and is often associated with geological sources, but in some locations anthropogenic inputs, such as the use of arsenical insecticides and the combustion of fossil fuels, can be extremely important additional sources. Arsenic occurs in natural waters in oxidation states III and V, in the form of arsenous acid (H_3AsO_3) and its salts, and arsenic acid (H_3AsO_5) and its salts, respectively (Sawyer et al., 2003).

The toxic effects of arsenic depend specially on oxidation state and chemical species, among others. Inorganic arsenic is considered carcinogenic and is related mainly to lung, kidney, bladder, and skin disorders (ATSDR, 2003a). The toxicity of arsenic in its inorganic form has been known for decades under the following forms: acute toxicity, subchronic toxicity, genetic toxicity, developmental and reproductive toxicity (Chakraborti et al., 2004), immunotoxicity (Sakurai et al., 2004), biochemical and cellular toxicity, and chronic toxicity (Mudhoo et al., 2011; Schwarzenegger et al., 2004). Drinking water is one of the primary routes of exposure of inorganic arsenic (Mudhoo et al., 2011; National Research Council, 2001). Ingestion of groundwater with elevated arsenic concentrations and the associated human health effects are prevalent in several regions across the world. Arsenic toxicity and chronic arsenicosis is of an alarming magnitude particularly in South Asia and is a major environmental health disaster (Bhattacharya et al., 2007; Chakraborti et al., 2004; Kapaj et al., 2006). Chronic arsenic ingestion from drinking water has been found to cause carcinogenic and noncarcinogenic health effects in humans (ATSDR, 2003a; Mudhoo et al., 2011; USEPA 2008, 2010a, 2010b). The growing awareness of arsenic-related health problems has led to a rethinking of the acceptable concentration in drinking water (Sawyer et al., 2003). Following a thorough review and in order to maximize health risk reduction, the USEPA in 2001 decided to reduce the drinking water maximum contaminant limit (MCL) to 0.010 mg/L, which is now the same as the WHO guidelines (USEPA, 2005a).

The adverse effects of arsenic in groundwater used for irrigation water on crops and aquatic ecosystems are also of major concern. The fate of arsenic in agricultural soils is less characterized compared to groundwater. However, the accumulation of arsenic in rice field soils and its introduction into the food chain through uptake by the rice plant is of major concern mainly in Asian countries (Bhattacharya et al., 2007; Duxbury et al., 2003). In foods, the major source of arsenic is mainly fish and seafood. The organic arsenic in food and seafood appears to be much less toxic than the inorganic forms (Uneyama et al., 2007). The presence of arsenic in fish has been detected in several species such as; sardine, chub mackerel, horse mackerel (Vieira et al., 2011) blue fish, carp, mullet tuna, and salmon (Castro-González & Méndez-Armenta, 2008). The results show that arsenic concentration is low in most fish, being always its highest concentration in muscle (Vieira et al., 2011). The JECFA established a PTWI for inorganic arsenic as 0.015 mg/kg body weight (FAO/WHO, 2005, JECFA 2004). Organo-arsenic intakes of about 0.05 mg/kg body weight/day seemed not to be associated to hazardous effects (Uneyama et al., 2007).

3. Assessment of exposure to heavy metals

Human exposure is defined by WHO as the amount of a substance in contact, over time and space, with the outer boundary of the body (WHO, 2000). The assessment of human exposure to contaminant chemicals in the environment can be measured by two major methods, each based on different data profiles, thus permitting the verification and validation of the information. One approach involves environmental monitoring i.e., determining the chemical concentration scenario. The second methodology is based on estimations of exposure through the use of biomarkers (Peterson, 2007).

Biomarkers are relevant indices in human health studies and are defined by the National Institute of Health (NIH) as a characteristic that is objectively measured and evaluated as an indicator of normal biological processes, pathogenic processes, or pharmacologic responses to a therapeutic intervention" (NIH, 2001). Biomarkers may be used at any level within biological organization (eg. molecular, cellular, or organ levels). These tools may be used to identify exposed individuals or groups, quantify the exposure, assess the health risks, or assist in diagnosis of environmental or occupational disease (Aitio et al., 2007).

A crucial measure for the assessment of exposure to hazardous chemicals, such as those from waste sites is evaluation of potentially exposed populations. This step also includes the degree, incidence extent, and routes of potential exposure. A most significant direct approach to assess exposure to hazardous substances within potentially exposed populations is to determine chemicals or their metabolic products on some biological fluids such as blood or urine, with certain defined levels being a reliable indicator of metal exposure.

However, long term storage of some toxic metals takes place in hard tissues such as teeth and bones. Additionally, samples of keratinous tissue components such as hair and nails are commonly used for routine clinical screening and diagnosis of longer-term exposure of metals. For example, the levels of lead in bones, hair, and teeth increase with age, suggesting a gradual accumulation of lead in the body. Therefore, contamination of food with lead and the possibility of chronic lead intoxication through the diet need constant monitoring

(Janssen, 1997). In addition, during mineralization of teeth cadmium and lead may persist within the matrix (Fischer, 2009).

Most of ingested arsenic is rapidly excreted via the kidney within a few days. However, high levels of arsenic are retained for longer periods of time in the bone, skin, hair, and nails of exposed humans (Mandal et al., 2003). Studies of arsenic speciation in the urine of exposed humans indicate that the metabolites comprise 10–15% inorganic arsenic and monomethylarsonic acid and a major proportion (60–80%) of dimethylarsenic acid (Bhattacharya et al., 2007). Recent studies have found monomethylarsonous acid and dimethylarsinous acid in trace quantities in human urine (Bhattacharya et al., 2007; Mandal et al., 2003).

Potential biomarkers include DNA and protein adducts, mutations, chromosomal aberrations, genes that have undergone induction and a host of other "early" cellular or subcellular events thought to link exposure and effect. Silins & Högberg (2011) in their review focus on three classes of biomarkers (exposure, effect and susceptibility). Biomarkers of exposure include measurements of parent compound, metabolites or DNA or protein adducts, and reflect internal doses, the biologically effective dose or target dose. Biomarkers of effects could be changes on a cellular level, such as altered expression of metabolic enzymes, and may also include markers for early pathological changes in complex disease developments, such as mutations and preneoplastic lesions. Biomarkers of susceptibility indicate an often constitutive ability of an individual to respond to specific exposures. The three categories of biomarkers cited above were exemplified by Nordberg (2010) in studies of health effects after heavy metal exposures.

Progress in the fields of genomics and proteomics is also reported, and more recent attention is focussed on proteomics technologies involved in finding new and relevant biomarkers for metal assessment. For example, preclinical changes in people exposed to heavy metals were recently monitored by proteomics biomarkers. In addition to urine and blood analysis proteomic profiling of serum samples, one representing the metal-exposed group and the other a control group, revealed three potential protein markers of preclinical changes in humans chronically exposed to a mixture of heavy metals (Kossowska et al., 2011). In this scope, and using these new tools, the effects of arsenic on human health were also illustrated (Vlaanderen et al., 2010).

Other symptoms associated with heavy metal exposure may also be evaluated such as effects on human skin damage, namely stress signals. For example, heavy metals down-regulated the phosphorylation levels of HSP27, and the ratio of p-HSP27 and HSP27 may be a sensitive marker or additional endpoint for the hazard assessment of potential skin irritation caused by chemicals and their products (Zhang et al., 2010).

Middendorf & Williams (2000) have critically reviewed early indicators of cadmium damage in kidneys, such as a low-molecular-weight protein (2-microglobulin), usually reabsorbed by the proximal tubules. Glycosuria, aminoaciduria, and the reduced ability of the kidney to secrete PAH are also indicators of nephrons damage by cadmium. An increase in urinary excretion of low- and high-molecular-weight proteins occurs as damage increases, reflecting the decline in glomerular filtration rate. This review also underlines that cadmium renal damage may occur after many years in workers removed from exposure in factories where nickel/cadmium was excessive.

More recently, some cellular functions have been used as biomarkers. For example, the autophagy pathway was proposed as a new sensitive biomarker for renal injury induced by cadmium (Chargui et al., 2011).

Non-invasive or a minimally invasive monitoring techniques are nowadays preferred, although these assays may require further improvement and validation. For example, the use of the buccal micronucleus assay as a biomarker of DNA damage is a contribution for epidemiological studies (Ceppi et al., 2010). Previously, children hand rinsing was used as a biomarker of short term exposure to As (Shalat et al., 2006). This method, added to the determination of total arsenic analyses in next morning urine was described by those authors for children using playground equipments treated with CCA.

In addition to the biomarkers mentioned above, various other groups of indicators have become widely used and play a significant role in trend analysis of exposures and chemical management response strategies. For example, higher plants, fungi, lichens, mosses, molluscs, and fish are important biomonitors for heavy metals contamination within the environment.

Another key point for human health risk evaluation is the mode of action analysis (MOA), defined by USEPA (2005b) as "a sequence of key events and processes, starting with interaction of an agent with a cell, proceeding through operational and anatomical changes, and resulting in cancer formation". The description of the adverse reactions in animal bioassays may provide relevant information for a better understanding of human health risk. In a recent review Thompson and co-workers (2011) focused on this parameter to illustrate the role of hexavalent chromium on human health assessment. Moreover, the relevance of animal testing data to humans is well established. However, the differences in metabolism between species, added to some intra-specific differences (e.g. gender, nutritional status, age, genetic predisposition, and frequency of exposure) are some limitations. In order to overlap these differences, a safety margin must be considered.

Finally, the complexity and number of available potential biomarkers for heavy metals exposure may be led to the development of improved prognostic and diagnostic tools.

4. Heavy metals analytical methods

4.1 Quantitative determination

Various approaches are described in the literature for detailed analysis of heavy metals in environmental, biological and food samples. Analytical methods frequently require sample preconcentration and/or pretreatment for the destruction of the organic matrix such as wet digestion, dry ashing, and microwave oven dissolution or extraction. Research has been carried out in sample collection, preservation, storage, pre-treatment, quantitative determination, speciation and microscopic analysis. Most of the new information about chemistry of heavy metals results mainly from continuing improvements in speciation and microscopic trace element analysis (Ortega, 2002). It is a tremendous challenge to develop sensitive and selective analytical methods that can quantitatively characterize trace levels of heavy metals in several types of samples (Rao, 2005). Table 1 summarizes the optical and the electrochemical methods applied for heavy metals determination (Karadjova et al., 2007; Draghici et al., 2010).

Technique	Principle	type of analysis	Applications
Atomic absorption spectrometry (AAS)	absorption of radiant energy produced, by a special radiation source, by atoms in their electronic ground state	-single element; -multielement analysis (2-6 elements)	widely used
Inductively coupled plasma with atomic emission spectrometry (ICP-AES)	measures the optical emission from excited atoms	simultaneous multielement analysis	widely used method for environmental analysis
Inductively coupled plasma with mass spectrometry (ICP-MS)	- argon plasma used as ion source; –used for separating ions based on their mass-to charge ratio	simultaneous multielement analysis	-widely used; -isotope determination
Atomic fluorescence spectrometry (AFS)	measures the light that is reemitted after absorption	single element	-mercury, arsenic, and selenium; -complementary technique to AAS
X-ray fluorescence (XRF)	-X-rays –primary excitation source; -elements emit secondary X-rays of a characteristic wavelength	simultaneous determination of most elements	-non-destructive analysis; -less suitable for analysis of minor and trace elements
Neutron activation analysis (NAA)	-conversion of stable nuclei of atoms into radioactive ones; -measurement of the characteristic nuclear radiation emitted by the radioactive nuclei	simultaneous multielement analysis	-most elements can be determined; - highly sensitive procedure
Electrochemical methods	-controlled voltage or current; -polarography; -potentiometry; - stripping voltammetry;	consecutive analysis of different metal ions	-analysis for transition metals and metalloids (total content or speciation analysis)

Table 1. Most usual methods applied for heavy metals determination (adapted from Draghici et al., 2010)

Atomic absorption spectrometry (AAS) and atomic emission spectrometry (AES) are the most widely used techniques for heavy metals quantitative analysis in environmental samples.

Several AAS can be distinguished depending on the mode of sample introduction and atomization. Flame (FAAS), graphite furnace (GFAAS), hydride generation (HGAAS), and cold vapor (CVAAS) systems have been described extensively (Ortega, 2002). FAAS and GFAAS are applicable for quantitative analysis of nearly 70 and 60 elements, respectively. Detection limits of GFAAS are approximately 100 times lower than those for FAAS. In HGAAS, the analyte is reduced to its volatile hydride and this technique is only applicable for the elements forming covalent gaseous hydrides, Ge, As, Se, Sn, Sb, Te, Bi, and Pb. Finally, CVAAS applies solely to Hg as it is the only analyte that has an appreciable atomic vapour pressure at room temperature (Ortega, 2002).

AES measures the optical emission from excited atoms to determine analyte concentration. Nowadays, Inductively Coupled Plasma Atomic Emission Spectrometry (ICP-AES) has clearly superseded FAAS because it is a truly multi-element technique.

Inductively coupled plasma-mass spectrometry (ICP-MS), a more recent technology, can also be used for rapid ultratrace multielement analysis. It consists of an ICP ion source, a quadrupole or magnetic sector mass filter, and an ion detection system. The detection sensitivity of ICP-MS is generally better than the graphite furnace AAS. One important feature is that it can detect and quantify small variations on isotopic compositions in geological and environmental samples (Zhang & Zhang, 2003). However, trace element quantification in biological and clinical samples present analytical complications associated with these sample types, such as non-spectroscopic interferences from the complex salt- and protein-rich matrix.

Atomic fluorescence spectrometry is a single-element technique that measures the light that is reemitted after absorption. It is a complementary technique to AAS that allows the determination of mercury, arsenic and selenium (after mineralization of the samples) using a specific atomic fluorescence spectrometer equipped with hydride generation (Biziuk & Kuczynska, 2007). The limits of detection are about 0.5 μg/L.

Radiochemical methods such as X-ray fluorescence spectrometry and neutron activation analysis are also strictly connected with atomic structure.

X-ray fluorescence analysis, one of the oldest nuclear techniques, is based on subjecting the sample to electromagnetic radiation of sufficient energy to remove electrons from the inner orbitals (Biziuk & Kuczynska, 2007). The fluorescence X-radiation is characteristic for each element and thus enables determination of elements with high selectivity. This radiation, however, has a low energy, that easily can be absorbed by the sample matrix; therefore, this technique is more suitable for very thin, very flat, and homogenous samples. USEPA published a standard method for elemental analysis using a field X-ray fluorescence analyzer (Poley, 1998). Applications include the *in situ* analysis of metals in soil, sediments, air monitoring filters, and lead in paint. Fluorescence radiation can also be obtained after bombardment of atoms with protons or charged particles produced by accelerator (Particle-Induced X-ray Emission; PIXE) (Biziuk & Kuczynska, 2007).

The sensitivity of X-ray spectrometry is lower than that of the neutron activation method (NAA). NAA is a non-destructive technique that is, in general, appropriate for materials that are difficult to convert into a solution for analysis. The required amount of samples is *ca.*, maximally, 200 mg and is simply packaged in an irradiation container (quartz, polyethylene, or aluminium foil), sealed, and irradiated with neutrons for a time determined by the half-life of the radionuclide or the composition of the sample (Biziuk & Kuczynska, 2007). NAA can be applied for analysis of several heavy metals by measuring the gamma activities of their activated radioisotopes such as: ^{76}As;^{115}Cd; ^{122}Sb, ^{124}Sb; and ^{203}Hg (Ortega, 2002; Chéry, 2003). The limits of detection may as low as 0.1 ng/g.

Another group of detection techniques is the electroanalytical methods. This group has gained considerable ground in the environmental and health analysis because of the simplicity, rapidity, and relative low cost of the techniques. Many of them exhibit excellent detection limits coupled with a wide dynamic range. They usually enable the determination of metals concentration at the level of their occurrence in the environment (Szyczewski, 2009). Measurements can generally be made on very small samples, typically in the microliter volume range. The principal methods include polarography, potentiometry and voltammetry. Stripping voltammetric analysis (especially the differential pulse anodic stripping voltammetry and adsorptive stripping voltammetry) is the most common and interesting option for the quantitation of heavy metals. Advantages of this technique include its sensitivity (10^{-10} mol/L in some cases) and accuracy; typically, minimal pretreatment of the sample is required. One major difficulty in the application of electroanalytical techniques to complex real-world samples has been the susceptibility of the electrode surface to fouling by surface active material in the sample. Metals commonly analyzed with this technique include Al, Fe, Cr, Co, Mo, Cd, Pb, Zn, Cu, and Ni, although others have also been reported. Typical results compare well with those obtained by GFAAS.

International organisation such as USEPA (http://www.epa.gov/), European Environment Agency (EEA; http://www.eea.eu.int/), WHO (http://www.who.int/peh/site map.htm), Occupational Safety and Health Administration (OSHA; http://www.osha.gov/), The National Institute for Occupational Safety and Health (NIOSH; http://www.cdc.gov/niosh/homepage.html), National Institute of Standards and Technology (NIST; http:// nvl.nist.gov/) and national structures established sampling and analytical techniques for pollutants determinations in different matrixes, different types of limits of pollutants in different matrixes and other regulations. Specialised laboratories use previously mentioned analytical methods but is also entitled to use other validated techniques.

4.2 Speciation analysis

The chemical species of an element are the specific forms of an element defined as to molecular, complex, or nuclear structure, or oxidation state (Ortega, 2002). The main analytical challenges concern speciation determination of redox and organometallic forms of arsenic and antimony, protein-bound cadmium, organic forms of lead (i.e. alkyllead compounds), organomercury compounds, inorganic platinum compounds, inorganic and organometallic compounds of selenium, organometallic forms of tin, and redox forms of chromium and vanadium. Recently, speciation analysis plays a unique role in the studies of biogeochemical cycles of chemical compounds, determination of toxicity and ecotoxicity of selected elements, quality control of food products, control of medicines and pharmaceutical products, technological process control, research on the impact of technological installation on the environment, examination of occupational exposure and clinical analysis (Kot & Namiesnik, 2000; Michalski, 2009). The fields of health and nutrition benefit tremendously from the information that speciation analysis provides (Rao & Talluri, 2007).

Chromatographic methods (liquid chromatography (LC), ion chromatography (IC) and gas chromatography (GC) and capillary electrophoresis (CE) are the most popular separation techniques which are mainly combined with AAS, AES, ICP-AES or ICP-MS (X. Zhang & C. Zhang, 2003). Table 2 presents the more relevant separation methods and hyphenated techniques for metal speciation.

Technique	Principle	Type of analysis	Applications
Liquid chromatography (LC)	repartition of the analyte between a stationary phase and a mobile liquid one	simultaneous multielement analysis	-environmental metal speciation; - hyphenated techniques for speciation: LC-AAS, LC-AES, LC-ICP-AES, LC-ICP-MS
Gas chromatography (GC)	repartition of the analyte between a stationary phase and a mobile gas one	simultaneous multielement analysis	-volatile or thermally stable compounds (Hg, Sn, Pb alkyl compounds); - techniques for speciation: GC-AAS, GC-AES, GC-MS
Ion chromatography (IC)	LC technique which uses ion- exchange resins	simultaneous multielement analysis	-lack of selectivity control; -hyphenated techniques for metal speciation: IC-AAS, IC-ICP-AES, IC-ICP-MS
Capillary electrophoresis (CE)	differential migrationof charged analytes along a capillary filled with a suitable conducting electrolyte	simultaneous multielement analysis	-cations, organic and inorganic compounds of the same metal, metalloids; - hyphenated techniques: CE-MS, CE-ICP-MS

Table 2. More relevant separation methods and hyphenated techniques for metal speciation.

Most of the current approaches to As, Pb and Hg speciation analysis rely on complete (or partial) extraction of species, with or without previous de-fatting and clean up of crude extracts, followed by high performance liquid chromatographic (HPLC) or CE separation and element-selective detection (Karadjova et al., 2007). Widely used extractants are water, methanol (MeOH)–water and MeOH–chloroform. HPLC separations or CE with ICP-MS detection are mostly used, while HGAAS detection for As and Pb is gradually declining because of poorer sensitivity (*ca.* 10-fold) (Leermakers et al., 2006; Mattusch & Wennrich, 2005). Volatile compounds of Pb, Hg, Sn and Se may be also detected by gas chromatography coupled with AAS, AES or mass spectrometric detection.

Concerning speciation studies for cadmium, several methods have been applied being the most used in soils IC followed by FAAS or ICP-AES (Ortega, 2002). For protein-bound cadmium speciation, size-exclusion chromatography and ICP-MS are the preferred methods (Rao & Talluri, 2007).

Ultraviolet and visible molecular absorption spectrometry depends on the chemical form of the element and gives information about its speciation. It is based on the formation of coloured compounds with appropriate reagents, and on the absorption of characteristic electromagnetic wavelength by this compound. Formations of metal–organic complex are well characterized (Biziuk & Kuczynska, 2007). The use of specific complexing agents and solid phase extraction has improved the technique's selectivity and lowered its limits of detection to the sub-μg/L level. It is the cheapest method for the speciation determination of Al(III), V(V), Cr(VI), Fe(II), Se(IV), Sn(IV), Pt(II), Pt(IV) and Tl(III) (Szyczewski, 2009). Examples include Cr (III) and Cr(VI) species in soil extracts (Jankiewicz & Ptaszyński, 2005) and water samples (Michalski, 2005).

Electro-analytical techniques find their main application in the investigation of dissolved species in environmental samples. They are species selective rather than element selective that can be deployed *in situ* with minimal sample perturbation. If the main targets of speciation analysis are grouped into redox states, metal(loid) complexes and organometal(loid) compounds, analytes in all three areas can be determined by electroanalysis (Town et al., 2003).

5. Case study: The wood preservative chromated copper arsenate

Chromated copper arsenate (CCA) has been used extensively in the past as a chemical wood preservative, and several risks for human and environmental health have been associated with its widespread use. CCA type C (34.0% As_2O_5, 47.5% CrO_3 and 18.5% CuO, w/w), was the most frequently used chemical formulation due to the products durability, performance, and leach resistance. The high durability of CCA-treated wood, added to the persistence of CCA residues from chemical industries within the environment (water, soil, food crops) thus creating a great danger to the public health, including cancer. Furthermore the disposal of CCA-treated wood remains a public health problem, due to elevate arsenic levels released into the environment. For this reason a better understanding of chemical-induced target toxicity on both humans, and other animals is progressively becoming an important part of the impact of hazardous substances on human health.

5.1 Inherent toxicity associated to chemical components in CCA

The characterization of the components of CCA is relevant to better understand the hazards of CCA-treated wood on human health. In this mixture, arsenic and copper act as insecticide, and fungicide, respectively. In addition, chromium plays a key role in the fixation of copper and arsenic to the wood. The toxicity of chromium, copper and arsenic compounds was reviewed by Katz & Salem (2005) in different taxa of animals, and humans. The effects of CCA on aquatic and agricultural environment were also mentioned by these authors. Both arsenic and hexavalent chromium are hazardous chemicals, and detailed arsenic effects on human health were described at the beginning of this chapter.

Cr(VI) has been classified as a human carcinogen by inhalation routes of exposure (IARC, 1990). Although hexavalent chromium may occur naturally in the environment, it is commonly generated by production industries (eg. stainless steel, painting, welding, leather tanning, and electroplating, among others). Previously, an elegant review performed by Costa (1997) underlined the hazards of chromium compounds on animals and human systems, and organs (e.g. respiratory, gastrointestinal, immune, liver, and kidney). More recently, a great number of laboratory and epidemiological studies were reviewed focussing on the health hazards induced by hexavalent chromium-based chemicals (Singh et al., 1999; Thompson et al., 2011). An increased incidence of lung cancer was described in those studies on workers exposed to chromate dust (Tokar et al., 2011). In addition, several adverse changes on haematological parameters were noted in tannery workers (Ramzan et al., 2011).

Copper is a naturally occurring element and a well recognized essential nutrient for human health, since it is involved in several biological processes. It is present within a wide range of food sources such as beef/calf liver, shrimp, nuts, avocados, and beans (ATSDR, 2004). Relevant aspects of whole body copper metabolism, cell and molecular basis for copper homeostasis were recently reviewed by De Romaña and co-workers (2011). In addition, as a brief summary, copper essentiality and toxicity were also reported, and, although acute or chronic copper poisoning is not common, adverse reactions on liver after chronic copper exposure were underlined in this review. The potential health hazards associated to varying levels of copper intake was also recently described (Stern, 2010).

Acute nephrotoxicity of CCA compounds per se, $Na_2Cr_2O_7$, Na_3AsO_4 and $CuSO_4$ was previously described on rats by Mason and Edwards (1989). Although these authors had reported the synergistic effect of different dosage of those compounds, experimental evidences on the nephrotoxicity of CCA on mice have also been described. For example, a set of experiments was designed to study the effects of arsenic pentoxide and chromium trioxide on kidneys, based on histopathology, and histochemistry. In addition, chromium and arsenic analyses (ICP-MS and GFAAS) were used for evaluation. Acute tubular necrosis and the individual effects of those compounds were reported after administration of CCA solution (Matos et al., 2009a, 2009b, 2010).

The sensitizing activity of CCA, namely lymphocyte proliferation was reported in mice using the local lymph node assay (Fukuyama et al., 2008).

5.2 Human exposure to chromated copper arsenate

Human contact with CCA is mainly due to environmental and/or occupational exposures. It occurs during the handling of treated wood and related equipment. Skin exposure and ingestion are the main routes of absorption, and inhalation is another probable route (Cocker et al., 2006). This investigation correlates exposure data based on urinary arsenic and chromium from workers.

Consequently, concerns have been raised owing to the high levels of arsenic and chromium concentrations in CCA treated wood, due to the potential human contact in occupational environments and to the ecological exposure (Chou et al., 2007; Zartarian et al., 2006). In this perspective, concerns about the safety of children have prompted more attention. In fact, children's exposure to these hazardous compounds may occur through hand-to-mouth playing activities. These include incidental ingestion of residues and dermal contact with the soil or sand beneath structures made of CCA-treated wood. Owing to this problem, a model was used in order to estimate children's absorbed dose of arsenic from CCA, using dermal contact and ingestion of soil (The probabilistic Stochastic Human Exposure and Dose Simulation model for wood preservatives - SHEDS-Wood) (Barraj et al., 2007; Xue, et. al., 2006; Zartarian et al., 2006).

6. Conclusion

Heavy metals have been proved to be toxic to both human and environmental health. Owing to their toxicity and their possible bioaccumulation, these compounds should be subject to mandatory monitoring. Several suitable separation and detection methods are available for laboratories engaged daily in routine analysis of a large number of biological or environmental samples. Also, the rapid development of molecular biological methods is bringing valuable advantages to the analytical field. Governments should promote harmonized data collection, research, legislation and regulations, and consider the use of indicators. Each of the two assessment methods outlined above (determining the chemical concentration scenario and the use of biomarkers) provide useful data helping to set standards and guideline values designed to protect human and environmental health from heavy metals contaminants. Exposure measurements are essential for the protection of high risk populations and subgroups. Furthermore, governments should, when setting acceptable levels or criteria related to chemicals, take into consideration the potential enhanced exposures and/or vulnerabilities of children.

7. Acknowledgment

The authors would like to thank to Fundação para Ciência e Tecnologia for the financial support of this work through the project PTDC/AGR-AAM/102316/2008 (COMPETE and co-financed by FEDER). Centro de Materiais Cerâmicos e Compósitos (CICECO) from Aveiro University (Portugal) is also acknowledged.

8. References

Agency for Toxic Substance and Disease Registry (ATSDR). (2003a). Toxicological Profile for Arsenic U.S. Department of Health and Humans Services, Public Health Humans Services, Centers for Diseases Control. Atlanta.

Agency for Toxic Substance and Disease Registry (ATSDR). (2003b). Toxicological Profile for Mercury U.S. Department of Health and Humans Services, Public Health Humans Services, Centers for Diseases Control. Atlanta.

Agency for Toxic Substances and Disease Registry (ATSDR). (2004). Toxicological Profile for Copper. U.S. Department of Health and Humans Services, Public Health Service, Centers for Diseases Control. Atlanta.

Agency for Toxic Substance and Disease Registry (ATSDR). (2007). Toxicological Profile for Lead U.S. Department of Health and Humans Services, Public Health Humans Services, Centers for Diseases Control. Atlanta.

Agency for Toxic Substance and Disease Registry (ATSDR). (2008). Draft Toxicological Profile for Cadmium U.S. Department of Health and Humans Services, Public Health Humans Services, Centers for Diseases Control. Atlanta.

Aitio, A., Bernard, A., Fowler, B.A. & Nordberg, G.F. (2007). Biological monitoring and biomarkers. In: *Handbook on the Toxicology of Metals*, Nordberg, G.F., et al. (Eds.), pp. 65-78, Academic Press/Elsevier, 3rd ed., ISBN 0-123694132, USA.

Apostoli, P. & Catalani, S. (2011). Metal ions affecting reproduction and development. *Metal Ions in Life Science*, 8, 263-303.

Barraj, L.M., Tsuji, J.S. & Scrafford, C.G. (2007). The SHEDS-Wood Model: incorporation of observational data to estimate exposure to arsenic for children playing on CCA-treated wood structures. *Environmental Health Perspectives*, 115, 781-786.

Bhattacharya, P., Welch, A.H., Stollenwerk, K. G., McLaughlin, M.J., Bundschuh, J. & Panaullah, G. (2007). Arsenic in the environment: Biology and Chemistry, *Science of the Total Environment*, 379, 109–120.

Biziuk, M. & Kuczynska, J. (2007). Mineral Components in Food – Analytical Implications, In: *Mineral Components in Foods*, Szefer P. And Nriagu J.O. (Eds), pp. 1-31, Taylor & Francis Group, ISBN 978-0-8493-2234-1, Boca Raton, FL.

Castro-González, M.I. & Méndez-Armenta, M. (2008). Heavy metals: Implications associated to fish consumption. *Environmental Toxicology & Pharmacology*, 26, 263-271.

Ceppi, M., Biasotti, B., Fenech, M., & Bonassi, S. (2010). Human population studies with the exfoliated buccal micronucleus assay: statistical and epidemiological issues. *Mutation Research*, 705, 11-19.

Chakraborti, D., Sengupta, M.K., Rahaman, M.M., Ahamed, S., Chowdhury, U.K. & Hossain M.A. (2004). Groundwater arsenic contamination and its health effects in the Ganga–Megna–Brahmaputra Plain. *Journal of Environmental Monitoring*, 6, 74–83.

Chargui, A., Zekri, S., Jacquillet, G., Rubera, I., Ilie, M., Belaid, A., Duranton, C., Tauc, M., Hofman, P., Poujeol, P., El May, M.V. & Mograbi, B. (2011). Cadmium-induced autophagy in rat kidney: an early biomarker of subtoxic exposure. *Toxicology Science*, 121, 31-42.

Chéry, C. C. (2003). Gel Electrophoresis for Speciation Purposes, In: *Handbook of Elemental Speciation: Techniques and Methodology*, Cornelis, R., Caruso, J. Crews, H. & Heumann, K. (Eds), pp. 224-239, John Wiley & Sons Ltd, ISBN: 0-471-49214-0, West Sussex, England.

Clarkson, T. (2006). The toxicology of mercury and its chemical compounds. *Critical Reviews in Toxicology*, 36, 609–662.

Cocker, J., Morton, J., Warren, N., Wheeler, J.P., & Garrod, A.N. (2006). Biomonitoring for chromium and arsenic in timber treatment plant workers exposed to CCA wood preservatives. *Annals of Occupational Hygiene*, 5, 517-525.

Costa, M. (1997). Toxicity and carcinogeneicity of Cr(VI) in animal models and humans. *Critical Review in Toxicology*, 27, 431-442.

Chou, S., Colman, J., Tylenda, C., & De Rosa, C. (2007). Chemical-specific health consultation for chromated copper arsenate chemical mixture: port of Djibouti. *Toxicology & Industrial Health,* 23, 183-208.

De Romaña, D.J., Olivares, M., Uauy, R. & Araya, M. (2011). Risks and benefits of copper in light of new insights of copper homeostasis. *Journal of Trace Elements in Medicine and Biology*, 25, 3–13.

Draghici, C., Coman, G., Jelescu, C., Dima, C. & Chirila, E. (2010). Heavy metals determination in environmental and biological samples, In: Environmental Heavy Metal Pollution and Effects on Child Mental Development- Risk Assessment and Prevention Strategies, NATO Advanced Research Workshop, Sofia, Bulgaria, 28 April-1 May 2010.

Duxbury, J.M, Mayer, A.B., Lauren, J.G. & Hassan, N. (2003). Food chain aspects of arsenic contamination in Bangladesh: effects on quality and productivity of rice. *Journal of Environmental Science Health Part A, Environmental Science Engineering & Toxic Hazard Substance Control*, 38, 61–69.

European Commission (2006). Regulation (EC) No 1881/2006. JO L364, 20.12.06, pp. 5-24.

ExtoxNet. (2003) Cadmium contamination of food, Available from http://ace.orst.edu/info/extoxnet/faqs/foodcon/cadmium.htm2003

FAO/WHO Expert Committee on Food Additives, Arsenic. (2005). Available from http://www.inchem.org/documents/jecfa/jeceval/jec_159.htm

Fischer, A., Wiechuła, D., Postek-Stefańska, L. & Kwapuliński, J. (2009). Concentrations of metals in maxilla and mandible deciduous and permanent human teeth. *Biology of Trace Elements Research*, 132, 19–26.

Figueroa, E. (2008). Are more restrictive food cadmium standards justifiable health safety measures or opportunistic barriers to trade? An answer from economics and public health. *Science of the Total Environment*, 389, 1-9.

Fukuyama, T., Ueda, H., Hayashi, K., Tajima, Y., Shuto, Y., Kosaka, T. & Harada, T. (2008). Sensitizing potential of chromated copper arsenate in local lymph node assays differs with the solvent used. *Journal of Immunotoxicology*, 5, 99-106.

Grandjean, P., Weihe, P., White, R.F., Debes, F., Araki, S., Yokoyama, K., Murata, K., Sorensen, N., Dohl, R. & Jorgensen, P.J. (1997). Cognitive deficit in 7-year-old children with prenatal exposure to methylmercury. *Neurotoxicology & Teratology*, 19, 417-428.

Guney, M., Zagurya, G.J., Doganb, N. & Onayb, T.T. (2010). Exposure assessment and risk characterization from trace elements following soil ingestion by children exposed to playgrounds, parks and picnic areas. *Journal of Hazardous Materials*, 182, 656–664.

Harrison, N. (2001). Inorganic contaminants in food, In: Food Chemical Safety Contaminants, Watson, D.H. (Ed.), pp. 148-168, Ltd, first Edition, Woodhead Publishing ISBN 1-85573-462-1, Cambridge.

International Agency for Research on Cancer (IARC). (1990). Chromium, nickel and welding. IARC Monographs Evaluation on Carcinogenic Risks Human, 49, 1–648.

Janssen, M.M.T. (1997). Contaminants, In: *Food Safety and Toxicity*, Vries, J. (Ed.), pp. 61-71, CRC Press LLC, ISBN 0-8493-9488-0, first edition, Boca Raton, USA.

Jankiewicz, B. & Ptaszyński, B. (2005). Determination of chromium in soil of łódź gardens. *Polish Journal of Environmental Studies* 14, 869-875.

Joint FAO/WHO Expert Committee on Food Additives (JECFA). (2004). Safety evaluation of certain food additives and contaminants. WHO Food Additives Series No 52.

Jomova, K. & Valko, M. (2010). Advances in metal-induced oxidative stress and human disease. *Toxicology*, 283, 65-87.

Kapaj, S., Peterson, H., Liber, K. & Bhattacharya, P. (2006). Human health effects from chronic arsenic poisoning – a review. *Journal of Environmental Science Health Part A, Environmental Science Engineering Toxic Hazard Substance Control*, 41, 2399-2428.

Karadjova, I.B., Petrov, P.K, Serafimovski, I., Stafilov, T. & Tsalev, D.L. (2007). Arsenic in marine tissues – The challenging problems to electrothermal and hydride generation atomic absorption spectrometry. *Spectrochimica Acta Part B*, 62, 258-268.

Katz, S.A. & Salem, H. (2005). Chemistry and toxicology of building timbers pressure-treated with chromate copper arsenate: a review. *J. of Applied Toxicology*, 25, 1-7.

Khlifi, R. & Hamza-Chaffai, A. (2010). Head and neck cancer due to heavy metal exposure via tobacco smoking and professional exposure: A review. *Toxicology & Applied Pharmacology*, 248, 71-88.

Kossowska, B., Dudka, I., Bugla-Płoskońska, G., Szymańska-Chabowska, A., Doroszkiewicz, W., Gancarz, R., Andrzejak, R. & Antonowicz-Juchniewicz, J. (2010). Proteomic analysis of serum of workers occupationally exposed to arsenic, cadmium, and lead for biomarker research: A preliminary study. *Science of the Total Environment*, 408, 5317-5324.

Kot, A. & Namiesnik, J. (2000). The role of speciation in analytical chemistry. *Trends in Analytical Chemistry*, 19, 69-79.

Leermakers, M., Baeyens, W., De Gieter, M., Smedts, B., Meert, C., De Bisschop, H.C., Morabito, R. & Quevauviller, P.H. (2006). Toxic arsenic compounds in environmental samples: speciation and validation, *Trends in Analytical Chem*istry, 25, 1-10.

Mandal, B.K., Ogra, Y. & Suzuki, K.T. (2003). Speciation of arsenic in human nail and hair from arsenic-affected area by HPLC-inductively coupled argon plasma mass spectrometry. *Toxicology &Applied Pharmacology*, 189, 73-83.

Mason, R.W., & Edwards, I.R. (1989). Acute toxicity of combinations of sodium dichromate, sodium arsenate and copper sulphate in the rat. *Comparative Pharmacology & Toxicology*, 93, 121-125.

Matos, R.C., Vieira, C., Morais, S., Pereira, M.L., & Pedrosa de Jesus, J.P. (2009a). Nephrotoxicity of CCA-treated wood: a comparative study with As_2O_5 and CrO_3 on mice. *Environmental Toxicology & Pharmacology*, 27, 259-263.

Matos, R.C., Vieira, C., Morais, S., Pereira, M.L., & Pedrosa de Jesus, J.P. (2009b). Nephrotoxicity effects of the wood preservative chromium copper arsenate on mice: histopathological and quantitative approaches. *Journal of Trace Elements in Medicine & Biology*, 23, 224-230.

Matos, R.C., Vieira, C., Morais, S., Pereira, M.L., & Pedrosa de Jesus, J.P. (2010). Toxicity of chromated copper arsenate: A study in mice. *Environmental Research*, 110, 424-427.

Mattusch, J. & Wennrich, R. (2005). Novel analytical methodologies for the determination of arsenic and other metalloid species in solids, liquids and gases. *Mikrochimica Acta*, 151, 137-139.

Michalski, R. (2005). Trace level determination of Cr(III)/Cr(VI) in water samples using ion chromatography with UV detection. *Journal of Liquid Chromatography & Related Technologies*, 28, 2849-2862.

Michalski, R. (2009). Applications of ion chromatography for the determination of inorganic cations. *Critical Reviews in Analytical Chemistry*, 39, 230–250.

Middendorf, P.J. & Williams, P.L. (2000). Nephrotoxicity: Toxic Responses of the Kidney, In: *Principles of Toxicology Environmental & Industrial Applications*, Williams, P.L., James, R.C., Roberts, S.M. (Eds), pp. 129-143, John Wiley & Sons, Inc., ISBN 0-47129321-0, New York.

Ming-Ho, Y. (2005). *Environmental Toxicology: Biological and Health Effects of Pollutants*, Chap. 12, CRC Press LLC, ISBN 1-56670-670-2, 2nd Edition, BocaRaton, USA.

Mudhoo, A., Sharma, S.K., Garg, V.K. & Tseng, C-H. (2011). Arsenic: an overview of applications, health, and environmental concerns and removal processes. *Critical Reviews in Environmental Science & Technology*, 41, 435–519.

Murata, K., Grandjean, P. & Dakeishi, M. (2007). Neurophysiological evidence of methylmercury neurotoxicity. *Am.J.Int.Med.*, 50, 765-771.

National Institute of Health. (2001). Biomarkers Definitions Working Group. Biomarkers and Surrogate endpoints: preferred definitions and conceptual framework. *Clinical Pharmacology & Therapeutics*, 69, 89-95.

National Research Council. (2001). Arsenic in drinking water—Update. Washington DC, National Academy Press.

Nordberg, G.F. (2010). Biomarkers of exposure, effects and susceptibility in humans and their application in studies of interactions among metals in China. *Toxicology Letters*, 192, 45-49.

Oehlenschläger, J. (2002). Identifying heavy metals in fish In: *Safety and Quality issues in fish processing*, Bremner, H.A. (Ed), pp. 95-113, Woodhead Publishing Limited, 978-1-84569-019-9, Cambridge.

Ortega, R. (2002). Analytical Methods for Heavy Metals in the Environment: Quantitative Determination, Speciation, and Microscopic Analysis, In: *Heavy Metals in the Environment*, Sarkar, B. (Ed), pp. 35-68, Marcel Dekker Inc., ISBN 0-8247-0630-7, New York.

Peterson, P.J. (2007) Assessment of Exposure to Chemical Pollutants in Food and Water, In: *Mineral Components in Foods*, Szefer P. And Nriagu J.O. (Eds), pp. 413-431, Taylor & Francis Group, ISBN 978-0-8493-2234-1, Boca Raton, FL.

Poley, G.J. (1998). Environmental Technology Verification Report. Field Portable X-ray Fluorescence Analyzer. Washington, DC: USEPA, EPA/600/R-97/145.

Ramzan, M., Malik, M.A., Iqbal, Z., Arshad, N., Khan, S.Y. & Arshad, M. (2011). Study of hematological indices in tannery workers exposed to chromium in Sheikhupura (Pakistan). *Toxicology & Industrial Health*, Apr 19. [Epub ahead of print].

Rao, R.N. & Talluri, M.V.N.K. (2007). An overview of recent applications of inductivelycoupled plasma-mass spectrometry (ICP-MS) in determination of inorganic impurities in drugs and pharmaceuticals. *Journal of Pharmaceutical & Biomedical Analysis*, 43, 1–13.

Rao, T.P., Metilda, J. & Gladis, M. (2005). Overview of analytical methodologies for sea water analysis: Part I—Metals. *Critical Reviews in Analytical Chemistry*, 35, 247–288.

Reilly, C. (2007). Pollutants in Food —Metals and Metalloids, In: *Mineral Components in Foods*, Szefer P. And Nriagu J.O. (Eds), pp. 363-388, Taylor & Francis Group, ISBN 978-0-8493-2234-1, Boca Raton, FL.

Sakurai, T., Kojima, C., Ochiai, M., Ohta, T. & Fujiwara, K. (2004). Evaluation of in vivo acute immunotoxicity of a major organic arsenic compound arsenobetaine in seafood. *International Immunopharmacology*, 4, 179–184.

Sawyer, C.N., McCarty, P.L. & Parkin, G.F. (2003). *Chemistry for environmental and Engineering and Science* (fifth Edition), Mc Graw Hill, ISBN 0-07-248066-1, NY.

Schwarzenegger, A., Tamminen, T., & Denton, J.E. (2004). Public health goals for chemicals in drinking water arsenic. Office of Environmental Health Hazard Assessment, California Environmental Protection Agency.

Shalat, S.L., Solo-Gabriele, H.M., Fleming, L.E., Buckley, B.T., Black, K., Jimenez, M., Shibata, T., Durbin, M., Graygo, J., Stephan, W. & Van De Bogart, G. (2006). A pilot study of children's exposure to CCA-treated wood from playground equipment. *Science of Total Environment*, 367, 80-88.

Silins, I. & Johan Högberg, J. (2011). Combined toxic exposures and human health: biomarkers of exposure and effect. *International Journal of Environmental Research & Public Health*, 8, 629-647.

Singh, J., Pritchard, D.E., Carlisle, D.L., Mclean, J.A., Montaser, A., Orenstein, J.M. & Patierno, S.R. (1999). Internalization of carcinogenic lead chromate particles by cultured normal human lung epithelial cells: formation of intracellular lead-inclusion bodies and induction of apoptosis. *Toxicology & Applied Pharmacology*, 161, 240–248.

Stern, B.R. (2010). Essentiality and Toxicity in Copper Health Risk Assessment: Overview, Update and Regulatory Considerations. *Journal of Toxicology & Environmental Health- Part A*, 73, 114-127.

Szyczewski, P., Siepak, J. , Niedzielski, P. & Sobczyński, T. (2009). Research on heavy metals in Poland. *Polish Journal of Environmental Studies*, 18, 755-768.

Tokar, E.J., Benbrahim-Tallaa, L. & Waalkes, M.P. (2011). Metal ions in human cancer development. *Metal Ions on Life Science*, 8, 375-401.

Thompson, C.H., Haws, L.C., Harris, M.A., Gatto, N. M. & Proctor, D. M. (2011). Application of the U.S. EPA mode of action framework for purposes of guiding future research: a case study involving the oral carcinogenicity of hexavalent chromium. *Toxicological Sciences*, 119, 20–40.

Town, R.M., Emons, H. & Buffle, J. (2003). Speciation Analysis by Electrochemical Methods, In: *Handbook of Elemental Speciation: Techniques and Methodology*, Cornelis, R., Caruso, J. Crews, H. & Heumann, K. (Eds), pp. 421-460, John Wiley & Sons Ltd, ISBN: 0-471-49214-0, West Sussex, England.

Uneyama, C., Toda, M., Yamamoto, M. & Morikawa, K. (2007). Arsenic in various foods: Cumulative data. *Food Additives & Contaminants*, 24, 447-534.

United States Environmental Protection Agency (USEPA). (2005a). Arsenic in drinking water fact sheet. 10.07.2011, Available from http://www.epa.gov/safewater/arsenic.html.

United States Environmental Protection Agency (USEPA). (2005b). Guidelines for carcinogen risk assessment EPA/630/P-03/001F.

United States Environmental Protection Agency (USEPA). (2008). Risk-Based Concentration Table, Available from http://www.epa.gov/reg3hwmd/risk/human/index.htm

United States Environmental Protection Agency (USEPA). (2009). Integrated Risk Information System (IRIS), Washington, DC 20005, Available from http://www.epa.gov/ncea/iris/.

United States Environmental Protection Agency (USEPA). (2010a). Mid-Atlantic Risk Assessment, available from http://www.epa.gov/reg3hwmd/risk/human/rbconcentration_table/usersguide.htm

United States Environmental Protection Agency (USEPA). (2010b). Risk-Based Concentration Table. Region 3 Fish Tissue Screening Levels.

Vieira, C., Morais, S., Ramos, S., Delerue-Matos, C. & Oliveira, M.B.P.P. (2011). Mercury, cadmium, lead and arsenic levels in three pelagic fish species from the Atlantic Ocean: intra- and inter-specific variability and human health risks for consumption. *Food & Chemical Toxicology*, 49, 923-932.

Vlaanderen, J., Moore, L. E., Smith, M. T., Lan, Q., Zhang, L., Skibola, C. F., Rothman, N. & Vermeulen, R. (2010). Application of OMICS technologies in occupational and environmental health research; current status and projections. *Occupational & Environmental Medicine*, 67, 136-43.

WHO. (2004a). Guidelines for drinking-water quality. Sixty-first meeting, Rome, 10-19 June 2003. Joint FAO/WHO Expert Committee on Food Additives, Avaible from http://ftp.fao.org/es/esn/jecfa/jecfa61sc.pdf

WHO. (2004b). Evaluation of certain food additives contaminants. Sixty-first report of the joint FAO/WHO Expert Committee on Food Additives. WHO Technical Report Series, No. 922.

WHO. (2006). Evaluation of certain food contaminants. Sixty-fourth report of the Joint FAO/WHO Expert Committee on Food Additives. WHO Technical Report Series, No. 930.

WHO/IPCS. (2000) Human Exposure Assessment, Environmental Health Criteria 214, WHO, Geneva.

Xue, J., Zartarian, V. G, Ozkaynak, H., Dang, W., Glen, G., Smith, L. & Stallings, C. (2006). A probabilistic arsenic exposure assessment for children who contact chromated copper arsenate (CCA)-treated playsets and decks, Part 2: Sensitivity and uncertainty analyses. *Risk Analysis*, 26, 533-541.

Zartarian, V., Jianping, X., Özkaynak, H., Dang, W., Glen, G., Smith, L., & Stallings, C. (2006). A Probabilistic Arsenic Exposure Assessment for Children Who Contact CCA-Treated Playsets and Decks. Part 1: Model Methodology, Variability Results, and Model Evaluation. *Risk Analysis*, 26, 515-531.

Zhang, I. & Wong, M.H. 2007. Environmental mercury contamination in China: sources and impacts. *Environment International*, 33, 108-121.

Zhang, X. & Zhang, C. (2003). Atomic Absorption and Atomic Emission Spectrometry, In: *Handbook of Elemental Speciation: Techniques and Methodology*, Cornelis, R., Caruso, J. Crews, H. & Heumann, K. (Eds), pp. 241-257, John Wiley & Sons Ltd, ISBN: 0-471-49214-0, West Sussex, England.

Zhang, Q., Zhang, L., Xiao, X., Su, Z., Zou, P., Hu, H., Yadong Huang, Y. & Qing-Yu, H. (2010). Heavy metals chromium and neodymium reduced phosphorylation level of heat shock protein 27 in human keratinocytes. *Toxicology In Vitro*, 24, 1098-1104.

11

Health Impacts of Noise Pollution Around Airports: Economic Valuation and Transferability

Michael Getzner and Denise Zak
Vienna University of Technology,
Centre of Public Finance and Infrastructure Policy,
Austria

1. Introduction

Air transportation generates numerous economic and social welfare benefits. Airports and their expansions are associated with direct, indirect, induced effects as well as catalytic impacts on regional and national economies (Arndt et al., 2009; Braun et al., 2010). Mobility and accessibility are important factors determining competitiveness of (regional and national) economies in an increasingly globalised world. On the other hand there are numerous environmental and health impacts related to the growing demand for air transport. Since the projected annual growth rates of numbers of passengers are about 5% in the next 20 to 25 years (Mahashabde et al., 2011), the continuing growth of the aviation sector has raised questions of appropriate valuation and treatment of external costs (e.g. human and environmental health). In the context of transport markets, a distinction of externalities into positive (external benefits) and negative (external costs) is appropriate. Large infrastructure projects like airports cause various external effects, associated especially with the provision of transport services and facilities, the need of constructing transport infrastructure as well as related production of vehicles or raw materials (Schipper et al. 2001). Air traffic and associated ground side traffic contribute to local and global noise and air pollution.

Despite a large body of research on the economic effects the demand for more information about the economic effects of pollution and noise exposure is increasing. Effects on human and environmental health as well as on property values, land use planning constraints and spatial and social polarization are issues of importance, requiring further scientific work (Eurocontrol, 2007). Noise pollution is a negative externality, which is defined as an unwanted by-product of production as well as consumption processes that have adverse effects on third-part individuals and communities. Since there is no explicit market for environmental goods like quiet, the economic valuation of noise damages is not simple or straightforward (Nelson, 2008). As an example, monetary values for all relevant external effects, more precisely environmental impacts, global warming and accidents are aimed to be covered by the ExternE methodology, whereas health impacts constitute the largest part of the estimated damage costs (Bickel & Friedrich, 2005). Generating values is necessary at least for three purposes; finding a basis of a possible internalization of external costs, inclusion as an input in cost-benefit appraisals, and defining mitigation or regulation measures in terms of cost-effectiveness (Eurocontrol, 2003).

Noise affects communities around airports; causing nuisance and health effects like sleep deprivation (Lu & P. Morrell, 2006). The World Health Organization recognizes community noise (also referred to as environmental, domestic or residential noise) as a public health problem and published guidelines to combat excessive noise pollution in 1999 (Berglund et al., 1999). In an extension the World Health Organization focuses on the health effects of night-time noise exposure for Europe (World Health Organization [WHO], 2009). Auditory and non-auditory effects on human health are related to noise exposure, with the latter effects being less well established (Clark & Stansfeld, 2007). These adverse effects on human health cause costs that are of relevant concern for the affected individuals and the entire economic system. Especially treatment costs of diseases and health problems (stationary and ambulant hospital treatments, medication and consultations), productivity losses in occupational settings (sickness absence, lost output, non-productive time and invalidity) and immaterial costs due to losses in quality of life are pivotal. Effects on housing prices and rents are also important economic dimensions. Residences in noise polluted areas are subject to value decreases and occasionally cost-intensive adjustments for noise insulation facilities (Sommer, 2002).

The linkage of clinical health effects and noise is complex. A direct relation between noise exposure and certain clinical symptoms is difficult to determine because of a range of interdependencies and influencing factors (European Commission [EC], 2005).

Based on this background, the research question for our paper is twofold: First, we want to examine the recent methodological developments on the valuation of airport-related external noise costs. Special attention is paid to benefit/cost transfer and the method's implications. Second, we discuss empirical results and possible transferability of our results, and draw conclusions. The structure of the paper is the following: Section 2 provides a short review of valuation techniques with the focus on the valuation of property values and willingness-to-pay methods to reduce health-related noise pollution of air transport. Section 3 provides a comprehensive discussion of the scientific literature on valuation results and the relation of health problems to noise pollution around airports. Section 4 summarizes the empirical results in the light of transferability from the study sites to potential policy sites. Finally, section 5 discusses the summaries and concludes.

2. Environmental valuation techniques: Overview on methodology

From the viewpoint of methodology there are many potential techniques assessing the economic values of externalities and environmental impacts. As will be shown in detail, valuing the environment and - in an extended perspective - (statistical) life and health is a challenging task to undertake. One option is to examine households' preferences for certain environmental amenities via the housing market, assuming that the status of environmental quality is revealed through residential choices and decisions.

Lancaster (1966) employed a new model of consumer theory, assuming that goods are not the direct objects of utility as it was common in traditional approaches. Consumers' utility derives on the basis of the inherent characteristics or properties of the good instead.

Housing is commonly treated as a heterogeneous and composite good. This good is not only defined by its attributes like size, house type or number of rooms, but also by location characteristics, summarizing accessibility, neighborhood, environmental quality, traffic effects and local public goods (Cheshire & Sheppard, 1995). While the vicinity of public transportation, roads and airports can be experienced as amenity in terms of mobility it is also related to negative externalities (Boyle, 2001).

For the economic valuation of health effects and environmental impacts of noise exposure at airports two methods are especially widely used: hedonic pricing and contingent valuation. The essential part of these techniques is the determination of the (marginal) willingness to pay (WTP) for an avoidance or reduction of these effects (den Boer & Schroten, 2007).

2.1 Hedonic pricing and contingent valuation

Valuation of environmental amenities cannot be realized through markets (alone) due to their public good character. Accordingly, an indirect method for valuing is necessary to assume and utilize a link of a certain amenity (or disamenity) and residential property values (McMillan et al., 1980). Rosen (1974) developed theories of consumer behavior and proposed the hedonic method as a useful tool for economic valuation (Lipscomb, 2003) on the hedonic assumption that individuals value the characteristics of different goods on grounds of their attributed utility. Rosen considered a model for using hedonic prices to assess the values of attributes for differentiated goods in terms of demand and supply perspective. Hedonic prices were defined as implicit prices, which are revealed by economic agents through market behavior (Rosen, 1974; Freeman, 1979). In theory, housing prices can be understood among others as a reflection of the money value of environmental quality to the individual or home owner. Assuming that the individual's utility function is weakly separable, the marginal rate of substitution between two goods is not dependent on the quantity of all other goods. Therefore the estimation of a demand curve for environmental quality without considering the prices of other goods is feasible within the hedonic pricing method (Freeman, 1981). Another important assumption is weak complementarity (Hanley & Spash, 1993).

Estimations of the effects of amenities and disamenities on housing values have been derived from hedonic models (Nelson, 2004). In the case of airport noise it is assumed that properties exposed to noise nuisance - ceteris paribus - sell at lower prices, reflecting preferences for quieter residences (Day, 2001). Despite the wide application of this method various problems exist and there is an ongoing critical debate. On a theoretical level Ekeland et al. (2002) question the using of market data for the demand function in the sense of Rosen (1974). In the hedonic price equation as well as in the demand curve the decision on independent variables and omitted variables is crucial. Multi-collinearity of included variables is also problematic. Segmentation of housing markets also has to be taken into account (Hanley & Spash, 1993). McMillan et al. (1980) point out that the property value measure does not necessarily reflect the true willingness to pay of households, when different household classes exist. This is due to the fact that house characteristics are inflexible, and that households are limited in their mobility (e.g. relocation costs), and that households have incomplete information on health effects of noise pollution.

The welfare implications of changes in goods that are not traded on markets can theoretically be implied by this model of market equilibrium. Further developments and extensions of the hedonic property value approach like the accounting for spatial effects have been established (Kuminoff et al., 2010) as well as including geographical attributes (Collins & A. Evans, 1994).

Contingent valuation relies on the stated preferences approach (Hanley & Barbier, 2009). Placing a monetary value on noise pollution and the consequences of environmental damages in a direct way is difficult. The lack of markets results from the non-rival or non-excludable nature of these damages. Market prices therefore cannot reflect social costs (benefits) appropriately. Preferences are therefore not fully captured by market transactions, if externalities exist (Hanemann, 1994). Economic values for non-market resources are estimated based on the information collected in survey questions (Smith, 2009). Consumers are directly asked for their (marginal) willingness to pay (WTP) or willingness to accept (WTA) (Hanley & Spash, 1993). The WTA or WTP measures captured within contingent valuation surveys are understood to reflect respondent's preferences monetarily, corresponding to welfare measures in the sense of the Hicksian consumers' surplus. The choice between WTA or WTP measures for a given context remains controversial (Atkinson & Mourato, 2008). Contingent valuation is widely used in cost-benefit analysis and environmental impact assessment, although it has been the target of a broad range of criticism towards validity and reliability (Venkatachalam, 2004).

There are inherent weaknesses and strengths in both approaches. In the context of health effects of noise pollution around airports, the main advantage of the hedonic pricing method (HPM) is that actual behavior of consumers in the housing market is observed, whereas the contingent valuation (CV) method is based on statements on the willingness to pay for of a chosen sample. A critique on CV is that the hypothetical WTP might be higher than the real WTP. A weakness of HPM is that the price of noise has to be calculated at an expense of modeling assumptions (Bjørner et al. 2003). Imperfect information is another problem within HPM studies (Delucchi et al. 2002). Furthermore hedonic pricing usually values environmental impacts on humans (noise, air pollution) but basically leaves out non-use values such as existence values of environmental amenities.

2.2 Benefit transfer

In many planning efforts, it is not feasible to conduct primary valuation studies due to budgetary constraints. Benefit transfer might therefore seem to be an economical alternative. The general idea of benefit transfer is that parameters or results of valuations obtained at study sites can be transferred to policy sites (Nellthorp et al., 2007).1 Environmental value transfer is mainly transposition of estimated values on one study site, valued by market-based and non-market based economic valuation method, to another. Considerations on cost-effectiveness are the most important reason for the further use of previous research results. Using already existing calculated results is therefore an attractive alternative due to time and resource consuming original research (Brouwer, 2000).

The application of environmental value transfer ranges from water quality improvements (Barton, 2002; Bliem et al., 2011), air quality (Rozan, 2004), and health-risk reductions (Brouwer & Bateman, 2005) to airport noise nuisance case studies (Johnson & Button, 1997).

[1] For overviews of benefit transfer see e.g. Wilson and Hoehn, 2006; Lindhjem and Navrud, 2008.

Basically, there are two approaches, namely unit value transfer and function transfer. The former can be subdivided into simple unit transfer and unit transfer with income adjustments, the latter into benefit function transfer and meta-analysis. Simple unit transfer is the easiest form, assuming that the same utility (and disutility) can be experienced on study and policy sites so that directly transferring the mean benefit estimate is possible. This approach is not feasible for transfer between countries, which differ in income levels, standard of living, and regulatory and economic frameworks. Consequently, unit transfer with income adjustments (e.g. purchase power parity) as an alternative has been established. By transferring entire benefit functions, more information is transferred effectively. Problems occur due to the limitations of observations from only one study or a small number of sites, especially in the exclusion of variables and in the demand as well as in the bid function (Navrud, 2002). A way of assessing different outcomes of different studies is meta-analysis, a statistical analysis of empirical findings. Based on average or global data, meta-analysis generates a value function (Brouwer, 2000). However, in most studies of benefit transfer, even with very similar conditions at the study and policy sites, substantial differences in values still remain unexplained.

Various problems arise in transferring benefits from study to policy sites. Benefit transfers can be applied within and between regions, as well as between countries. Generally, when conducting benefit transfer, it is more likely that the valued good and the population affected will be similar, the closer the study site is to the policy site in terms of geography and socio-political context. In transferring values internationally, especially issues regarding currency conversion, the variation in measurable characteristics (e.g. income) and the complex quantification of differences in culture and shared experiences are relevant (Ready & Navrud, 2006). Rosenberger and Stanley (2006) differentiate between three potential sources of error within benefit transfer. (1) Measurement error results from judgements and assumptions of the underlying primary studies. (2) Generalization error is inversely related to correspondence between study and policy sites. (3) Publication selection bias eventually refers to selection criteria for research results and that the chosen empirical literature cannot represent an unbiased sample of evidence.

Monetarization of aircraft and airport related noise nuisance has gained high interest and stimulated a continuing debate in the scientific community. Case-specific studies, deploying revealed and stated preference methods have produced several insights and results. However, broad use of diverse approaches and techniques implies many difficulties for benefit transfers. On the one hand different theoretical assumptions of stated and revealed preference methods aggravate possible benefit transfers, which are reflected in inherent limitations in terms of general applicability. The disparity of values resulting from the use of the two methodological groups per se as well as within the methods is more problematic (Johnson & Button, 1997).

3. Empirical evidence: Economic values for air traffic noise pollution

Aircraft noise is supposed to produce a variety of economic and psychosocial effects (see in detail the section 2.4 below on health effects). Exposure to noise may affect quality of life and environmental amenity, performance and property values (S. Morrell et al., 1997). The analysis of the relationship of this environmental impact on housing prices is a common methodology and can be examined in different ways.

Noise can be defined as unwanted or undesirable sound and is perceived as an environmental stressor (Stansfeld & Matheson, 2003; Haralabidis et al., 2008). Noise is typically measured by decibels (dB), a measure of the intensity of sound pressure levels. This logarithmic scale is weighted by the frequency sensitivities of the human ear referred to as A-weighting. The scale ranges from 0, the human audibility threshold, up to 130, the pain threshold. Noise exposure levels above 40 dB(A) have an influence on individual's well-being and levels above 60 dB(A) are associated with health problems. On this scale everyday noise ranges from 45 dB(A) to 115 dB(A). Road traffic causes noise levels of over 55 dB(A), and 32% of the European Union population is permanently exposed to this kind of noise pollution. Airport and air-traffic noise exceeding 55 dB(A) affects three million people in the European Union. Airport noise is therefore the second most important source of noise nuisance (Barreiro et al., 2005).

In order to study economic impacts and the perception of noise definition and measurement techniques are required. A variety of measures for aircraft noise can be distinguished. The "noise exposure forecast", the "noise and number index" (NNI) and "annual energy mean sound level" (Ldn) have been three standard measures (McMillen, 2004). Data on noise exposure has been difficult to compare because of different national noise indices and noise standards (Nijland & van Wee, 2005). In Europe the NNI measuring the amount of noise incidents and their maximum levels throughout a day and aggregating it into a statistic, has been substituted by the Leq (Boes & Nüesch, 2011). "Leq" means "level of equivalent sound" and measures the summation of energy or number of noise events, the levels of exposure to and the time average of sound over a certain period (Bell, 2001). The day-night level (DNL or Ldn) describes the equivalent sound levels over a 24 hour period. Nighttime noise levels are increased by an adjustment factor of 10 dB (A), reflecting the higher disturbance compared to day-time noise exposure. Similarly to Ldn a day-evening-night level Lden is used with a different adjustment factor of 5 dB (A) for evening noise (Passchier-Vermeer & Passchier, 2000). While the valuation methods have remained almost unchanged over the last two decades the development of methodologies concerning noise measurement as well as the linkage of noise and annoyance has proceeded (Rich & Nielsen, 2004). According to the hedonic pricing method, findings of these studies are often presented in terms of the "Noise Depreciation Index" (NDI), which is also known as "Noise Depreciation Sensitivity Index" (NDSI). This measure defines the average house value decrease, when it comes to a 1 dB increase in aircraft noise (Dekkers & van der Straaten, 2008). In the monetary valuation of airport noise the choice of a certain threshold value, other noise sources and the accessibility to the airport need to be taken into consideration (Lijesen et al., 2010).

3.1 Hedonic pricing

In a recent study Dekkers and van der Straaten (2008) include aircraft, railway and road traffic noise in their hedonic study on housing prices around Amsterdam Airport Schiphol (for a summary of empirical studies see Table 1). A threshold value of 45 dB (A) is chosen due to the assumption that aircraft noise nuisance is perceived more disturbing than other noise sources. Data on house prices and date of sales (period 1999-2003) as well as structural housing characteristics are collected. Aircraft noise is computed by modeled flight paths, covering an area of 70 by 55 kilometers for the 2002-2004 period and of 55 by 55 kilometers for the 1999-2001 period. As a result aircraft noise has the largest effect on house prices with a stated NDI of 0.77, which means that a 1 dB (A) increase in aircraft noise leads to a decrease in average house values of 0.77%. In this analysis aircraft noise is assumed to be a continuous variable. Therefore the marginal benefit curve is a continuous function and easier comparable with the marginal cost curve. The marginal and total benefits of aircraft noise reduction are determined. Based on regression results the marginal benefit of 1 dB noise reduction amounts to €1,459 per house. Using an interest rate of 7% (comprised of 4% basic interest and 3% risk compensation) a marginal benefit of noise pollution reduction of €102/dB/house/year is calculated. This brings about an annual total benefit of 1 dB noise reduction of €574 million around the airport examined. In addition the authors emphasize the dependence of the marginal WTP for noise reduction on income, other household characteristics and preferences for environmental quality.

Ahlfeldt and Maenning (2007) also analyze land values in Berlin based on a hedonic model. The empirical results show that areas within the Tempelhof air corridor sell at approximately 9% discount due to noise pollution, while no significantly negative impacts are ascertained for Tegel Airport.

Cohen and Coughlin (2008) use a hedonic price approach including spatial effects to identify the impacts of noise on residential housing prices near Hartsfield-Jackson Atlanta International airport, often referred to as the world's busiest passenger airport. For the analysis two data sources are combined. The noise contour map for the airport's surroundings and sale price data of single-family dwellings including detailed housing characteristics, both for the year 2003, are used. The dwellings are located in and near the noise boundaries. Houses in areas exposed to a day-night sound noise levels of 70-75 dB sell for 20.8% less than houses in areas with a noise level below 65 dB. However, no statistically significant relationships between the effects of noise at this airport on the property values of the small city of College Park can be found, as Lipscomb (2003) shows.

In a case study of Winnipeg International Airport, covering sales data of 1,635 single detached houses an NDI estimate of 1.3 for 1985/1986 is detected (Levesque, 1994). Uyeno et al. (1993) distinguish between detached family houses, condominiums and vacant land in their hedonic analysis for Vancouver International Airport in 1987. The computed NDSI is 0.65 for detached houses and 0.9 for condominiums. For vacant land they find a statistically significant difference, implying an even higher impact compared to the other categories.

In contrast to other study results Pennington et al. (1990) cannot find a statistically significant noise impact from Manchester International Airport in the period 1985-1986, taking relevant neighborhood and house characteristics into account. Pommerehne (1988) compares the application of the hedonic technique and contingent valuation method to assess aircraft and road noise impacts for the city of Basle. A sample of 223 dwellings are analysed, including single and multi family houses, sole residential houses and houses with commercial and residential use. In the case of aircraft noise a mean WTP of 22.3 SFr per household/month for the hedonic analysis is found to reduce noise.

The impact of noise and air pollution on rents in Geneva is analyzed by Baranzini and Ramirez (2005). Three different databases are included in the analysis; a geographical information system, statistical data on the Geneva rental market and environmental data stemming from the "Geneva cantonal office for the protection against noise". Their results cover values for numerous sources of noise with separate results for airport noise, distinguishing between public and private sector tenants, and day (Ld measure) and day-evening-night noise levels (Lden measure). In the private rental sector the property price impact in terms of Ld per additional 10 dB(A) is 6.6%, while rents in the public sector are about 8% lower. Considering Lden for the airport area an impact of approximately 12% per additional 10 dB(A) is observed. Summarizing the results, with an impact on rents of about 1% per additional dB(A) the effect of airport noise is slightly higher than the impact of other noise sources of 0.7%.

Hedonic pricing and spatial econometrics are combined by Salvi's (2008) study on property values for Zurich Airport area. A data set is used, which includes the average aircraft noise emissions measured by different Leq metric variants. The choice of a threshold of 50 dB(A) for the noise contour zone and a second data set of 3737 single-family homes (included in the final sample) sold between 1995-2005 in the Canton of Zurich lead to a NDI of 0.97.

The research of Espey and Lopez (2000) also takes the impact of proximity to the airport on property values into account. A random sample of 1,417 single-family, owner-occupied houses of different census tracts near the airport is drawn and structural and environmental characteristics of these homes are collected. Data on noise is provided by annual noise exposure maps, which include the noise contours for the 65, 70 and 75 Ldn noise areas. Their hedonic analysis indicates that houses in areas with noise levels of 65 dB and above sell for approximately 2.4% less than homes located below this threshold. Contrary to earlier empirical findings, proximity to the Reno-Sparks airport can be treated as a disamenity with a value difference of 2.6% for equivalent houses one versus two miles apart from the airport. McMillen (2004) observes house transactions for single-family houses and assessment data in 1997 for Chicago O'Hare Airport, focusing on an area covering a 2 mile band of the defined noise contour line. The values of houses near the airport subject to noise levels from 65 dB are about 9% lower than comparable houses in less noise polluted areas.

A broader approach is used by van Praag and Baarsma (2005) who try to value noise pollution and value depreciation around Amsterdam Airport by means of an extended hedonic method, integrating subjective questions about well-being and happiness into their model.2 An equation is estimated, defining happiness as a function of household income, age, family size, noise perception and presence of noise insulation. Income and percentage change in noise levels are determining factors of the shadow price. Moreover this work has stimulated the discussion about adequate monetary compensation schemes for aircraft noise nuisance. Lijesen et al. (2010) transfer the results of the above-mentioned study from the Dutch noise index Ku (Kosten Unit) into dB values. The monthly WTA of an increase in noise exposure from 53 dB to 55 dB of a household with a net income of €1,500 per month equals 2.24%, a further rise in noise from 55 dB to 58 dB is 1.58% of household income.

In their survey on noise nuisance around Amsterdam Schiphol Airport the results of Lijesen et al. (2010) indicate that aircraft noise has the largest impact on housing prices, followed by rail and road traffic noise. Data on housing sales (1999-2003) and characteristics, variables on

[2] Recently the use of these happiness surveys has become more important in welfare economics, since happiness indicators can reflect (personal) welfare more accurately than income (cf. e.g. Layard, 2006; Bruni, 2007; Frey, 2008).

the housing environment (for example population density, distance to the next railway station) as well as transport noise sources are included. The calculated NDI is 0.8, i.e. a 1 dB decrease of noise leads to an increase of house values of 0.8% corresponding to an average value increase of €1,880 per household. Projected for the entire region of the analysis, a reduction of noise by 1 db (A) means a total benefit of €574 million.

Lu (2011) evaluated employment effects and the social costs of noise and aircraft engine emissions at the Taiwanese Taoyuan International Airport. For the estimation of annual noise costs an average NDI of 0.6 is assumed, accounting for the number of residences in each noise zone of the noise contour and the annual average house rents. These aggregate costs are allocated to individual flights on the basis of the marginal noise nuisance of the incremental effect of an extra flight on the day-night sound level. Total annual noise costs of approximately €12 million are estimated for the year 2008.

Jud and Winkler (2006) combine hedonic and event study models to assess the announcement effect of a new airport hub at Greensboro airport in North Carolina on housing prices. Noise is correlated with several property market aspects like traffic congestion and air pollution. Separating noise from other determinants of property values is considered problematic by the authors. They emphasize that the ex post perspective of most studies - in other words after the property market has adjusted to the increased noise exposure level - has to be seen critically. The announcement effect of an increase in noise intensity and frequency due to airport expansions is therefore focused. While no actual noise changes can be observed using this combination of methodologies, the announcement of significant change in airport traffic is assumed to be related to airport proximity and affects surrounding properties. The sample is drawn from housing sales occurring from 1997-2004, focusing on the change in property values prior and post the announcement, but before the construction or operation of the new airport facility. Within a 2.5 mile band around Greensboro airport the noise discount was 0.2% before the announcement, compared to a decrease of housing prices of 9.4% afterwards. Thus, a 9.2% increase in the discount is made out following the announcement. The difference in values of properties located more distant (within a 2.5- 4 mile band) to the airport decreases by 5.7%, comparing the noise discount of 2.7% before and 8.4% after the announcement.

Another event study (Pope 2008) focuses on the impact of a noise disclosure in the housing market surrounding Raleigh-Durham International Airport in North Carolina, highlighting the problem of information asymmetry between sellers and potential buyers. The airport authority sent a notification letter and a noise contour map to all homeowners living in 55 to 70 dB noise zones around the airport as well as to real estate agents. The primary data used are single-family house transactions between 1992 and 2000 in Waker County North Carolina. Only the sales of house within the defined noise zones requiring disclosure and within a one mile buffer zone around this area, serving as a kind of natural control group, are included in the analysis. Controlling for spatial and temporal confounders, a further decrease in residential property values of 2.9% in the zone of severe noise exposure (65-70 Ldn) is made out, while no effect of the noise disclosure on house prices in low noise areas can be observed. This study demonstrates that the availability of information for buyers has a potential impact on the implicit price of airport noise. One possible explanation is that there was a lack of information prior to the disclosure and that the estimated marginal value of airport noise is affected by the information status.

Study	Location	Date of Price Observation	Valuation technique	Empirical findings
Lu (2011)	Taiwan Taoyuan International Airport	2008	hedonic pricing	average NDI 0.6
Lijeson et al. (2010)	Amsterdam	1999-2003	hedonic pricing	NDI 0.8
Dekkers/ van der Straaten (2008)	Amsterdam Schiphol	1999-2003	hedonic pricing	NDI 0.77
Cohen&Coughlin (2008)	Atlanta	2003	hedonic pricing	noise discount of 20.8%
Salvi (2008)	Zurich	1995-2005	hedonic pricing/ spatial econometrics	NDI 0.97
Pope (2008)	Raleigh–Durham International Airport	1992-2000	hedonic pricing/ event study	price discount of 2.9%
Ahlfeldt& Maenning (2007)	Berlin Tegel/ Berlin Tempelhof	2005	hedonic pricing	noise discount of 9%
Jud& Winkler (2006)	Greensboro Airport	1997-2004	hedonic pricing/ event study models	noise discount of 9.2% noise discount of 5.7%
Baranzini& Ramirez (2005)	Geneva	2003	hedonic pricing	discount on rents of 1% per dB(A)
Nelson (2004)	US/ Canadian Airports		meta-analysis of 20 hedonic pricing studies	NDI 0.51-0.67 NDI 0.8-0.9
Schipper (2004)/ Schipper et al. (1998)	US/Canada/ UK/ Australia		meta-analysis of 19 hedonic pricing studies	mean NDI 0.48
McMillen (2004)	Chicago O`Hare	1997	hedonic pricing	noise discount of 9%
Lipscomb (2003)	Atlanta	1997-2000	hedonic pricing	statistically insignificant
Espey&Lopez (2000)	Reno-Sparks Airport	1991-1995	hedonic pricing	noise discount of 2.4%
Levesque (1994)	Winnipeg	1985/ 1986	hedonic pricing	NDI 1.3
Uyeno et al. (1993)	Vancouver	1987	hedonic pricing	NDI 0.65 for detached houses, NDI 0.9 for condominiums
Pennington et al. (1990)	Manchester	1985/ 1986	hedonic pricing	statistically insignificant
Pommerehne (1988)	Basle	1983/ 1984	hedonic pricing	mean WTP 22.3 SFr

Table 1. Summary of hedonic pricing studies

Nelson (2004) considered the relationship between airport noise and property values in terms of NDI estimates. The author conducts a meta-analysis of 20 hedonic property value studies for 23 US and Canadian Airports, covering 33 NDI estimates. The effect of airport noise on US housing prices is 0.51-0.67% per additional decibel, while the noise discount amounts to 0.8-0.9% for Canadian property values. Another meta-analysis by Schipper et al. (1998) surveys 19 published and unpublished hedonic studies, providing 30 NDI estimates and finds a mean NDI of 0.48 for published works that include other price influencing factors (Schipper, 2004).

Table 1 summarizes the most relevant hedonic price studies; the NDI which may be transferred to other contexts than the ones of the respective studies since it is dimensionless seem to range from 0.48 to 1.3, with a broad average around 0.8 to 0.9.

3.2 Contingent valuation

Few stated preference studies on aircraft noise have been conducted (Navrud, 2004). Pommerehne (1988) uses both techniques for the valuation of noise impacts for Basle to validate the contingent valuation method and test the compatibility of the methods. Thus 223 households were not directly asked for their willingness-to-pay for a noise reduction by a half, but were told to be part of a large survey on environmental problems guided by the University of Basle. Information then followed, describing households about the possibilities of relocation to identical dwellings, located in areas where traffic noise is reduced by half and takeover of the associated moving costs by a special fund. Actual net rents and maximum tolerable increase in rents for the new dwelling were questioned, preventing strategic behavior and enhancing realistic decision-making by the households. The results indicate a mean WTP of SFr 32.3 per household and month in the case of aircraft noise.

Caplen (2000) uses a contingent valuation framework to examine the maximum willingness to pay (WTP) to prevent and minimum willingness to accept to allow an increase (by 10%) in the frequency of aircraft flights for Southampton International Airport. Focusing on the southern end of the runway, the study was completed in 1998. The sample consisted of 150 questionnaires and 116 were returned. For an increase in daytime-flights the author finds a mean WTP of £3.35 and a mean WTP of £9.11 for an increase in night-flights.

Marmolejo Duarte (2008) tries to identify the marginal value of quiet by evaluating the acoustical impact of Barcelona's airport expansion. 309 respondents of this contingent valuation survey stated an averaged WTP of €8.95 per person and month. Feitelson et al. (1996) discuss the impact of aircraft noise succeeding airport expansions on the WTP for residences. Home owners and tenants near a major hub airport are asked in a telephone survey for their WTP for residences without aircraft noise disturbance and then questioned for their WTP, when the same residence is exposed to various noise levels, measured in Ldn. In comparison to residences without any noise exposure the difference of valuation for those properties subject to severe and frequent noise is 2.4-4.1% of the housing prices per Ldn and for tenants this noise premium is 1.8-3.0% of the rent per Ldn. Noise can be seen as multi-attribute-externality and the results reveal that the WTP structures of households are kinked, which means that at a certain threshold of noise nuisance the households are unwilling to pay anything for the residence. The following Table 2 summarizes and provides an overview of the existing recent empirical works.

Study	Location	Valuation technique	Empirical findings
Marmolejo Duarte (2008)	Barcelona	contingent valuation	averaged WTP of 8.95€/ person/month
Caplen (2000)	Southhampton	contingent valuation	mean WTP £3.35/ month day-time flights mean WTP £9.11/ month night-time flights
Feitelson et al. (1996)	major hub airport	contingent valuation	noise discount of 2.4-4.1% of housing price per Ldn; 1.8-3% of rent per Ldn
Pommerehne (1988)	Basle	contingent valuation	mean WTP 32.3 SFr

Table 2. Summary of contingent valuation studies

3.3 Epidemiological studies: Health impacts and long-term health effects of chronic aircraft noise exposure

Noise related health effects can be distinguished into auditory and non-auditory, with the latter being further subdivided into socio-psychological and physical effects. There are sleep disturbance, disturbance in performance and daily activities, annoyance and mental health problems (fear, depression, frustration) and stress-related physical phenomena (Health Council of the Netherlands [HCN], 1999). Noise exposure directly causes physiological responses such as increased blood pressure and heart rate. Chronic noise nuisance may aggravate these reactions and foster long-term and subsequent illnesses or symptoms. Noise provokes annoyance, if the exposed individual feels disturbed. The stated physical responses may be induced by annoyance reactions (Clark & Stansfeld, 2007). Annoyance is a central psychological factor within noise effect research (Quehl & Basner, 2006). Within this chapter, we focus on the non-auditory impacts of airport noise exposure.

Kaltenbach et al. (2008) conducted a selective literature review of epidemiological studies (period of 2000-2007) focusing on illnesses, learning disorders and annoyance resulting from aircraft noise. In residential areas an outdoor day-time noise equivalent noise levels of 60 dB (A) and night time exposure of 45 dB (A) are associated with an increase in incidence of hypertension. A level of above 45 dB (A) leads to a higher prescription frequency of blood pressure-lowering medication and so a dose-dependent connection to aircraft noise can be assumed. School children are affected particularly, because daytime outdoor noise exposure levels above 50 dB (A) result in relevant learning difficulties and disorders. Annoyance of affected population is also a pivotal factor. According to a study for Frankfurt airport, 25% of local residents feel highly annoyed at day-time continuous sound levels of 53 dB(A).

Jarup et al. (2008) assessed the relation of aircraft and road traffic noise respectively and hypertension by analyzing blood pressure measurements, health and lifestyle data of 4,861 residents near six European airports.3 Results indicate that the risk of hypertension is related to long term noise exposure, particularly for night-time aircraft noise exposure. A similar association is found for daily average road traffic noise produced in the airport surroundings.

[3] This work is part of the HYENA study (hypertension and exposure to noise near airports), a four year key action project on environment and health (2002-2006). For more information see: http://www.hyena.eu.com/

In a longitudinal study, Eriksson et al. (2007) analyze the relation of the incidence of hypertension and aircraft noise around Stockholm Arlanda Airport. Between 1992-1994 and 2002-2004 a cohort of 2,754 men was surveyed. Residential aircraft noise exposure was measured in terms of Leq and divided into categories with levels above a threshold of 50 dB (A). 2,027 men completed a follow-up examination and had no former treatment of hypertension and a blood pressure below 140/90 mm Hg at enrollment. Restricted to this sample, analyses result in the association of the risk of hypertension and long-term noise exposure. Accounting for confounders, the incidence of hypertension in middle-aged Swedish men in particular is associated with aircraft noise exposure. The impact of aircraft noise on general health status and use of medication for residents near Amsterdam Schiphol is analyzed by Franssen et al. (2004). A postal questionnaire was completed by 11,812 residents in 1996/1997, comprising questions about respiratory complaints, sleep disturbance, annoyance, general health status, medication use, residential satisfaction and perceived risk, covering an area of 25 km around the airport with noise exposure levels from Lden 50 dB (A). Late evening noise exposure is associated with the intake of non-prescribed sleep medication and sedatives. For vitality related health complaints, e.g. headaches or tiredness, an association is found. Results suggest that the general health status may be poorer and the risk for cardiovascular diseases is higher at aircraft noise exposure levels above 50 dB (A).

An association of prescription prevalence of cardiovascular and antihypertensive drugs and night-time noise exposure is determined, linking prescription data of 809,379 insured persons and noise data (threshold 40 dB (A)) in the vicinity of Cologne-Bonn Airport. Aircraft noise increases the prevalence rate of the stated medication, particularly in cases where a conjunction with anxiolytic medication is given (Greiser et al., 2007).

Knipschild (1977a) links the data of 6,000 participants of a community cardiovascular survey and aircraft noise exposure of Amsterdam Airport Schiphol. Respondents are divided into two subgroups, with the first group of residents exposed to an NNI (noise and number index) exceeding 37 and the second exposed to NNI in a range of 20-30. Comparing the residents of both noise zone subgroups, in areas exposed to higher noise levels the share of residents suffering from cardiovascular impairment is 50% higher. People living in areas with higher noise levels are more often in medical treatment for hypertension and heart trouble. The author finds that the prevalence of cardiovascular disease is higher in high noise areas. Therefore evidence suggests that cardiovascular disease and aircraft noise are related causally.

The frequency of consultation of general practitioners in high noise areas surrounding Schiphol airport indicates another association: 19 practitioners provided the data (diagnosis, drug use, age, sex, address) of all their patients of one week and it is shown that in areas exceeding NNI levels of 33 the total contact rate is higher (2-3 times higher than in areas with NNI below 20). Accounting for confounders (gender, age, socioeconomics), results indicate that aircraft noise leads to an increase in the contact rate with general practitioners for psychological and diverse psychosomatic problems (Knipschild, 1977b).

The association of medication use and aircraft noise is studied by Knipschild and Oudshoorn (1977). Two villages near Schiphol airport, one not exposed to noise and the other one exposed to differing noise levels (basically no noise exposure, from 1969 exposure levels above an NNI of 35 and in a last timeframe at 1973 only exposed to daytime noise exposure) by analyzing purchase data of pharmacies in the period of 1967-1974. While the drug consumption remained unchanged in the control village, the use of antacids on prescription and cardiovascular medication increased in the six year period to almost twice its initial amount in the noise exposed area. Due to a similar increase in the use of antihypertensive drugs it is concluded that aircraft noise is a risk factor for hypertension. The consumption of sedatives and hypnotics increased in the period of high noise exposure (1969-1972) and decreased when the government regulated night-time flights. Aircraft noise can be a causal factor for sleep disturbance and mental disorders.

For the analysis of the frequency of various illnesses and medication use respectively, data of questionnaires filled in by doctors and patients is evaluated by Vallet et al. (1999). In a comparison of 275 exposed and 374 non-exposed residents in the proximity of Roissy Airport, defined by national noise contours (French measure indice psophique), associations between the level of noise exposure and use of neuro-psychiatric, sedative, anti-ulcerous and anti-acid medication are identified after adjustments for socioeconomic criteria. Aircraft noise is therefore associated with anxiety as well as annoyance. In the noisier areas a significant increase in sick leaves can be observed. No significant correlation is found for an increase in blood pressure.

Another study examines the relationship of hypertension and community exposure to aircraft noise in the vicinity of Arlanda Airport, comprising two random samples of 266 residents in noise exposed areas in the airport's surroundings and another 2693 living in other parts of Stockholm. Individual characteristics are considered in a questionnaire, also accounting for history of hypertension. After adjusting for confounders (age, gender, smoking, education) the prevalence odds ratio for hypertension is 1.6 for residents exposed to energy averaged noise levels above 55 dB (A) and 1.8 for those with noise levels exceeding 72 dB (A). Aircraft noise may increase the risk of hypertension and therefore might be a risk factor for cardiovascular disease (Rosenlund et al., 2001).

Mental and physical effects on residents near Futenma and Kadena military airfields exposed to a range of Ldn levels of 55 to above 70 are surveyed by a self-reported questionnaire (7095 valid answers). Significant dose-response relationships are found for nervousness, depressiveness and vague complaints as well as in terms of respiratory, digestive and mental instability. With increasing noise levels these responses elevate (Miyakita et al., 2002). A recent Italian study tries to assess the impact on psychiatric disorders, comparing personnel interview data of 71 participants (aged 18-75) in the immediate vicinity of Elma's airport and of 284 subjects of a matched non-exposed control group. Noise is measured in distance to the airport terms and therefore statements about intensity of the exposure or noise-sensitivity are not feasible. However, higher lifetime prevalence rates for "generalized anxiety disorder" and "anxiety disorder not otherwise specified" are reported for the exposed residents, indicating a higher risk for anxietal syndromes (Hardoy et al., 2005).

The association between road and air traffic noise exposure (occupational and community) and blood pressure as well as ischemic heart disease has also been subject to a meta-analysis. Van Kempen et al. (2002) analyze 43 epidemiologic studies published in the period of 1970-1999, finding that aircraft noise is positively associated with cardiovascular medication, the consultation of general practitioners and angina pectoris.

Children are supposed to be vulnerable to environmental impacts like noise pollution particularly. The RANCH project aims to examine exposure-effect relations between chronic noise exposure and children's health and cognition. It is the largest study funded by the European Commission focusing on aircraft and road traffic noise, covering three European countries.4 Influences of air and road traffic on children's cognition and health status as well as on mental health are assessed within this framework. In a cross-national and cross-sectional survey 2,844 school children (aged 9-10) in the vicinity of three major airports of the Netherlands, Spain and the UK were surveyed. Data of noise contour zones and on-site measurements were also used. Questionnaires and standardized test were conducted in the classrooms, and additional information was collected from parents. For analysis, data was pooled and exposure-effect relationships were developed for the whole sample. Linear associations between aircraft noise exposure and impaired performance in reading comprehension and recognition memory were detected, while a non-linear association in terms of annoyance was identified. For the analysis of mental health status a "Strength and Difficulties Questionnaire" was utilized. Aircraft noise levels were classified in ranges from 30-77 dB (A). After full adjustment no association on children's overall mental health status in terms of conduct and emotional problems or prosocial behaviour were measured, but an association of aircraft noise and hyperactivity was identified (Stansfeld et al., 2005; Stansfeld et al., 2009).

The effects of noise exposure on school children living adjacent to London Heathrow Airport with respect to cognitive performance, stress responses and mental health were studied by Haines et al. (2001a). The comparison of the health status as well as cognitive performance of 340 children (aged 8-11) at four schools located in high noise exposure areas (defined by Leq exceeding 66 dB (A)) and four control schools in less exposed areas (Leq below 57 dB (A)), including questionnaires of 21 teachers and 284 parents, revealed several associations. Chronic exposure to high levels of aircraft noise was consistently and strongly associated with higher annoyance levels. The association of poorer performances in reading comprehension as well as long-term memory recognition may be an indication of possible cognitive function impairments related to aircraft noise. In terms of reading comprehension, the association could not be attributed to socio-demographic factors, noise annoyance or noise interference. With respect to mental health, no associations between noise exposure and depression, anxiety, hyperactivity and conduct problems could be established.

Haines et al. (2001b) analyze data of 451 school children (aged 8-11) attending 10 schools in West London areas with noise levels above Leq 63 and compared them to data of 10 control schools exposed to Leq levels below 57 dB (A)). They found associations regarding annoyance levels and impaired reading performance. Psychological morbidity and hyperactivity were weakly associated with aircraft noise, while no associations were confirmed in the spheres of memory, stress responses or attention.

Elevated psychophysical stress (expressed in rest blood pressure and concentrations of epinephrine and norepinephrine) as well as lower quality of life was determined for 9-11 year old children, comparing data of 217 children before and after the operation of a new Munich airport over a two year period. Children in quieter areas (Leq 55 after and Leq 53

---

[4] For more information on this project and further publications see http://www.wolfson.qmul.ac.uk/RANCH_Project/

prior to opening) were matched to those living in noisier surroundings (Leq 62 after and Leq 53 prior to the opening), using socioeconomic data. Quality of life was measured by KINDL index, including psychological, physical, social and functional daily life (G.W. Evans et al., 1998).

Van Kempen's (2010) conducted a cross-sectional study around Schiphol Airport on the association of transportation noise and neurobehavioral effects, 553 primary school children (aged 9-11) completed tests on reading comprehension, perceptual skills, attention, memory as well as motor system (in terms of paper-and-pencil tests and "Neurobehavioral Evaluation System" test) to assess cognitive performance. In addition a questionnaire on health and behavioural indicators and socioeconomic status was answered by the caregivers. In the case of aircraft noise, higher noise levels in the school and residential environment lead to a significant elevation of errors in more difficult tasks within the tests. Therefore it can be concluded that performance of less complex tasks is not susceptible to the impacts of noise.

A meta-analysis of 13 epidemiological studies on noise and blood pressure of children in urban environments published in the last 30 years focuses on methodological issues. Drawing general conclusions was impeded due to differences in study design, blood pressure and noise measurement as well as accounting for socioeconomic confounders. However, a tendency that aircraft noise is positively associated with children's blood pressure was indicated (Paunović et al., 2011).

Babisch and van Kamp (2009) carried out a meta-analysis, covering 20 studies referring to aircraft noise on the basis of commercial and 8 of military activity, whilst differentiating between effects on children and adults. In conclusion, no empirically supportable, generalized exposure-response relationship due to methodological and noise data difficulties could be ascertained, although there was sufficient evidence that an association between aircraft noise and the use of cardiovascular medication and blood pressure is existent

4. Implications for transferability of values and results

The current paper has reviewed and summarized the existing (empirical) literature on the economic effects of noise pollution around airports. Transferring these diverse results is not straightforward, but the review shows that there is a broad common ground on which conclusions for new policy sites can be drawn. Regarding property values, hedonic pricing studies as well as contingent valuation surveys are commonly used for the association of airport noise related impacts on housing values. Generalization and transferability are limited due to methodological differences between the studies. Especially the differing use of noise measures, noise contours and the individual national noise standards has impeded comparability of results. The choice of a certain noise threshold, referring to the complexity and of the definition of noise exposure, is crucial and aggravates comparability and transferability.

Another difference is the consideration of spatial confounders and variables on housing characteristics. Hedonic as well as contingent valuation studies have shown decreases in residential property values. There are only a few contingent valuation studies, so their general applicability might be limited. Nevertheless, results of both methodological approaches are dependent on theoretical assumptions, subjects, and areas, and there are also studies that cannot find statistically significant results.

Taking all arguments together, it is safe to assume an average NDI of around 0.8 to 0.9 with a range of 0.5 to 1.3. This means that property values decrease by 0.8 to 0.9% with a 1 dB(A) increase in noise levels, above a certain threshold of 45 dB(A). Socioeconomic factors, however, should be taken into account, bearing in mind that often residents of lower socioeconomic status live in noise polluted areas in the vicinity of airports.

We find that the NDI - even in the light of the manifold differences between the study sites - delivers measures robust enough to value properties around airports even without employing original (primary) research. Merely all studies find significant negative impacts of air traffic noise pollution on property values, in a comparable way. Conducting cost-benefit analysis for extensions or new construction of airports, together with science based noise maps, thus allows at least for computing a reasonable and robust range of total costs of noise pollution. The WTP studies reviewed support the hedonic pricing results, but are seemingly more context-dependent (i.e. influences by the study design and the survey technique).

Health effects by themselves are reported by epidemiologic studies, focusing on incidence, prevalence and risk of symptoms and certain illnesses. Evidence is available for effects on adults and children. Empirical findings differ in terms of study design, samples, methodological assumption, noise measures and adjustments of outcomes. Various associations on health related noise effects have been identified. Hypertension risk and incidence are associated with aircraft noise (Jarup et al., 2008; Eriksson et al., 2007; Knipschild & Oudshoorn, 1977). Risk for cardiovascular diseases increases with noise levels (Rosenlund et al., 2001; Knipschild, 1977a), in particular for night-time noise exposure (Greiser et al., 2007). There is also a link of the intake of sedatives and noise nuisance at night, which may be associated with negative effects on sleep quality (Franssen et al., 2004). In terms of mental health, associations between aircraft noise disturbance and the risk of long-term syndromal anxietal states are found (Hardoy et al., 2005; Vallet et al., 1999). Annoyance is related to airport noise, both for adults and children (Vallet et al., 1999; Kaltenbach et al., 2008; Haines, 2001b). Effects on children's health are primarily cognitive, as there are associations regarding reading comprehension and memory (Stansfeld et al., 2005; Stansfeld et al., 2009; Haines, 2001a). Stress and quality of life are affected similarly and there are also weak associations for hyperactivity as well as psychological morbidity (Haines, 2001b; G.W. Evans et al., 1998). Dose-response relations that explicitly link the dose or input variable (noise) and a specific response or outcome (health problem, symptom, illness) in a population are needed (Berry & Flindell, 2009), but significant dose-response functions are still not available for most health impacts.

Despite the bulk of evidence for adverse impacts on human health, there are also ambiguous findings. For example, van Kempen et al. (2006) investigated heart rate and blood pressure of school children within a cross-national RANCH framework and found an association between noise exposure at school and at home and blood pressure for the Dutch sample , but not for the British sample. Night-time aircraft noise changes do not have disturbing effects on sleep necessarily due to the adaption of residents to noise intrusions (Fidell et al., 2000).

Several studies are also considered with the association of perinatal influences of aircraft noise in terms of low birth weight and premature birth (e.g. Knipschild et al., 1981; Matsui et al., 2003; Rehm & Jansen, 1978). Due to methodological limitations and a lack of adjustments for possible confounders, conclusions cannot be drawn (S. Morrell et al., 1997; Amt für Gesundheit, 2008).

With respect to mental health, no direct association can be established due to operationalization difficulties basically, notwithstanding existing evidence for an apparent increased prevalence of anxiety and depression among residents living in airport surroundings (van Kamp & Davies, 2008). Most of the empirical works reviewed adjust their findings for socioeconomic and other health determinants, so this could be classified as an attempt to foster robustness of results.

Regarding the transferability of health effects, the studies exhibit significant negative health effects of air traffic noise pollution. For "policy sites" without original (primary) data, it is safe to assume similar health effects. For valuing these, however, it is important to assess the number of residents affects by certain noise levels, and value these, for instance, by treatment costs, or costs of the specific diseases. Usually, national frameworks for conducting cost-benefit analysis in the transport sector are well equipped with money values for these health effects. The current paper has to leave out a detailed discussion regarding adequate money values for these noise-related health effects. Under the assumption of fully informed households, discounted property values measured, e.g., by means of hedonic pricing may reflect the individual's assessment of health risks. Therefore, property values include the valuation of some of the health impacts around airports.

However, as many scientific studies have only recently established the linkages between noise and several health problems, it cannot readily be assumed that individuals indeed hold all relevant information to assign money values to health effects, and then incorporate these into property values. Thus, hedonic prices only reflect parts of the health effects, presumably rather nuisance than more serious problems such as reading difficulties of children, or high blood pressure. It has to be left open in the current paper which share of total health costs are reflected in hedonic prices.

5. Conclusion

The present chapter attempts to assess the economic impacts of various health impacts caused by noise pollution. International scientific literature and empirical findings are reviewed in order to assess evidence for potential health impacts of noise pollution in airport's surroundings and to analyze transferability of results.

Hedonic pricing studies reporting NDI estimates and noise discounts for residential property values, rents, vacant land and condominiums demonstrate decreasing prices in zones located in airport's vicinity. Resident's willingness to pay and willingness to accept changing flight times, frequencies and various levels of noise exposure reflect people's perception of noise as an environmental disamenity.

Demand for robust and statistically reliable correlations on the likelihood of health effects occurring under environmental noise levels is increasing, especially in terms of an adequate basis of decision-making for policy authorities. For the quantification and derivation of economic costs policy makers could use dose-response relationships (Berry & Flindell, 2009), which attribute environmental inputs like noise to a specified health related output variable.

In the light of expanding expenditures and further expected pressure for national health care systems, health effects fostered by increasing demand in the air transportation sector can be substantial.

Aircraft and airport activity related noise remains a concern in terms of public health. Further research is required to capture the complex correlation of airport related noise exposure and the effects on human health appropriately. Summing up, the detrimental effect of air traffic noise pollution on property values - reflecting only parts of economic values of health problems - is about 0.8 to 0.9% per dB(A) as the most relevant noise index. Negative health effects are well proven, however, the valuation of these much more depends on the regional, legal and socio-economic context of the concrete airport subject to economic studies.

6. Acknowledgements

The writing of this paper was financially supported by a research project funded by ZIT (Zentrum für Innovation und Technologie, Vienna) under project No. 517495. We also thank the anonymous reviewers for their comments. All errors are, of course, the responsibility of the authors.

7. References

Ahlfeld, G.M. & Maenning, W. (2008). Assessing external effects of city airports: Land values in Berlin, *Hamburg Contemporary Economic Discussions*, No.11, University of Hamburg

Amt für Gesundheit Frankfurt (2008). Fluglärm und Gesundheit. Ergebnisse epidemiologischer Studien- Literaturüberblick. Amt für Gesundheit, Frankfurt

Arndt, A.; Braun, T.; Eichinger, A. & Pansch, H. (2009). Economic catalytic impacts of air transport in Germany - The influence of connectivity by air on regional economic development. *Presented at the 13th Air Transport Research Society Conference*, Abu Dhabi, June 2009

Atkinson, G. & Mourato, S. (2008). Environmental Cost-Benefit Analysis. *Annual Review of Environment and Resources*, Vol. 33, Issue 3, 317-344

Babisch, W. & van Kamp, I. (2009). Exposure-response relationship of the association between aircraft noise and the risk of hypertension. *Noise & Health*, Vol. 11, Issue 44, 161-168

Baranzini, A.; Ramirez, J.V. (2005). Paying for quietness: The impact of noise on Geneva rents, *Urban Studies*, Vol. 42, No. 4, 633-646

Barreiro, J.; Sánchez, M. & Viladrich-Grau, M. (2005). How much are people willing to pay for silence? A contingent valuation study. *Applied Economics*, Vol. 37, Issue 11, 1233-1246

Barton, D.N. (2002), The transferability of benefit transfer: contingent valuation of water quality improvements in Costa Rica. *Ecological Economics*, Vol. 42, Issues 1-2, 147-164

Bell, R. (2001). The impact of airport noise on residential real estate. The Appraisal Journal, Vol. LXIX, No.3, 312-321

Berglund, B.; Lindvall, T. & Schwela, D.H. (Eds.) (1999). Guidelines for community noise. World Health Organization, Geneva

Berry, B.F./ Flindell, I.H. (2009). Estimating Dose-Response relationships between noise exposure and human health impacts in the UK. BEL: 2009 - 001, Final Project Report, 13.07.2011.

Bickel, P. & Friedrich, R. (Eds.) (2005). ExternE: Externalities of energy. Methodology 2005 Update. Universität Stuttgart- Institut für Energiewirtschaft und Rationelle Energieanwendung , European Commission, Luxembourg

Bjørner, T.B.; Kronbak, J. & Lundhede, Th. (2003). Valuation of Noise Reduction- Comparing results from hedonic pricing and contingent valuation. Amternes og Kommunernes Forskningsinstitut (AKF), Report No.51, 08.05.2011, available from http://www.akf.dk/udgivelser_en/2003/noise_reduction/

Bliem, M.; Getzner, M.& Rodiga-Lassnig, P. (2011). Temporal stability of individual preferences for river restoration in Austria using a choice experiment. Mimeo, Vienna University of Technology.

Boes, S. & Nüesch, S. (2011). Quasi-experimental evidence on the effect of aircraft noise on apartment rents. *Journal of Urban Economics*, Vol. 69, Issue 2, 196-204

Boyle, M.A. & Kiel, K.A. (2001). A Survey of House Price Hedonic Studies of the Impact of Environmental Externalities. *Journal of Real Estate Literature*, Vol. 9, No.2, 117-144

Braun, T.; Klophaus, R. & Lueg-Arndt, A. (2010). Wider economic benefits of air transport: estimating consumer surplus for Germany. *Proceedings of 12th World Conference of Transport Research*, Lisbon, July 2010

Brouwer, R. (2000). Environmental value transfer: state of the art and future prospects. *Ecological Economics*, Vol. 32, Issue 1, 137-152

Brouwer, R. & Bateman, I.J. (2005). Benefits transfer of willingness to pay estimates and functions for health-risk reductions: a cross-country study. *Journal of Health Economics, Vol.* 24, Issue 3, 591–611

Bruni, L. (2007). *Economics and happiness – framing the analysis.* Oxford University Press, Oxford

Caplen, J.G.F. (2000). Southampton international airport: an environmental approach. *Eco - Management and Auditing,* Vol. 7, Issue 1, 43-49

Cheshire, P. & Sheppard, S. (1995). On the Price of Land and the Value of Amenities.*Economica New Series,* Vol. 62, No. 246, 247-267

Cohen, J.P. & Coughlin, C.C. (2008). Spatial hedonic models of airport noise, proximity, and housing prices. *Journal of Regional Science,* Vol. 48, No.5, 859-878

Clark, C. & Stansfeld, S.A. (2007). The Effect of Transportation Noise on Health and Cognitive Development: A Review of Recent evidence. *International Journal of Comparative Psychology,* Vol. 20, No.2-3, 145-158

Collins, A. & Evans, A. (1994). Aircraft noise and residential property values: an artificial neural network approach. *Journal of Transport Economics and Policy,* Vol. 28, No.2, 179–199

Day, B. (2001). The theory of hedonic markets: obtaining welfare measures for changes in environmental quality using hedonic market data. Economics of the environment

Consultancy, 31.05.2011, available from: http://eprints.ucl.ac.uk/17583/1/17583.pdf

Dekkers, J. & van der Straaten, W. (2008). Monetary valuation of aircraft noise; a hedonic analysis around Amsterdam Airport. *Tinbergen Institute Discussion Paper TI 2008-064/3*, Amsterdam

Delucchi, M.A.; Murphy, J.J.; McCubbin, D.R. (2002). The health and visibility cost of air pollution: a comparison of estimation methods. *Journal of Environmental Management*, Vol. 64, Issue 2, 139-152

Den Boer, L.C. & Schroten, A. (2007). Traffic noise reduction in Europe. Health effects, social costs and technical and policy options to reduce road and rail traffic noise. CE Delft

Ekeland, I.; Heckman, J.J. & Nesheim, L. (2002). Identifying hedonic models. *American Economic Review*, Vol. 92, Issue 2, 304–309

Eriksson, C.; Rosenlund, M.; Pershagen, G.; Hilding, A.; Östenson, C.G. & Bluhm, G. (2007). Aircraft Noise and Incidence of Hypertension. *Epidemiology*, Vol. 18, No. 6, 716-721

Espey, M. & Lopez, H. (2000). The impact of airport noise and proximity on residential property values. *Growth and Change*, Vol. 31, Issue 3, 408–419

Eurocontrol (2007). Environmental effects around airports, toward new indicators? EUROCONTROL Experimentation centre, EEC Note 09/07, Synthesis Report

Eurocontrol (2003). Attitudes towards and values of aircraft annoyance and noise nuisance. Survey Report EEC/SEE/2003/002, Eurocontrol

European Commision (2005). Position paper on the effectiveness of noise measures. WG-HSEA 18-02-2005 EU Working Group on Health& Socio-Economic Aspects, European Commision, Bruessels

Evans, G.W.; Bullinger, M. & Hygge, S. (1998). Chronic noise exposure and physiological response: a prospective study of children living under environmental stress. *Psychological Science*, Vol. 9, No. 1, 75-77

Feitelson, E.I; Hurd, R.E. & Mudge, R.R. (1996). The impact of airport noise on willingness to pay for residences. *Transportation Research Part D: Transport and Environment*, Vol.1, Issue 1, 1-14

Fidell, S.; Pearsons, K.; Tabachnick, B.G. & Howe, R. (2000). Effects on sleep disturbance of changes in aircraft noise near three airports. *Journal of Acoustical Society of America*, Vol. 107, Issue 5, 2535-2547

Franssen, E.A.M.; van Wiechen, C.M.A.G.; Nagelkerke, N.J.D & Lebret, E. (2004). Aircraft noise around a large international airport and its impact on general health and medication use. *Journal of Occupational & Environmental Medicine*, Vol.61, No.5, 405-413

Freeman, A.M. (1981). The benefits of environmental improvement: theory and practice. 2. print, Johns Hopkins Univ. Press, Baltimore, Md. [u.a.]

Freeman, A.M. (1979). Hedonic prices, property values and measuring environmental benefits: A survey of the issues. *The Scandinavian Journal of Economics*, Vol. 81, No. 2, Measurement in Public Choice, 154-173

Frey, B.S. (2008). Happiness - a revolution in economics. MIT Press, Cambridge

Greiser, E.; Greiser, C.& Janhsen, K. (2007). Night-time aircraft noise increases prevalence of prescriptions of antihypertensive and cardiovascular drugs irrespective of social class—the Cologne-Bonn Airport study. *Journal of Public Health*, Vol. 15, No.5, 327-337

Haines, M.M.; Stansfeld, S.A.; Job, R.F.; Berglund, B. & Head, J. (2001a): Chronic aircraft noise exposure, stress responses, mental health and cognitive performance in school children. *Psychological Medicine*, Vol. 31, Issue 2, 265- 277

Haines M.M.; Stansfeld, S.A; Brentnall, S.; Head, J.; Berry, B.; Jiggins, M. & Hygge, S. (2001b). The West London Schools Study: the effects of chronic aircraft noise exposure on child health. *Psychological Medicine*, Vol.31, Issue 8, 1385-1396

Hanemann, W.M. (1994). Valuing the environment through contingent valuation. *The Journal of Economic Perspectives*, Vol. 8, No. 4, 19-43

Hanley, N. & Barbier, E.B. (2009): Pricing Nature. Cost-benefit analysis and environmental policy. Elgar, Cheltenham [u.a.]

Hanley, Nick & Spash, C.L. (1993). Cost-benefit Analysis and the environment. Elgar, Aldershot [u.a.]

Haralabidis, A.S.; Dimakopoulou, K.; Vigna-Taglianti, F.; Giampaolo, M.; Borgini, A.; Dudley, M.L.; Pershagen, G.; Bluhm, G.; Houthuijs, D.; Babisch, W.; Velonakis, M.; Katsouyanni, K. & Jarup, L. (2008). Acute effects of night-time noise exposure. *European Heart Journal*, Vol. 29, Issue 5, 658-664

Hardoy, M.C.; Carta, M.G.; Marci, A.R.; Carbone, F.; Cadeddu, M.; Kovess, V.; Dell'Osso, L. & Carpiniello, B. (2005). Exposure to aircraft noise and risk of psychiatric disorders: the Elmas survey. In: *Social Psychiatry Psychiatric Epidemiology*, Vol. 40, No.1, 24– 26

Health Council of the Netherlands: Public health impact of large airports. Publication No. 1999/14, Health Council of the Netherlands, 1999

Jarup, L.; Babisch, W.; Houthuijs, D.; Pershagen, G.; Katsouyanni, K.; Cadum, E.; Dudley, M.L; Savigny, P.; Seiffert, I.; Swart, W.; Breugelmans, O.; Bluhm, G.; Selander, J.; . Haralabidis, A.S.; Dimakopoulou, K.; Sourtzi, P.; Velonakis, M. & Vigna-Taglianti, F. (2008). Hypertension and Exposure to Noise Near Airports: the HYENA Study. *Environmental Health Perspectives*, Vol. 116, No.3, 329-333

Johnson, K. & Button, K. (1997). Benefit transfer: are they a satisfactory input to benefit cost analysis? An airport noise nuisance study. *Transportation Research Part D*, Vol.2, No.4, 223-231

Jud, D.G. & Winkler, D.T. (2006). The announcement effect of an airport expansion on housing prices. *Journal of Real Estate Finance and Economics*, Vol. 33, Issue 2, 91-103

Kaltenbach, M.; Maschke, C. & Klinke, R. (2008). Gesundheitliche Auswirkungen von Fluglärm. Übersichtsarbeit. *Deutsches Ärzteblatt*, Jg. 105, Heft 31-32, 548-557

Knipschild, P. (1977a). Medical effects of aircraft noise: community cardiovascular survey. *International Archives of Occupational and Environmental Health*, Vol. 40, No.3, 185-190

Knipschild, P. (1977b). Medical effects of aircraft noise: general practice survey. *International Archives of Occupational and Environmental Health*, Vol. 40, No.3, 191-197

Knipschild, P. & Oudshoorn, N. (1977). Medical effects of aircraft noise: drug survey. *International Archives of Occupational and Environmental Health*, Vol. 40, No.3, 197-200

Knipschild, P.; Meijer, H. & Salle', H. (1981). Aircraft noise and birth weight. *International Archives of Occupational and Environmental Health*, Vol. 48, No. 2, 131-136

Kuminoff, N.V.; Parmeter, C. F &/ Pope, J.C (2010). Which hedonic models can we trust to recover the marginal willingness to pay for environmental amenities? *Journal of Environmental Economics and Management*, Vol. 60, Issue 3, 145-160

Lancaster, K.J.: (1966). A new approach to consumer theory. *The Journal of Political Economy*, Vol. 74, No. 2, 132-157

Layard, R. (2006). Happiness - lessons from a new science. Penguin Press, London

Levesque, T.J. (1994). Modelling the effects of airport noise on residential housing markets: A case study of Winnipeg International Airport. *Journal of Transport Economics and Policy*, Vol. 28, No. 2, 199-210

Lijesen, M.; van der Straaten, W.; Dekkers, J.; van Elk, R. & Blokdijk, J. (2010). How much noise reduction at airports? *Transportation Research Part D: Transport and Environment*, Vol. 15, Issue 1, 51-59

Lipscomb, C. (2003). The impacts of an airport and local infrastructure on housing prices in a small urban city. *Review of Urban and Regional Development Studies*, Vol. 15, No. 3, 255-273

Lindhjem, H., Navrud, S. (2008). How reliable are meta-analyses for international benefit transfers? Ecological Economics 66 (2-3), 425-435.

Lu, C. & Morrell, P. (2006). Determination and applications of environmental costs at different sized airports - aircraft noise and engine emissions. *Transportation*, Vol. 33, Issue 1, 45-61

Lu, C. (2011). The economic benefits and environmental costs of airport operations: Taiwan Taoyuan International Airport. Forthcoming in *Journal of Air Transport Management*, Vol. 18, Issue 6, November 2011, 360-363, doi:10.1016/j.jairtraman.2011.02.006

Mahashabde, A.; Wolfe, P.; Ashok, A.; Dorbian, C.; He, Q.; Fan, A.; Lukachko, S.; Mozdzanowska, A.; Wollersheim, C.; Barett, S.R.H;/ Locke, M. & Waitz, I. (2011). Assessing the environmental impacts of aircraft noise and emissions. *Progress in Aerospace Sciences*, Vol. 47, Issue 1, 15-52

Marmolejo Duarte, C. (2008). Willingness to pay for noise reduction in residential areas affected by airport traffic: the case of Barcelona. *Proceedings of 15th Annual Congress of the European Real Estate Society*, Cracow, June 2008

Matsui, T.; Matsuno, T.; Ashimine, K.; , Hiramatsu, K.; Osada, Y. & Yamamoto, T. (2003). The Okinawa Study : Effect of chronic Aircraft Noise exposure on birth weight, prematurity and intrauterine growth retardation. *Proceedings of the 8th International Congress on Noise as a Public Health Problem*, Rotterdam, June/July 2003

McMillen, D. (2004). Airport expansions and property values: the case of Chicago O'Hare airport. *Journal of Urban Economics*, Vol. 55, Issue 3, 627-640

McMillan, M.L.; Reid, B.G. & Gillen, D.W. (1980). An extension of the hedonic approach for estimating the value of quiet. *Land Economics*, Vol. 56, No. 3, 315-328

Miyakita, T.; Matsui, T., Ito, A.; Tokuyama, T.; Hiramatsu, K.; Osada, Y. & Yamamoto, T. (2002). Population based questionnaire survey on health effects of aircraft noise on residents living around U.S. airfields in the Ryukyus- part I: an analysis of 12 scale scores. *Journal of Sound and Vibration*, Vol. 250, Issue 1, 129-137

Morrell, S.; Taylor, R. & Lyle, D. (1997). A review of health effects of aircraft noise. *Australian and New Zealand Journal of Public Health*, Vol. 21,No. 2, 221-236

Navrud, S. (2004). The Economic Value of noise within the European Union- a review and analysis of studies. *Proceedings of Acustica 2004, Ibero-American Congress on Environmental Acoustics*, September 2004, Guimaraes, Portugal

Navrud, S. (2002). The state-of-the-art on economic valuation of noise. Final report to the European Commission DG on Environment, 29.06.2011, available from http://www.cevreselgurultu.cevreorman.gov.tr/dosya/background_information/noise_monetisation_EU_WG_HSAE.pdf

Nellthorp, J.; Birstow, A. & Day, B. (2007). Introducing willingness-to-pay for noise changes into transport appraisal: an application of benefit transfer. *Transport Reviews*, Vol.27, No. 3, 327-353

Nelson, J.P. (2004). Meta-analysis of airport noise and hedonic property values. Problems and prospects. *Journal of Transport Economics and Policy*, Vol. 38, Part 1, 1-28

Nelson, J.P. (2008): Hedonic property value studies of transportation noise: aircraft and road traffic. In: *Hedonic methods in housing markets: Pricing environmental amenities and segregation*, Baranzini, A.; Ramirez, J. & Schaerer, C. & Thalmann, P. (Eds.), 57-82, Springer, New York

Nijland, H. A. & van Wee, G. P. (2005). Traffic noise in Europe: A comparison of calculation methods, noise indices and noise standards for road and railroad traffic in Europe. *Transport Reviews*, Vol. 25, Issue 5, 591—612

Passchier-Vermeer, W. & Passchier, W.F. (2000). Noise exposure and public health. *Environmental Health perspectives*, Vol.108, Supplement 1, 123-131

Paunović, K.; Stansfeld, S.A.; Clark, C. & Belojević, G. (2011). Epidemiological studies on noise and blood pressure in children: Observations and suggestions. *Environment International*, Vol. 37, Issue 5, 1030-1041

Pennington, G.; Topham, N. & Ward, R. (1990). Aircraft noise and residential property values adjacent to Manchester International Airport. *Journal of Transport Economics and Policy*, Vol. 24, No. 1, 49-59

Pommerehne, W.W. (1988). Measuring environmental benefits: a comparison of hedonic technique and contingent valuation. In: *Welfare and efficiency in public economics*, Bös, D.; Rose, M. & Seidl, C. (Eds.), 363-400, Springer, Berlin [u.a.]

Pope, J.C. (2008). Buyer information and the hedonic: the impact of a seller disclosure on the implicit price for airport noise *Journal of Urban Economics*, Vol. 63, Issue 2, 498-516

Quehl, J. & Basner, M. (2006). Annoyance from nocturnal aircraft noise exposure: laboratory and field-specific dose–response curves. *Journal of Environmental Psychology*, Vol. 26, Issue 2, 127-140

Rehm S. & Jansen G. (1978). Aircraft noise and premature birth. *Journal of Sound and Vibration*, Vol. 59, Issue 1, 133-135

Ready, R. & Navrud, S. (2006). International benefit transfer: Methods and validity tests*Ecological Economics*, Vol. 60, Issue 2, 429-434

Rich, J.H. & Nielsen, O.A. (2004). Assessment of traffic noise impacts. *International Journal of Environmental Studies*, Vol. 61, Issue 1, 19 -29

Rosen, S. (1974). Hedonic prices and implicit markets: product differentiation in pure competition. *The Journal of Political Economy*, Vol. 82, No. 1, 34-55

Rosenberger, R.S. & Stanley, T.D. (2006). Measurement, generalization, and publication: sources of error in benefit transfers and their management. *Ecological Economics*, Vol. 60, Issue 2, 372-378

Rosenlund, M.; Berglind, N.; Pershagen, G.; Jarup, L. &, Bluhm, G. (2001). Increased prevalence of hypertension in a population exposed to aircraft noise. *Occupational and Environmental Medicine*, Vol. 58, Issue 12, 769-773

Rozan, A, (2004). Benefit Transfer: A comparison of WTP for air quality between France and Germany. *Environmental and Resource Economics*, Vol. 29, No. 3, 295-306

Salvi, M. (2008). Spatial estimation of the impact of airport noise on residential housing prices *Swiss Journal of Economics and Statistics*, Vol. 44, Issue 4, 577-606

Schipper, Y. (2004). Environmental costs in European aviation. *Transport Policy*, Vol. 11, Issue 2, 141-154

Schipper, Y.; Rietveld, P. & Nijkamp, P. (2001). Environmental externalities in air transport markets. *Journal of Air transport Management*, Vol. 7, Issue 3, 169-179

Schipper, Y.; Nijkamp, P. & Rietveld, P. (1998). Why do aircraft noise value estimates differ? *Journal of Air Transport Management*, Vol. 4, Issue 2, 117–124

Smith, V.K. (2009). Fifty years of contingent valuation. In: *Handbook on contingent valuation*, Alberini, A. & Kahn, J.R. (Eds.), 7-66, Elgar, Cheltenham [u.a.]

Sommer, H. (2002). Verkehrsbedingte Lärmkosten in der Schweiz. Presented at „15 Jahre Lärmschutzverordnung"conference , Olten, April 2002

Stansfeld, S.A.; Berglund, B.; Clark, C.; Lopez-Barrio, I.; Fischer, P.; Öhrström, E.; Haines, M.M.; Head, J.; Hygge, S.; van Kamp, I. & Berry, B.F. (2005). Aircraft and road traffic noise and children's cognition and health. Results from a cross sectional study. *The Lancet*, Vol. 365, Issue 9475, 1942-1949

Stansfeld, S.A.; Clark, C.; Cameron, R.M.; Alfred, T.; Head, J.; Haines, M.M.; van Kamp, I; van Kempen, E. & Lopez-Barrio, I. (2009). Aircraft and road traffic noise exposure and children's mental health. *Journal of Environmental Psychology*, Vol. 29, Issue 2, 203-207

Stansfeld, S.A. & Matheson, M.P. (2003). Noise pollution: non-auditory effects on health. *British Medical Bulletin*, Vol. 68, Issue 1, 243–257

Uyeno, D.; Hamilton, S.W. & Biggs, A.J.G. (1993). Density of residential land use and the impact of airport noise. *Journal of Transport Economics and Policy*, Vol. 27, No. 1, 3-18

Vallet, M.; Cohen, J.M.; Mosnier, A. & Trucy, D. (1999). Airport noise and epidemiological study of health effects: a feasibility study. *Proceedings of Internoise 99*, Fort Lauderdale, Florida, December 1999

van Kamp, I. & Davies, H. (2008). Environmental noise and mental health: Five year review and future directions. *Proceedings of 9th International Congress of the Intenational Commission on the biological effects of Noise (ICBEN): Noise as a Public Health Problem*, Mashantucket, Connecticut, July 2008

van Kempen, E.; van Kamp, I.; Lebret, E.; Lammers, J.; Emmen, H. & Stansfeld, S. (2010). Neurobehavioral effects of transportation noise in primary schoolchildren: a cross-sectional study. *Environmental Health*, Vol. 9, Issue 1, 1-13

van Kempen, E.; Kruize, H.; Boshuizen, H.C.; Ameling, C.B.; Staatsen, B.A.M. & de Hollander, A.E.M. (2002). The association between noise exposure and blood pressure and ischemic heart disease: A meta-analysis. *Environmental Health Perspectives*, Vol. 110, No. 3 , 307-317

van Kempen, E.; van Kamp, I.; Fischer, P.; Davies, H.; Houthuijs, D.; Stellato, R.; Clark, C. & Stansfeld, S.A. (2006). Noise exposure and children's blood pressure and heart rate: the RANCH project. *Journal of Occupational and Environmental Medicine*, Vol. 63, Issue 9, 632-639

van Praag, B.M.S. & Baarsma, B.E. (2005). Using Happiness surveys to value intangibles: the case of airport noise. *The Economic Journal*, Vol. 115, Issue 500, 224-246

Venkatachalam, L. (2004). The contingent valuation method: a review. *Environmental Impact Assessment Review*, Vol. 24, Issue 1, 89–124

World Health Organization (2009). Night noise guidelines for Europe. WHO Regional Office Europe, Copenhagen

Wilson, M. A., Hoehn, J. P. (2006). Valuing environmental goods and services using benefit transfer: The state-of-the art and science. *Ecological Economics*, Vol. 60, Issue 2, 335-342

12

Interaction Between Exposure to Neurotoxicants and Drug Abuse

Francisca Carvajal, Maria del Carmen Sanchez-Amate,
Jose Manuel Lerma-Cabrera and Inmaculada Cubero
University of Almeria/Department of Neuroscience and Health Sciences, Almeria, Spain

1. Introduction

Humans are continuously exposed to a variety of environmental neurotoxicants. Over the past 30 years, at least 100,000 chemicals, including pesticides, food additives, drugs, and cosmetics, have been registered for commercial use in the United States (Muir & Howard, 2006). Twenty years ago, about 750 chemicals had shown neurotoxic effects in laboratory animals (Anger, 1984). Actually, the number is thought to exceed a thousand, although no authoritative estimate of the real number of neurotoxicants is available (Grandjeand & Landrigan, 2006).

About two-thirds of all agricultural use of xenobiotics involves herbicides and about one-eighth involves insecticides; approximately 20% of usage is fungicides, fumigants, and other pesticides (United States Environmental Protection Agency [U.S. EPA], 2001). Organophosphate insecticides represent 50% of all the insecticide use worldwide. In fact in Europe, the use of pesticide on crops exceeds 140.000 metric tons (The use of plant protection products in the European Union. Data 1992–2003. Eurostat statistical books [http://epp.eurostat.ec.europa.eu/cache/ITY_OFFPUB/KS-76-06-669/EN/KS-76-06-669-EN.PDF]). Although European policies to reduce pesticide use have been introduced, according to EU statistical data for 1992-2003, annual pesticide consumption has not decreased. Estimates made by the World Health Organization (WHO) indicate that three million acute organophosphate poisonings and over 200,000 deaths may occur annually in the world (Ferrer & Cabral, 1995; WHO, 1990). Thus, exposure to neurotoxic compounds has become in a serious public health problem worldwide.

Numerous reports have indicated a link between xenobiotic exposure and human health, including disturbances in the CNS (for a review, see Costa et al., 2008). Moreover, numerous studies have reported long-term neurological and neurobehavioral sequelae following a pesticide poisoning event (Delgado et al., 2004; Rosenstock et al., 1991; Steeland et al., 1994). Thus, humans exposed to acute or chronic levels of organophosphate (OP) compounds, a potent neurotoxic widely employed in industry, households and agriculture for pest control, exhibit long-term alterations in neuropsychological performance and cognitive processes, such as processing speed, visual attention, visuoperceptual abilities, memory impairment and problem solving (Farahat et al., 2003; Fiedler et al., 1997; Roldan-Tapia et al., 2004, 2006;

Steenland et al., 1994). Also, emotional deficits have been found after exposure to OPs (Savage et al., 1998; Yokoyama et al., 1998). Pesticide exposure has been correlated with emotional disturbances such as anxiety increases, depression and suicide risk (London et al., 2005; Roldan-Tapia et al., 2006).

On the other hand, the use of pesticides in agriculture has been linked with several dopamine-associated CNS disorders including Parkinson´s Disease (PD) (Dick, 2006) and Attention-Deficit/Hyperactivity Disorder (ADHD) (Bouchard et al., 2010). Specifically, pesticide exposure is a risk factor for PD (Ascherio et al., 2006; Brown et al., 2006; Dick, 2006) and recent studies have shown that it may contribute to ADHD prevalence (Bouchard et al., 2010). Given that dopamine (DA) has been identified as the critical neurotransmitter in the reward circuit mediating substance abuse (for a review, see Di Chiara & Bassareo, 2007), exposure to certain environmental neurotoxicants might influence the development of drug addiction. There are numerous reports associating neurotoxicant exposure and dopaminergic disorders such as PD and ADHD in the literature; however studies examining any potential effects of neurotoxicants on drug addiction are just recently being conducted and published, in spite of the fact that drug abuse is an important public health problem leading to serious negative consequences for individuals and society. Estimates of the total overall costs of substance abuse in the United States, including health- and crime-related costs, exceed $600 billion annually (Office of National Drug Control Policy, 2004). This includes approximately $235 billion for alcohol abuse (Rehm et al., 2009). Thus, these data stresses the need for new scientific research aimed toward the assessment of neurochemical and neurobiological mechanisms underlying exposure to neurotoxicants and drug abuse.

2. Environmental neurotoxicants and drug abuse

In recent years, a growing body of clinical evidence has revealed that acute, intermittent or continuous exposure to a wide variety of chemically unrelated environmental pollutants (such as volatile organic chemicals, woods preservatives, solvents, or organophosphate pesticides) might result in the development of multiple chemical intolerance (Miller, 2001) and increased sensitivity to drugs of abuse (Newlin, 1994; Sorg & Hochstatter, 1999). The general population is exposed to multiple agents, either as intrinsically complex mixtures or as separate substances, such as specifics drugs. Since the behavior of any given chemical in the body is affected by other chemicals, there is a need to study the toxicological and behavioral effects of environmental neurotoxicant mixtures and drugs. Since both environmental neurotoxicants and drug abuse present a health hazard to the population, these studies should merit special attention. Moreover, such studies would open new perspectives to the promising and exciting scientific field that tries to bridge environmental health sciences, toxicology and drug research.

A large variety of studies in animals (Mutti et al., 1988; Von Euler et al., 1991, 1993) and humans (Edling et al., 1997) have demonstrated that repeated volatile organic compound exposure have deleterious effects on the dopaminergic system. The most ubiquitous volatile organic compound is formaldehyde (Form). Acute exposure to formaldehyde can cause eye, nose, throat, and skin irritation, whereas long-term exposure has been linked to certain cancers as well as asthma (Daisey et al., 2003). Furthermore, numerous animal studies on the adverse effects of formaldehyde on behavioral responses to cocaine have revealed drug-pollutant cross-sensitization (Sorg et al., 1996, 1998, 2001).

In 1996, Sorg and her collaborators demonstrated that animals pretreated with repeated high-level formaldehyde inhalation (1h/day x 7days) showed a significantly enhanced locomotor response to cocaine compared to controls, an indicator that specific limbic pathways may have been sensitized (Sorg et al., 1996). However, the same pattern of exposure, but with low-level formaldehyde doses failed to cause behavioral sensitization to cocaine (Sorg et al., 1998) suggesting that formaldehyde effects on behavioral response to cocaine are dose-dependent.

Paradoxically, long-term low-level formaldehyde exposure (1h/day x 5days/week x 4 weeks) produced behavioral sensitization to later cocaine injection, suggesting altered dopaminergic sensitivity in mesolimbic pathways (Sorg et al., 1998). More specifically, this study has shown that repeated exposure to a relatively low-level volatile organic compound, formaldehyde, amplifies behavioral responses to cocaine. Taking together, these data suggests that the effect of formaldehyde on the cross-sensitization to cocaine depends both on the dose and on the pattern of exposure to this volatile organic compound (Sorg et al., 1998).

Furthermore, humans are routinely exposed to heavy metals through a variety of sources (air, food, water or soil). Thus, prolonged exposure to heavy metals, such as cadmium, copper, lead, nickel, and zinc can cause deleterious health effects in humans (for a review, see Järup, 2003). Mainly, heavy metal exposure can directly influence behavior by impairing mental and neurological function, influencing neurotransmitter production and use, and altering numerous metabolic body processes. The adverse effects of heavy metal exposure are well documented; however, few studies have been carried out to understand their effects on drug use. Next, we are going to describe the effect of two heavy metals (lead and manganese) over the incidence of drug abuse.

The symptoms of acute lead poisoning are headache, irritability, abdominal pain and various symptoms related to the nervous system. Additionally, populations exposed to environments with high lead concentrations may show an increase in the incidence of drug abuse (Ensminger et al., 1997). Experimental studies show that adult lead exposure decreases behavioral sensitivity to cocaine (Burkey et al., 1997; Nation et al., 1996). Animal studies have found evidence that chronic lead exposure in adulthood causes a delay in the development of cocaine-induced locomotor sensitization, as well as a decrease in the magnitude of the locomotor response (Nation et al., 1996). Operant responses, rather than only simple behavioral responses, such as locomotor activity, are also affected by lead exposure. Thus, chronic lead exposure caused cocaine-induced disturbance attenuation in fixed-interval responding (Burkey et al., 1997). In agreement with these data, there are studies showing attenuated cocaine-induced increases in extracellular dopamine levels in the nucleus accumbens region after chronic lead exposure (Nation & Burkey, 1994).

By contrast, the evidence suggests that, after perinatal lead exposure, early developmental lead exposure may increase sensitivity to the reinforcing effects of cocaine and heroin in adulthood (Nation et al., 2004). Several studies have shown that acute administration of cocaine to rats developmentally exposed to low levels of lead produces an attenuation of drug reinforcement according to a conditioned place preference (CPP) paradigm (Miller et al., 2000), and a drug discrimination preparation (Miller et al., 2001). A similar pattern of attenuation is evident in studies that examined the effects of developmental chronic low-level lead exposure on morphine-induced CPP (Valles et al., 2003). Thus, these studies suggest that lead exposure during development can cause long-term changes in the response that these individuals give to drugs of abuse in adulthood, probably reducing the reinforcing properties of drugs.

Consistent with these data, there is experimental evidence indicating that exposure to another heavy metal, manganese (Mn), has had effects on psychostimulant vulnerability too. Thus, Mn exposure in young adult rats leads to a reduced behavioral response to amphetamines (Vezer et al., 2007). Interestingly, Mn-exposed rats show opposite locomotor responsiveness when challenged with different doses of cocaine (Reichel et al., 2006). Specifically, postnatal Mn exposure causes increased locomotor activity in combination with lower doses of cocaine; and an attenuated locomotor response in combination with high doses of cocaine. These data suggests that Mn exposure can increase dopaminergic receptor sensitivity. In fact, postnatal Mn exposure caused persistent declines in DAT protein expression and [3H] dopamine uptake in the striatum and nucleus accumbens, as well as long-term reductions in striatal dopamine efflux into adulthood (McDougall et al., 2008).

Another set of experiments was carried out to study the effects of pesticides on drug-induced behavior. These studies have shown, for example, that the daily administration of a oral dose of herbicide 2,4-dichlorophenoxyacetic acid (2,4-D) during gestation and development up to post-natal day 23 (PND23) increases an animal's sensitivity to amphetamine (Duffard & Evangelista de Duffard, 2002).

Also, it has been shown that exposure to another pesticide, chlorpyrifos, causes alteration in several drug-induced responses. For example, tolerance to locomotor effects was shown after a dopaminergic agonist challenge with amphetamine 30 days after exposure to CPF (Lopez-Crespo et al., 2007). In a separate study, the motivational and reward properties of amphetamine were decreased in the place preference paradigm months after CPF administration (Sanchez-Santed et al., 2004). Based on these studies, it has been proposed that CPF intoxication may produce long-term hyposensitivity in the dopaminergic system. Recent studies have found that monoamine levels decreased dramatically in the nucleus accumbens 30 days after CPF exposure (Moreno et al., 2008). Other organophosphates, such as chlorphenvinphos, also cause changes in the dopaminergic system. Thus, behavioral studies have shown that 3 weeks after acute exposure to high doses of chlorphenvinphos (CVP), there is an hyposensitivity to behavioral responsiveness to amphetamine and scopolamine (Gralewicz et al., 2000; Lutz et al., 2000, 2005). Furthermore, exposure to chlorphenvinphos prevents behavioral sensitization to amphetamine (Lutz et al., 2006).

3. Environmental neurotoxicants and ethanol intake

As described in the previous section, several studies have shown the interaction between neurotoxicants and the abuse of certain drugs, such as cocaine, amphetamines or morphine. Given that ethanol (EtOH) is one of the most commonly used drugs worldwide, next we will present the specific literature referring to neurotoxicant exposure and its relationship to ethanol intake.

The great majority of people in modern society regularly consume ethanol. In fact, about 100 billion Euros on alcoholic beverages are spent annually by Europeans, which is reflected by the high rate of alcohol consumption per capita of 10 liters of pure ethanol per year. But, consuming and abusing these huge amounts of alcohol is clearly a problem, with enormous health and socioeconomic effects worldwide. According to the Alcohol-Related Disease Impact (ARDI) tool, from 2001–2005, there were approximately 79,000 deaths annually attributable to excessive alcohol use. Thus, excessive alcohol use is the 3rd leading lifestyle-related cause of death for people in the United States, after tobacco addiction and obesity (McGinnis & Foege, 1999). The economic cost of ethanol abuse is estimated at greater than $235 billion every year (Rehm et al., 2009), including health care costs, lost worker productivity, and crime.

Several studies have suggested a relationship between several neurotoxic agents and alcohol intake. First of all, we will focus on the interaction between lead exposure and alcohol intake. The exposure to this heavy metal has already been linked to reduced behavioral sensitivity to cocaine (Burkey et al., 1997; Nation et al., 1996). Also, populations exposed to environments with high lead concentrations may show an increase in the incidence of drug abuse (Ensminger et al., 1997). Epidemiological data has revealed that alcoholic industrial workers have higher blood lead levels than their non alcoholic colleagues, suggesting that alcoholic workers could be more susceptible to the toxic effects of lead (Cezard et al., 1992; Dalley et al., 1989).

Animal studies have found evidence that ethanol exposure for 8 weeks resulted in a marked increase in the accumulation of lead in the blood (Gupta & Gill, 2000a) and brain (Gupta & Gill, 2000b) of animals exposed to lead, making them more vulnerable to the toxic effects of lead. Thus, for example, levels of lead in the brain were approximately twice higher in lead and ethanol co-exposed animals than in animals exposed to lead alone (Gupta & Gill, 2000b). Another set of experimental studies has shown that mice treated chronically with lead exhibit some alterations in ethanol-induced behaviours, such as a reduction in ethanol-induced locomotor activity (Correa et al., 1999). In a self-administration task, dietary lead exposure led to lever pressing at a significantly lower rate than the control group (Nation et al., 1991). Apparently, lead toxicity reduces sensitivity to ethanol effects. Moreover, when subjects were exposed simultaneously to lead and ethanol, the level of dopamine decreased significantly, and was accompanied with increased norepinephrine levels (Flora & Tandom, 1987; Gupta & Gill, 2000b).

As with lead, simultaneous exposure to aluminium and ethanol also deplete brain dopamine (DA) and 5-hydroxytryptamine (5-HT) levels, when compared to rats given aluminium alone (Flora et al., 1991). Also, the concentration of aluminium in the blood and liver was significantly higher in rats exposed to both aluminium and ethanol than in those exposed only to aluminium. These results suggest that prolonged ethanol consumption may increase the rats' susceptibility to certain effects of aluminium.

3.1 The relationship between organophosphate exposure and ethanol intake

Decades ago, an interesting study showed that 114 agricultural workers suffering acute organophosphate intoxication developed intolerance to nicotine- and ethanol-containing beverages (Tabershaw & Cooper, 1966). Another epidemiological study, carried out by

Spiegelberg in 1961, described persistent intolerances for alcohol and nicotine among Germans who had manufactured chemical weapons, including organophosphate nerve agent, during World War II (Spiegelberg, 1961). These studies were the first to propose the existence of a relationship between organophosphate compound exposure and ethanol intake. In addition, more recently, clinical reports have shown that a significant percentage (66%) of Gulf War veterans reported that alcohol beverages, even a can of beer, made them feel ill (Miller, 2001). Unfortunately, there are not many epidemiological studies considering organophosphate exposure as a determinant of ethanol intake.

In agreement with clinical data, Overstreet and his colleges reported that Flinder rats, which had been bred for increased sensitivity to organophosphate poisoning, showed enhanced responses to ethanol or nicotine (Overstreet et al., 1996, 2001). Thus, Flinder Sensitive Line (FSL) rats exhibited a significantly greater ethanol-induced (Overstreet et al, 1990, 1996) and nicotine-induced hypothermic response (Overstreet et al, 1996; Schiller & Overstreet, 1993) compared to its parallel bred counterparts, the Flinder Resistant Line (FRL) rats. It suggests that FSL rats, selectively bred for increased cholinergic responses, also show an increased sensitivity to the effects of alcohol or nicotine.

Taken together, clinical and experimental evidence strongly points to the existence of important, but poorly understood, neurobiological interactions between organophosphate exposure and ethanol intake. Therefore, we investigated the impact of OP exposure on voluntary alcohol consumption from a molecular and a behavioral approach in an animal model. To that aim, we employed an experimental model in Wistar rats based on the administration of a single high dose (250 mg / kg) of the organophosphate chlorpyrifos (CPF). CPF is an OP used worldwide in the agricultural industry and in households as a pesticide (Pope, 1999; Richardson, 1995). The primary mechanism of acute toxic action of these compounds is acetylcholinesterase (AChE) inhibition, which results in acute cholinergic over stimulation at nicotine and muscarinic synapses of the peripheral, autonomic and central nervous system (Lotti, 2001; Richardson, 1995). Additionally, non-AChE targets such as the monoaminergic (Aldridge et al., 2003; Dam et al., 1999; Moreno et al., 2008), the gabaergic (Rocha et al., 1996; Sánchez-Amate et al., 2002), or the glutamatergic systems (Gultekin et al., 2007) have also been proposed as alternative mechanisms involved in the acute lethal action and/or side effects of short and long-term OP exposure.

After subcutaneous administration, CPF keeps acetylcholinesterase (AChE) activity mildly inhibited for weeks. This unique biochemical profile points to the long-lasting presence of the compound in the body (Bushnell et al., 1993; Pope et al., 1992). Since CPF-induced AChE inhibition is not associated with overt cholinergic toxicity (Bushnell et al., 1993; Pope et al., 1992), exposure to high doses of this OP has been used in animal research to investigate the neurobehavioral effects of OP exposure during a wide temporal window of approximately 8-12 weeks (Richardson, 1995). Thus, exposure to a single subcutaneous injection of CPF would provide an animal model to conduct extensive neurobehavioral testing during a long interval of approximately 8 weeks.

The two-bottle choice paradigm provides a convenient method for a rapid screening of alcohol preferences in rats. Thus, early paradigms assessing the reinforcing effects of alcohol typically used an oral preference paradigm where animals were allowed to drink alcohol or water. In fact, free choice procedures are widely employed for selection of rat lines with genetically determined high or low ethanol preference (Files et al., 1997; Sinclair et al., 1989).

Eight weeks after CPF administration, Wistar rats were allowed to drink ethanol in a two bottle paradigm (water vs. 8%-20% w/v ethanol) to evaluate if pre-exposure to the organophosphate caused them long-lasting avoidance. In this long-term drinking model, changes in alcohol-drinking behavior occur over time between CPF and vehicle-treated rats. Thus, the CPF pretreated rats showed lower ethanol consumption and ethanol preference than the control group at 8, 15, and 20% ethanol concentration (Carvajal et al., 2007). These results are consistent with clinical and experimental data showing that exposure to organophosphates might be linked to increased ethanol sensitivity and reduced voluntary consumption of ethanol-containing beverages in humans.

Since different factors might contribute to alcohol consumption, from week 4 to week 8 after CPF administration, an additional set of neurobiological, physiological, and behavioral responses to ethanol were evaluated. First, we analyzed whether CPF alters gustatory sensory processing as measured by taste preferences for sucrose, quinine and saccharin. CPF-pretreated rats showed the same taste preference pattern as vehicle-treated rats. Secondly, we verified that ethanol avoidance was not secondary to ethanol-induced flavor aversion disturbances since both CPF- and vehicle-treated rats showed a similar pattern of flavor avoidance in response to ethanol. Finally, we explored the sedative/hypnotic properties of alcohol as assessed by the righting reflex. These data showed that 4 weeks after poisoning, CPF-treated rats showed enhanced sensitivity to the sedative properties of ethanol not associated with altered blood ethanol levels.

It is possible that increased ethanol sensitivity is partially mediated by several CPF toxicity mechanisms (for more details, see Carvajal et al., 2007). As noted above, the main CPF action mechanism is acetylcholinesterase inhibition. For example, it was demonstrated that administering cholinesterase inhibitors, galantamine or desoxypeganine, reduces alcohol consumption in alcohol-preferring rats (Doetkotte et al., 2005; Mann et al., 2006). Also, CPF decreases nicotinic alpha-7nAch receptor density (Slotkin et al., 2004), with a known role in ethanol intake and ethanol-induced sedation (Bowers et al., 2005; de Fiebre and de Fiebre, 2005). In this regard, there have been significant studies showing, at least at the genetic level, that knockout mice lacking alpha-7nAchR receptor specifically show reduced ethanol intake and increased sedation to ethanol (Bowers et al., 2005; de Fiebre and de Fiebre, 2005). Finally, alternative noncholinesterasic CPF neurotoxicity mechanisms (Casida and Quistad, 2004) might also cause ethanol avoidance (for more details, see Carvajal et al., 2007). However, future experimental research is required to test more specifically the implication of these CPF toxicity mechanisms in ethanol avoidance.

In summary, administration of a single high dose of CPF to adult Wistar rats elicited long-lasting reduced voluntary ethanol drinking and increased sedation to ethanol without evidence of altered ethanol metabolism, which indicates that CPF-ethanol neurobiological interactions may exist. Thus, there is the interesting possibility that some OPs such as CPF might induce long-lasting neural disturbances in brain systems critically involved in neurobehavioral responses to ethanol.

Investigating specific brain targets has been proposed as an important tool for developing our understanding of behavioral, emotional and cognitive impairments caused by OP compounds (Gupta, 2004). Considering this, in another study we explore whether CPF exposure induces significant disturbances in basal and/or ethanol-evoked neural activity in a set of cholinoceptive brain regions critically involved with neurobiological responses to ethanol. For this purpose, brain regional c-fos expression in response to acute ethanol (1.5 or 3.0 g/kg, i.p.) or saline solution was assessed in adult male Wistar rats previously injected with either a single high dose of CPF (250 mg/kg, sc) or vehicle. Results showed that first, CPF exposure did not modify the regional c-fos expression in response to acute ethanol administration; and secondly, CPF administration reduces long-term basal c-fos expression in the arcuate hypothalamic nucleus.

The arcuate hypothalamic nucleus AgRP/NPY expressing cells have been hypothesized to have a key role in voluntary ethanol consumption (Kalra & Kalra, 2004; Thiele et al., 2003). Taking together this fact and the present observation that long-term CPF exposure blunts c-fos expression in this brain region, one tempting hypothesis is that CPF causes long-term inhibition of neural activity in AgRP/NPY expressing cells in the Arc leading to reduced voluntary ethanol consumption. However, future behavioral and molecular studies are required to understand more extensively the role of Arc neural disturbances in long-term and long-lasting CPF-induced ethanol avoidance.

Although experimental data shown here constitute only an initial exploration of the putative relationship between organophosphate exposure and ethanol intake, both preclinical and experimental literature, and the preliminary findings of this study, suggests that further research is warranted. The use of well controlled animal models aiming to characterize the neurobiological mechanisms of drug/pollutant interactions would open new perspectives to this new scientific field that bridges environmental health sciences, toxicology, and drug research (Miller, 2001). Also, such research may result in public health and prevention programs that produce significant improvements in the integrity of long-term cognitive and behavioral outcomes.

4. Conclusion

In this chapter, we have provided a brief overview of this new scientific field that bridges environmental health sciences, toxicology, and drug research. In recent years, a large variety of studies have shown that different environmental neurotoxicants can lead to vulnerability to drug abuse. However, neurobiological interactions between environmental pollutants and drugs of abuse are still poorly understood. In the particular case of pesticides, both clinical and experimental research have shown that exposure to organophosphates might be linked to increased ethanol sensitivity and reduced voluntary consumption of ethanol-containing beverages. However, the mechanisms by which organophosphates may exert their effects on ethanol intake have yet to be elucidated. Accordingly, further laboratory and epidemiological research into the role of pesticides, and specifically chlorpyrifos, exposure in alcohol intake is needed. These studies appear to demonstrate a link between environmental neurotoxicant exposure and drug addiction, although much work needs to be done to further identify and characterize the underlying mechanisms involved.

5. Acknowledgment

This work was supported by Spanish grants from the Ministerio de Ciencia y Tecnologia [PM/99-1046, SEJ2006-03629], Junta de Andalucia [CTS-280], and FEDER [UNAM05-23-006].

6. References

Anger, W.K. (1984). Neurobehavioral testing of chemicals: impact on recommended standards. *Neurobehavioral Toxicology and Teratology*, Vol.6, No.4, (March 1984), pp. 147-153, ISSN 0275-1380.

Aldridge, J.E.; Seidler, F.J.; Meyer, A.; Thillai, I. & Slotkin, T.A. (2003). Serotonergic systems targeted by developmental exposure to chlorpyrifos, effects during different critical periods, *Environmental Health Perspective*, Vol.111, No.14, (November 2003), pp. 1736–1743, ISSN 0091-6765

Ascherio, A.; Chen, H.; Weisskopf, M.C.; O'Reilly, E.; McCullough, M.L.; Calle, E.E.; Schwarzschild, M.A. & Thun M.J. (2006). Pesticide exposure and risk for Parkinson's disease, *Annals of Neurology*, Vol.60, No.2, (August 2006), pp. 197–203, ISSN 1531-8249

Bouchard, M.F.; Bellinger, D.C.; Wright, R.O. & Weisskopf, M.G. (2010). Attention-deficit/hyperactivity disorder and urinary metabolites of organophosphate pesticides, *Pediatrics*, Vol.125, No.6, (May 2010), pp. 1270-1277, ISSN 0031-4005

Bowers, B.J.; McClure-Begley, T.D.; Keller, J.J.; Paylor, R.; Collins, A.C. & Wehner, J.M. (2005). Deletion of the alpha7 nicotinic receptor subunit gene results in increased sensitivity to several behavioral effects produced by alcohol, *Alcoholism: Clinical and Experimental Research*, Vol.29, No.3, (March 2005), pp. 295–302, ISSN 0145-6008

Brown, T.P.; Rumsby, P.C.; Capelton, A.C.; Rushton, L. & Levy, L.S. (2006). Pesticides and Parkinson's disease—is there a link? *Environmental Health Perspectives*, Vol.114, No.2, (February 2006), pp. 156–164, ISSN 0091-6765

Burkey, R.T.; Nation, J.R.; Grover, C.A. & Bratton, G.R. (1997). Effects of chronic lead exposure on cocaine-induced disturbance of fixed-interval behavior, *Pharmacology, Biochemistry and Behavior*, Vol.56, No.1, (January 1997), pp. 117–121, ISSN 0091-3057

Bushnell, P.J.; Pope, C.N. & Padilla, S. (1993). Behavioral and neurochemical effects of acute chlorpyrifos in rats: Tolerance to prolonged inhibition of cholinesterase, *The Journal of Pharmacology and Experimental Therapeutics*, Vol.266, No.2, (August 1993), pp. 1007–1017, ISSN 0022-3565

Carvajal, F.; Lopez-Grancha, M.; Navarro, M.; Sanchez-Amate, M.C. & Cubero, I. (2007). Long-lasting reductions of ethanol drinking, enhanced ethanol-induced sedation, and decreased c-fos expression in the Edinger-Westphal nucleus in Wistar rats exposed to the organophosphate Chlorpyrifos, *Toxicological Science,* Vol.96, No.2, (April 2007), pp. 310-320, ISSN 1096-6080

Carvajal, F.; Sanchez-Amate, M.C. & Cubero, I. (2011). A single high dose of chlorpyrifos reduces long-term basal c-fos expression in the rat arcuate hypothalamic nucleus. In preparation

Casida, J.E. & Quistad, G.B. (2004). Organophosphate toxicology: safety aspects of nonacetylcholinesterase secondary targets, *Chemical Research in Toxicology*, Vol.17, No.8, (August 2004), pp. 983-998, ISSN 0893-228X.

Cezard, C.; Demarquilly, C.; Boniface, M. & Haguenoern, J.M. (1992). Influence of the degree of exposure on lead on relations between alcohol consumption and the biological indices of lead exposure, epidemiological study in a lead acid battery factory,

British Journal of Industrial Medicine, Vol.49, No.9, (September 1992), pp. 645–647, ISSN 0007-1072

Correa, M.; Miquel, M.; Sanchis-Segura, C. & Aragón, C. (1999). Effects of chronic lead administration on ethanol-induced locomotor and brain catalase activity, *Alcohol*, Vol.19, No.1, (August 1999), pp. 43-49, ISSN 0741-8329

Costa, L.G. ; Giordano, G.; Guizzetti, M. & Vitalone, A. (2008). Neurotoxicity of pesticides: a brief review, *Frontiers in Bioscience*, Vol.13, No.1, (January 2008), pp. 1240–1249, ISSN 1093-9946

Daisey, J.M.; Angell, W.J. & Apte, M.G. (2003). Indoor air quality, ventilation and health symptoms in schools: an analysis of existing information, *Indoor Air*, Vol.13, No.1, (March 2003), pp. 53–64, ISSN 0905-6947

Dalley, S.; Girre, C.; Hispard, E.; Tomas, G. & Fournier, L. (1989). High blood lead levels in alcoholics : wine vs. Beer, *Drug Alcohol Dependence*, Vol.23, No.1, (January 1989), pp. 45–48, ISSN 0376-8716

Dam, K.; Garcia, S.J.; Seidler, F.J. & Slotkin, T.A. (1999). Neonatal chlorpyrifos exposure alters synaptic development and neuronal activity in cholinergic and catecholaminergic pathways, *Developmental Brain Research*, Vol.116, No.1, (August 1999), pp. 9-20, ISSN 0165-3806

de Fiebre, N.C. & de Fiebre, C.M. (2005). Alpha7 nicotinic acetylcholine receptor knockout selectively enhances ethanol-, but not beta-amyloid induced neurotoxicity, *Neuroscience Letters*, Vol.373, No.1, (January 2005), pp. 42–47, ISSN 0304-3940

Delgado, E.; McConnell, R.; Miranda, J.; Keifer, M.; Lundberg, I.; Partanen, T. & Wesseling C. (2004). Central nervous system effects of acute organophosphate poisoning in a two-year follow-up, *Scandinavian Journal of Work, Environment & Health*, Vol.30, No.5, (October 2004), pp. 362–370, ISSN 0355-3140

Di Chiara, G. & Bassareo, V. (2007). Reward system and addiction: what dopamine does and doesn't do, *Current Opinion in Pharmacology*, Vol.7, No.1, (February 2007), pp. 69-76, ISSN 1471-4892

Dick, F.D. (2006). Parkinson's disease and pesticide exposures, *British Medical Bulletin*, Vol.79–80, No.1, (January 2007), pp. 219–31, ISSN 0007-1420

Doetkotte, R.; Opitz, K.; Kiianmaa, K. & Winterhoff, H. (2005). Reduction of voluntary ethanol consumption in alcohol-preferring alko alcohol (AA) rats by desoxypeganine and galanthamine, *European Journal of Pharmacology*, Vol.522, No.1-3, (October 2005), pp. 72–77, ISSN 0014-2999

Duffard, R. & Evangelista de Duffard, A.M. (2002). Environmental chemical compounds could induce sensitization to drugs of abuse, *Annals of New York Academy of Science*, Vol.965, (June 2002), pp. 305–313, ISSN 0077-8923

Edling, C.; Hellman, B.; Arvidson, B.; Andersson, J.; Hartvig, P.; Lilja, A.; Valind, S. & Langstrom, B. (1997). Do organic solvents induce changes in the dopaminergic system? Positron emission tomography studies of occupationally exposed subjects, *International Archives of Occupational and Environmental Health*, Vol.70, No.3, (August 1997), pp. 180–186, ISSN 0340-0131

Ensminger, M.E.; Anthony, J.C. & McCord, J. (1997). The inner city and drug use: initial findings from an epidemiological study, *Drug and Alcohol Dependence*, Vol.48, No.3, (December 1997), pp. 175–184, ISSN 0376-8716

Farahat, T.M.; Abdelrasoul, G.M.; Amr, M.M.; Shebl, M.M.; Farahat, M.M. & Anger, W.K. (2003). Neurobiological effects among workers occupationally exposed to organophosphorous pesticides, *Occupational and Environmental Medicine*, Vol.60, No.4, (April 2003), pp. 279-286, ISSN 1351-0711

Ferrer, A. & Cabral, R. (1995). Recent epidemics of poisoning by pesticides, *Toxicology Letters*, Vol.82–83, (December 1995), pp. 55–63, ISSN 0378-4274

Fiedler, N.; Kipen, H.; Kelly-McNeil, K. & Fenske, R. (1997). Long-term use of organophosphates and neuropsychological performance, *American Journal of Industrial Medicine*, Vol.32, No.5, (November 1997), pp. 487-496, ISSN 0271-3586

Files, F.J.; Denning, C.E.; Hyytia, P.; Kiianmaa, K. & Samson, H.H. (1997). Ethanol-reinforced responding by AA and ANA rats following the sucrose-substitution initiation procedure, *Alcoholism: Clinical and Experimental Research*, Vol.21, No.4, (June 1997), pp. 749–753, ISSN 0145-6008

Flora, S.J. & Tandon, S.K. (1987). Effect of combined exposure to lead and ethanol on some biochemical indices in the rat, *Biochemical Pharmacology*, Vol.36, No.4, (February 1987), pp. 537–541, ISSN 0006-2952

Flora, S.J.; Dhawan, M. & Tandom, S.K. (1991). Effects of combined exposure to aluminium and ethanol on aluminium body burden and some neuronal, hepatic and haematopoietic biochemical variables in the rat, *Human and Experimental Toxicology*, Vol.10, No.1, (January 1991), pp. 45-48, ISSN 0960-3271

Gralewicz, S.; Lutz, P. & Szymczak, W. (2000). Hyposensitivity to amphetamine following exposure to chlorphenvinphos protection by amphetamine preexposure, *Acta Neurobiologiae Experimentalis*, Vol. 60, No.2, (April 2000), pp. 203–208, ISSN 0065-1400

Grandjean, P. & Landrigan, P.J. (2006). Developmental neurotoxicity of industrial chemicals, *The Lancet*, Vol.368, No.9553, (December 2006), pp. 2167-2178, ISSN 0140-6736

Gultekin, F.; Ozturk, M. & Adogan, M. (2000). The effect of organophosphate insecticide chlorpyrifos-ethyl on lipid peroxidation and antioxicant enzymes (in vitro), *Archives of Toxicology*, Vol.74, No.9, (November 2000), pp. 533-538, ISSN 0340-5761

Gupta, V. & Gill, K.D. (2000a). Lead and ethanol coexposure: implications on the dopaminergic system and associated behavioral functions, *Pharmacology, Biochemistry and Behaviour*, Vol.66, No.3, (July 2000), pp. 465-474, ISSN 0091-3057

Gupta, V. & Gill, K.D. (2000b). Influence of ethanol on lead distribution and biochemical changes in rats exposed to lead, *Alcohol*, Vol.20, No.1, (January 2000), pp. 9-17, ISSN 0741-8329

Harwood, H.J.; Fountain, D. & Livermore, G. (1998). Economic costs of alcohol abuse and alcoholism, *Recent Development in Alcoholism*, Vol.14, pp. 307-30, ISSN 0738-422X

Järup, L. (2003). Hazards of heavy metal contamination, *British Medical Bulletin*, Vol.68, No.1, (December 2003), pp.167-182, ISSN 0007-1420

Kalra, S.P. & Kalra P.S. (2004). Overlapping and interactive pathways regulating appetite and craving, *Journal of Addictive Disease*, Vol.23, No.3, (July 2004), pp. 5-21, ISSN 1055-0887

London, L.; Flisher, A.; Wesseling, C.; Mergler, D. & Kromhout, H. (2005). Suicide and exposure to organophosphate insecticides, cause or effect? *American Journal of Industrial Medicine*, Vol.47, No.4, (April 2005), pp. 308–321, ISSN 0271-3586

Lopez-Crespo, G.; Carvajal, F.; Flores, P.; Sanchez-Santed, F. & Sanchez-Amate, M.C. (2007). Time-course of biochemical and behavioural effects of a single high dose of chlorpyrifos, *Neurotoxicology*, Vol.28, No.3, (May 2007), pp. 541–547, ISSN 0161-813X

Lotti, M. (2001). Clinical toxicology of anticholinesterase agents in humans. In: *Handbook of Pesticide Toxicology. Second edition*, R.I. Krieger, (Ed.), 1043-1085, Academic Press, ISBN 978-0-12-426260-7, San Diego.

Lutz, P.; Gralewicz, S.; Kur, B. & Wiaderna, D. (2005). Amphetamine- and scopolamine-induced locomotor activity following treatment with cholphenvinphos or chlorpyrifos in rats, *International Journal of Occupational Medicine and Environmental Health*, Vol.18, No.2, (April 2005), pp. 115–125, ISSN 1232-1087

Lutz, P.; Tomas, T.; Gralewicz, S. & Nowakowska, E. (2000). Long-term effects of acute exposure to chlorphenvinphos on behavioural responsiveness to amphetamine and scopolamine in rats, *International Journal of Occupational Medicine and Environmental Health*, Vol.13, No.3, (July 2000), pp. 215–222, ISSN 1232-1087

Lutz, P.; Wiaderna, D.; Gralewicz, S. & Kur, B. (2006). Exposure to chlorphenvinphos, an organophosphate insecticide, prevents from behavioural sensitization to amphetamine, *International Journal of Occupational Medicine and Environmental Health*, Vol.19, No.2, (April 2006), pp. 132–141, ISSN 1232-1087

Mann, K.; Ackermann, K.; Diehl, A.; Ebert, D.; Mundle, G.; Nakovics, H.; Reker, T.; Richter, G.; Schmidt, L.G.; Driessen, M.; Rettig, K.; Opitz, K. & Croissant, B. (2006). Galantamine: a cholinergic patch in the treatment of alcoholism: a randomized, placebo-controlled trial, *Psychopharmacology (Berl)*, Vol.184, No.1, (January 2006), pp. 115-21, ISSN 0033-3158

McDougall, S.A.; Reichel, C.M.; Farley, C.M.; Flesher, M.M.; Der-Ghazarian, T.; Cortez, A.M.; Wacan, J.J.; Martinez, C.E.; Varela, F.A.; Butt, A.E. & Crawford, C.A.(2008). Postnatal manganese exposure alters dopamine transporter function in adult rats: Potential impact on nonassociative and associative processes, *Neuroscience*, Vol.154, No.2, (June 2008), pp. 848-860, ISSN 0306-4522

McGinnis, J.M. & Foege, W.H. (1999). Mortality and Morbidity Attributable to Use of Addictive Substances in the United States, *Proceedings of the Association of American Physicians*, Vol.111, No. 2, (February 1999), pp. 109–118, ISSN 1525-1381

Miller, C.S. (2001). Toxicant-induced loss of tolerance, *Addiction*, Vol.96, No.1, (January), pp. 115-139, ISSN 0965-2140

Miller, D.K.; Nation, J.R. & Bratton, G.R. (2000). Perinatal exposure to lead attenuates the conditioned reinforcing properties of cocaine in male rats, *Pharmacology, Biochemistry and Behavior*, Vol.67, No.1, (September 2000), pp. 111–119, ISSN 0091-3057

Miller, D.K.; Nation, J.R. & Bratton, G.R. (2001). The effects of perinatal lead exposure to lead on the discriminative properties of cocaine and related drugs, *Psychopharmacology*, Vol.158, No.2, (November 2001), pp. 165–174, ISSN 0033-3158

Moreno, M.; Cañadas, F.; Cardona, D.; Suñol, C.; Campa, L.; Sanchez-Amate, M.C.; Flores, P. & Sanchez-Santed, F. (2008). Long-term monoamine changes in the striatum and nucleus accumbens alter acute chlorpyrifos exposure, *Toxicology Letters,* Vol.176, No.2, (January 2008), pp. 162-167, ISSN 0378-4274

Muir, D.C. & Howard, P.H. (2006). Are there other persistent organic pollutants? A challenge for environmental chemists, *Environmental Science and Technology*, Vol.40, No.23, (December 2006), pp. 7157–7166, ISSN 0013-936X

Mutti, A.; Falzoi, M.; Romanelli, A.; Bocchi, M.C.; Ferroni, C. & Franchini, I. (1988). Brain dopamine as a target for solvent toxicity: Effects of some monocyclic aromatic hydrocarbons, *Toxicology,* Vol.49, No.1, (April 1988), pp. 77–82, ISSN 0300-483X

Nation, J.R.; Dugger, L.M.; Dwyer, K.K.; Bratton, G.R. & Grover, C.A. (1991). The effects of dietary lead on ethanol-reinforced responding, *Alcohol and Alcoholism,* Vol.26, No.4, (July 1991), pp. 473-480, ISSN 0735-0414

Nation, J.R. & Burkey, R.T. (1994). Attenuation of cocaine-induced elevation of nucleus accumbens dopamine in lead-exposed rats, *Brain Research Bulletin*, Vol.35, No.1, (January 1994), pp. 101-104, ISSN 0361-9230

Nation, J.R.; Livermore, C.L. & Burkey, R.T. (1996). Chronic lead exposure attenuates sensitization to the locomotor-stimulating effects of cocaine, *Drug and Alcohol Dependence*, Vol.41, No.2, (June 1996), pp. 143–149, ISSN 0376-8716

Nation, J.R.; Smith, K.R. & Bratton, G.R. (2004). Early developmental lead exposure increases sensitivity to cocaine in a self-administration paradigm, *Pharmacology, Biochemistry and Behavior*, Vol.77, No.1, (January 2004), pp. 127–135, ISSN 0091-3057

Newlin, D.B. (1994). Drug sensitization, substance abuse, and chemical sensitivity, *Toxicology and Industrial Health*, Vol.10, No.4-5, (July-October 1994), pp. 463–480, ISSN 0748-2337

Office of National Drug Control Policy (2004). The Economic Costs of Drug Abuse in the United States, 1992-2002. Washington, DC: Executive Office of the President (Publication No. 207303). Available at www.ncjrs.gov/ondcppubs/publications/ pdf/economic_costs.pdf

Overstreet, D.H.; Rezvani, A.H. & Janowsky, D.S. (1990). Increased hypothermic responses to ethanol in rats selectively bred for cholinergic supersensitivity, *Alcohol and Alcoholism*, Vol.25, No.1, (January 1990), pp. 59-65, ISSN 0735-0414

Overstreet, D.H.; Miller, C.S.; Janowsky, D.S. & Russell, R.W. (1996). Potential animal model of multiple chemical sensitivity with cholinergic supersensitivity, *Toxicology*, Vol.111, No.1-3, (July 1996), pp. 119–134, ISSN 0300-483X

Overstreet, D.H. & Djuric, V. (2001). A genetic rat model of cholinergic hypersensitivity, implications for chemical intolerance, chronic fatigue, and asthma, *Annals of the New York Academy of Science*, Vol.933, (March 2001), pp. 92-102, ISSN 0077-8923

Pope, C.N.; Chakraborti, T.K.; Chapman, M.L. & Farrar, J.D. (1992). Long-term neurochemical and behavioural effects induced by acute chlorpyrifos treatment, *Pharmacology, Biochemistry and Behavior*, Vol.42, No.2 (June 1992), pp.251-256, ISSN 0091-3057

Pope, C.N. (1999). Organophosphorus pesticides, Do they all have the same mechanism of toxicity? *Journal of Toxicology and Environmental Health, Part B Critical Reviews*, Vol.2, No.2, (April-June 1999), pp. 161-181, ISSN 1093-7404

Rehm, J.; Mathers, C.; Popova, S.; Thavorncharoensap, M.; Teerawattananon Y. & Patra, J. (2009). Global burden of disease and injury and economic cost attributable to alcohol use and alcohol-use disorders, *The Lancet*, Vol.373, No.9682, (June 2009), pp. 2223–2233, ISSN 0140-6736

Reichel, C.M.; Wacan, J.J.; Farley, C.M.; Stanley, B.J.; Crawford, C.A. & McDougall, S.A. (2006). Postnatal manganese exposure attenuates cocaine-induced locomotor activity and reduces dopamine transporters in adult male rats, *Neurotoxicology and Teratology*, Vol.28, No.3, (May-June 2006), pp. 323–332, ISSN 0892-0362

Richardson, R.J. (1995). Assesment of the neurotoxic potential of chlopryrifos relative to other organophosphorus compounds: A critical review of the literature. *Journal of Toxicology and Environmental Health*, Vol.44, No.2, (February 1995), pp. 135-165, ISSN 0098-4108

Rocha, E.S.; Swanson, K.L.; Aravaca, Y.; Goolsby, J.E.; Maelicke, A. & Alburquerque, E.X. (1996). Paraoxon: Cholinesterase-independent stimulation of transmitter release and selective block of ligand-gated ion channels in cultured hippocampal neurons, *The Journal of Pharmacology and Experimental Therapeutics*, Vol.278, No.3, (September 1996), pp. 1175-1187, ISSN 0022-3565

Roldan-Tapia, L. & Sanchez-Santed, F. (2004). Neuropsychological sequelae of acute poisoning by pesticides containing cholinesterase inhibitors, *Revista de Neurologia*, Vol.38, No.6, (March 2004), pp. 591-597, ISSN 0210-0010

Roldan-Tapia, L.; Nieto-Escamez, F.A.; del Aguila, E.M.; Laynez, F.; Parron, T. & Sanchez-Santed, F. (2006). Neuropsychological sequelae from acute poisoning and long-term exposure to carbamate and organophosphate pesticide, *Neurotoxicology and Teratology*, Vol.28, No.6, (November-December 2006), pp. 694-703, ISSN 0892-0362.

Rosenstock, L.; Keifer, M.; Daniell, W.E.; McConnell, R. & Claypoole, K. (1991). Chronic central nervous system effects of acute organophosphate pesticide intoxication, *The Lancet*, Vol.338, No.8761, (July 1991), pp. 223-227, ISSN 0140-6736

Sánchez-Amate, M.C.; Dávila, E.; Cañadas, F.; Flores, P. & Sanchez-Santed, F. (2002). Chlorpyrifos Shares Stimulus Properties with Pentylenetetrazol as Evaluated by an Operant Drug Discrimination Task, Neurotoxicology, Vol.23, No.6, (December 2002), pp. 795-803, ISSN 0161-813X

Sanchez-Santed, F.; Cañadas, F.; Flores, P.; Lopez-Grancha, M. & Cardona, D. (2004). Long-term functional neurotoxicity of paraoxon and chlorpyrifos : behavioural and pharmacological evidence, *Neurotoxicology and Teratology*, Vol.26, No.2, (March-April 2004), pp. 305–317, ISSN 0892-0362

Savage, E.P.; Keefe, T.J.; Mounce, L.M.; Heaton, R.K.; Lewis, J.A. & Burcar, P.J. (1998). Chronic neurological sequelae of acute organophosphate pesticide poisoning, *Archives of Environmental Health*, Vol.43, No.1, (January-February 1998), pp. 38-45, ISSN 0003-9896

Schiller, G.D. & Overstreet, D.H. (1993). Selective breeding for increased cholinergic function: Preliminary study of nicotinic mechanisms. *Medical Chemistry Research*, Vol.2, No.8-9 (October 1993), pp. 578-583, ISSN 1054-2523

Sinclair, J.D.; Le, A.D. & Kiianmaa, K. (1989) The AA and ANA rat lines selected for differences in voluntary ethanol consumption, *Experientia*, Vol.45, No.9, (September 1989), pp. 798–805, ISSN 0014-4754

Slotkin, T.A.; Southard, M.C.; Adam, S.J.; Cousins, M.M. & Seidler, F. J. (2004). Alpha7 nicotinic acetylcholine receptors targeted by cholinergic developmental neurotoxicants: Nicotine and chlorpyrifos, *Brain Research Bulletin*, Vol.64, No.3, (September 2004), pp. 227–235, ISSN 0361-9230

Steenland, K.; Jenkins, B.; Ames, R.G.; O'Malley, M.A.; Chrislip, D.W. & Russo, J. (1994). Chronic neurologic sequelae of acute organophosphate pesticide poisoning, *American Journal of Public Health*, Vol.84, No.5, (May 1994), pp. 731–736, ISSN 0090-0036

Sorg, B.A.; Willis, J.R.; Nowatka, T.C.; Ulibarri, C.; See, R.E. & Westberg, H.H. (1996). Proposed animal neurosensitization model for multiple chemical sensitivity in studies with formalin, *Toxicology*, Vol.111, No.1-3, (July 1996), pp. 135-145, ISSN 0300-483X

Sorg, B.A.; Willis, J.R.; See, R.E.; Hopkins, B. & Westberg, H.H. (1998). Repeated low-level formaldehyde exposure produces cross-sensitization to cocaine: possible relevance to chemical sensitivity in humans, *Neuropsychopharmacology*, Vol.18, No.5, (May 1998), pp. 385-394, ISSN 0893-133X

Sorg, B.A. & Hochstatter, T. (1999). Behavioral sensitization after repeated formaldehyde exposure in rats. *Toxicology and Industrial Health*, Vol.15, No.3-4, (April-June 1999), pp. 346–355, ISSN 0748-2337

Sorg, B.A.; Tschirgi, M.L.; Swindell, S.; Chen, L. & Fang, J. (2001). Repeated formaldehyde effects in an animal model for multiple chemical sensitivity, *Annals of New York Academy of Sciences*, Vol.933, (March 2001), pp. 57–67, ISSN 0077-8923

Spiegelberg, V. (1961). Psychopathologisch-neurologische Schaden nach Einwirkung Synthetischer Gifte, In: *Wehrdienst und Gesundheit, vol. III* (Darmstadt, Wehr und Wissen Verlagsgesellshaft)

Tabershaw, I. & Cooper, C. (1966). Sequelae of acute organic phosphate poisoning. *Journal of Ocuppational Medicine*, Vol.8, No.1, (January 1966), pp.5-20, ISSN 0096-1736

Thiele, T.E.; Navarro, M.; Sparta, D.R.; Fee, J.R.; Knapp, D.J. & Cubero I. (2003). Alcoholism and obesity: overlapping neuropeptide pathways? *Neuropeptides*, Vol.37, No.6, (December 2003), pp. 321-337, ISSN 0143-4179

U.S. EPA (2002) Interim Reregistration Eligibility decision for chlorpyrifos. US EPA, Washington, DC, http://www.epa.gov/oppsrrd1/reregistration/status.html.

Valles, R.; Cardon, A.L.; Heard, H.M.; Bratton, G.R. & Nation, J.R. (2003). Morphine conditioned place preference is attenuated by perinatal lead exposure, *Pharmacology, Biochemistry and Behavior*, Vol.75, No.2, (May 2003), pp. 295–300, ISSN 0091-3057

Vezer, T.; Kurunczi, A.; Naray, M.; Papp, A. & Nagymajtenyi, L. (2007). Behavioral effects of subchronic inorganic manganese exposure in rats, *American Journal of Industrial Medicine*, Vol.50, No.11, (November 2007), pp. 841–852, ISSN 0271-3586

Von Euler, G.; Ogren, S.O.; Bondy, S.C.; McKee, M.; Warner, M.; Gustafsson, J.A.; Eneroth, P. & Fuxe, K. (1991). Subacute exposure to low concentrations of toluene affects dopamine mediated locomotor activity in the rat, *Toxicology,* Vol.67, No.3, (May 1991), pp. 333– 349, ISSN 0300-483X

Von Euler, G.; Ogren, S.O.; Li, S.M.; Fuxe, K. & Gustafsson, J.A. (1993). Persistent effects of subchronic toluene exposure on spatial learning and memory, dopamine-mediated locomotor activity and dopamine D2 agonist binding in the rat, *Toxicology,* Vol.77, No.3, (March 1993), pp. 223–232, ISSN 0300-483X

World Health Organization. (1990). Public health impact of pesticides used in agriculture. Geneva: WHO

Yokoyama, K.; Araki, S.; Murata, K.; Nishikitani, M.; Okumura, T.; Ishimatsu, S. & Takasu, N. (1998). Chronic neurobehavioral and central and autonomic nervous system effects of Tokyo subway sarin poisoning, *Journal of Physiology,* Vol.92, No.3-4, (June-August 1998), pp. 317-323, ISSN 0928-4257

13

Global Warming and Heat Stress Among Western Australian Mine, Oil and Gas Workers

Joseph Maté and Jacques Oosthuizen
Edith Cowan University, 270 Joondalup Dr, Joondalup, Western Australia, Australia

1. Introduction

The earth is currently experiencing a change in its climate which in some areas is resulting in warmer ambient temperatures. Globally the frequency and severity of heat waves have increased over the last few decades leading to an associated increase in the burden of morbidity and mortality associated with heat waves. Global temperatures are predicted to rise even further in the foreseeable future [1, 2].

Heat wave related research thus far has largely been focused on the health of the general population, in particular older people and little has been done to investigate its impact on occupational cohorts. Workers employed in outdoor occupations such as surface mining, construction and farming are deemed to be high risk groups, particularly those workers who are required to wear impermeable protective clothing and personal protective equipment (PPE) such as gloves and respirators [3]. During the 15 year period (1992-2006), 423 workers in the USA died as a result of occupational exposure to heat [4].

Three key factors influencing thermal balance among workers are: climatic conditions; metabolic demands; and clothing. Heat induced illnesses are related to and exacerbated by a combination of environmental work and clothing factors as well as sub-normal tolerance to heat, alcohol and drug abuse, dehydration (due to excessive sweating, diarrhoea, vomiting), being un-acclimatised to heat, electrolyte imbalance, and lack of sleep and fatigue [5]. When the body reaches a point where it can no longer maintain thermal equilibrium, core body temperature begins to rise and various forms of heat related illness (HRI) may develop. Types of HRI include heat oedema, heat cramps, heat syncope, heat exhaustion and 2 types of heat stroke (HS); Namely classical HS which results from extended exposure to hot environmental conditions and exertional HS which occurs sporadically in individuals with high metabolic output rates in combination (usually) with hot environmental conditions. Exertional HS has been reported in athletes, workers in the mining and construction industry, and military personnel [6].

Heat stroke generally occurs when core body temperature (T_c) exceeds 39°C. Symptoms include the cessation of sweating, red, hot, and dry skin, rapid and strong pulse, headache, dizziness, nausea and confusion, and this can lead to unconsciousness and death if left untreated [4]. The risk and severity of excessive heat strain varies widely among people.

In an occupational context heat strain is normally identified by various measures, including heart rate, core body temperature and the sudden onset of severe fatigue, nausea, dizziness and light-headedness. Generally people are at greater risk if they have experienced profuse sweating sustained over a number of hours, their net weight loss exceeds 3% of body weight, and their 24 hr urinary sodium excretion exceeds more than 50mmoles [7].

Repetitive exposure to hot working conditions usually enables workers to adapt to hot work environments leading to a reduction in heart rate and body temperature and an increase in sweating. Furthermore it has been demonstrated among heat acclimatised workers that core body temperature decreases by 0.1 – 0.5 °C during resting periods [8].

2. Ambient working environment

The expansion of Western Australia's resource industry has brought with it an increased number of personnel required on site [9]. As these industrial sites tend to be located in remote areas exposed to hot and sometimes humid conditions, the exposure of more personnel to extreme environmental conditions is inevitable. For example, miners have experienced WBGT exposures of 29.1°C to 31.5°C [10, 11] and a Basic Effective Temperature ranging between 26.6°C and 29.4°C [12]. Within the mining industry, particularly underground mining, the geothermal gradient contributes to ambient heat. With current mining trends, mines are becoming increasingly deeper, and as a result, so too are the thermal gradients. For example, in a South African mine, a geothermal gradient of 10 – 22°C$\cdot$km^{-1} has been recorded [13]. As such, a significant thermal environment is present thus requiring attention to improving the environmental strain experienced by personnel.

In addition to the heat gained by personnel in these hot environments, high metabolic heat loads associated with heavy working tasks have also been reported (Mate et al. 2007). For example, the task of shovelling has been measured to range from between 266 W$\cdot$m^{-2} and 407 W$\cdot$m^{-2} [14, 15], while drilling has been found to range from 217 W$\cdot$m^{-2} to 290 W$\cdot$m^{-2} [15, 16]. Shovelling at 266 W$\cdot$m^{-2} for a 75 kg individual without the capacity to cool could increase core body temperature (T_c) by ~0.1°C$\cdot$min^{-1}. According to the International Standards Organization 7243, such work intensities correspond to high and very high metabolic rates [17]. If heavy work intensities are performed during environmental conditions previously described, the onset of a heat-related illness can occur [18], causing symptoms ranging from central and/or peripheral fatigue [19-22], decreased focus/concentration, oedema of the periphery [23], up to a more serious and sometimes fatal heat stroke [23].

The beginning of the fly-in/fly-out (FIFO) work regime can be traced back to the middle of the last century where workers in the Gulf of Mexico were flown in long distances to work offshore on oil platforms [24]. Other industries began to use this FIFO method of labour for their work force requirements. Currently, approximately 49% of Western Australia's mining sites are operating on a FIFO basis [25]. This method of employment provides employers an opportunity to have personnel from all regions of Australia to fill vacancies. Having a diverse work force introduces unique heat stress concerns which would otherwise not be present in a traditional mining town scenario. For example, in the northern regions of Australia during the wet months (2010/2011), temperatures ranged on average from 33.0°C to 22.1°C while concurrently in Tasmania during the same season the hottest day time temperature was recorded to be 18.4°C with highs ranging from approximately 3.0 to 15.0°C to lows of -3.0 to 6.0°C [26].

If employees are flown in from such temperature extremes, the probabilities of experiencing heat stress injuries are more likely. It is not only the location of origin that is of concern, where workers go during the off phase of their swing and how long they stay there for could also cause problems. With swing shifts ranging anywhere between one week on and one week off up to four weeks on and two weeks off, the 'down' time is what is of interest. As will be discussed later in more detail in this chapter, the acclimation status of a worker influences their capacity to deal with occupational heat loads. Initially, at the start of the swing, workers may not be acclimated to the task and thus would be more susceptible to heat stress related injuries. As time on the swing progresses, physiological responses to the continuous heat insults enables a larger heat load to be tolerated. Once these insults are removed, such as during vacation to a cooler climate, the heat acclimated responses are less responsive and return the worker to a vulnerable state.

Usual physiological adaptations during heat acclimation, that occur irrespective of the acclimation modality, include: a reduction in resting heart rate in the heat [27], decreased resting core temperature [8], increase in plasma volume [28], decrease in rectal and skin temperature [29], change in sweat composition [30], reduction in the sweating threshold [31] and an increase in sweating efficiency [29].

The process of acclimation is dependent upon several variables such as duration and frequency of acclimating sessions, temperature, humidity and exercise intensity. For example, Yamazaki [27] used a 6 day acclimation protocol with participants exercising at 50% $\dot{V}O_{2max}$ in ambient conditions of 36°C and 50% RH. Buono et al. [8] had a protocol which required their participants to exercise for 7 consecutive days for four bouts of 25 min with a 5 min rest while treadmill walking (1.34 $m{\cdot}s^{-1}$ at a 3% grade) and cycling (75 W at 35°C at 75% RH). Shvartz and colleagues [29] used a bench step protocol which equated to a load equal to 85% $\dot{V}O_{2max}$ during ambient conditions of 21.5°C DB, 17.5°C WB, for 12 days. Two hour treadmill walks for 9 days in humid heat (37°C, 74% RH) was used by Garden et al. [32] for their acclimation protocol. Although there are many different acclimation protocols, there is a general consensus within literature that the greater the intensity of exercise during acclimation, the quicker observable responses will be elicited.

The effectiveness of acclimation is dependent upon the acclimating conditions. Ideally, individuals should be acclimated in environmental conditions and workloads similar to those they would typically experience [33]. For example, individuals who work in desert type conditions should be acclimated in hot and dry conditions whereas those who work in tropical conditions should be acclimated in hot and humid conditions [32, 34]. A study on working capacity under dry and humid heat loads was performed by Nag et al. [35]. One group of subjects were acclimated to dry and hot conditions (41.3 ± 0.6°C and 40 - 50% RH) while another group was acclimated to humid and hot conditions (39.2 ± 0.6°C and 70 - 80% RH) for 9 days. It was found that those individuals who were acclimated in humid conditions were able to perform more work in similar conditions than those who were acclimated under dry conditions. Regardless of the acclimation protocol, both groups increased their work performance compared to the unacclimated state.

The benefits of acclimation were eloquently demonstrated by Wyndham and colleagues [36] when they calculated the quantity of work that could be performed between acclimated and unacclimated men in a laboratory setting. It was concluded that unacclimated individuals would reach a critical body temperature (a $\overline{T}_b$ where voluntary cessation of exercise occurs) quicker (600 min) than acclimated individuals (750 min) at the same ambient T_{wb}, particularly when initial core temperature was already elevated. These changes in sensitivity by the various thermolytic responses facilitate a reduction in the net rate of net heat gain.

The process of acclimating requires between several days to weeks of continual exposure to specific environmental and working conditions. Resources such as heat chambers may not necessarily be available on work sites which may make the process difficult. Consideration must also be made for the decay in heat acclimation status, which can range from between 6 days to 4 weeks [33, 37].

Despite the physiological advantage of a lower resting rectal temperature (T_{re}), increased sweat rate, reduced sweating threshold, reduction in resting heart rate, and increased blood volume, the commitment to induce these physiological responses in acclimation is both time and labour intensive. Even though miners have a good level of acclimatization, as previously described, heat stress related illnesses are still experienced despite currently implemented heat stress interventions. This supports the need for further cooling methods to be employed in heat stressful occupations.

Work-related injuries related to fatigue may be caused by dehydration [38], physical exertion (due to intensity and/or duration) and/or an elevated body temperature [19]. The deleterious effect of dehydration on running memory and perceptual motor coordination functions was found to occur beyond 2% dehydration [39]. When observing the effects of 2% body dehydration on word recognition, serial addition and trail marking tests, performance was found to decrease with increases in dehydration [38]. Performing prolonged activities in the heat can result in altered brain activity. During prolonged exercise (such as during a 12 h work shift), fatigue is thought to occur in the synapses due to excessive use, decreased spinal excitability to inputs and reductions in motoneural output from the spine resulting in a reduction in peripheral feedback [21]. Associated with elevated body temperatures are alterations in the central nervous system to drive working muscles [40-42]. With a reduction in working musculature, the ability to perform tasks may increase the risk of injury. Additionally, visual acuity is impaired during elevated body temperatures [43] while a reduction in mental and simple tasks occurs between a temperature of 30 - 33°C WBGT [44]. It was also identified by Nielsen et al. [45] through alterations in electroencephalogram measurements in the frontal cortex during hyperthermia, that the ability to exercise was reduced. These findings indicate that there are some neurological perturbations occurring while body temperatures are elevated, which could explain the commonly observed reduction in work and coordination.

3. Physiology of heat stress

As core body temperature increases, blood circulating through the core of the body picks up heat energy and the warmer blood flows to the skin where the blood is cooled and heat is exchanged with the environment. The rate of heat loss through the skin depends upon the temperature differences between the skin and the environment. Furthermore, the skin secrets sweat that evaporates thus removing additional heat energy from the skin. This process is influenced by humidity and air movement over the skin. Clothing can hamper heat loss through this process. If the net heat gain is equal to heat loss then the storage rate of heat is 0 and the body is in equilibrium.

There are 3 key factors that influence thermal balance, these are; climatic conditions, work demands and clothing. Heat induced illnesses are related to and exacerbated by a combination of environmental work and clothing factors as well as sub-normal tolerance, alcohol and drugs abuse, dehydration (excessive sweating, diarrhoea and vomiting) being un-acclimatised and electrolyte imbalance [46].

The risk and severity of excessive heat strain varies widely among people. In an occupational context heat strain is normally identified by various measures, including heart rate, core body temperature and the sudden onset of severe fatigue, nausea, dizziness and light headedness. Generally people are at greater risk if they have experienced profuse sweating sustained over a number of hours, their net weight loss exceeds 3% of body weight and their 24 hr urinary sodium excretion exceeds more than 50mmoles [47].

3.1 Heat stress indices introduction

Thermoregulation of mean body temperature ($\overline{T}_b$) is continually in a state of adjustment as a result of metabolic processes and interactions with the environment [48]. The regulatory centre for $\overline{T}$b is located in the brain; more specifically, the preoptic anterior hypothalamus (PO/AH). In response to afferent signals from thermal receptors located throughout the body, the PO/AH integrates these signals and effector responses are initiated (sweating and/or increased skin blood perfusion during warm conditions) to restore $\overline{T}$b or body heat content (Hb). These thermolytic mechanisms will continue until a thermal homeostasis is restored, as seen by an absence of a rising $\overline{T}$b or core temperature (T_c).

Under conditions of thermal neutrality, the net change in Hb approximates zero. During conditions of uncompensable heat loads (conditions where heat gain is greater than heat loss), a rise in Tc is observed. Ultimately, it is the thermal gradient between the Tc and skin, and the skin and environment which determines the rate and direction of net heat gain or loss; this relationship is illustrated in Figure 1. This thermal heat exchange can be expressed by the following heat balance equation as adapted from [49]:

$$S = M \pm (R + C) \pm W - E \tag{1}$$

Where S = rate of net heat storage (either positive or negative)

M = metabolic heat production (always positive)

E = evaporative heat loss (always negative)

R = radiative heat exchange,

C = conductive heat exchange

W = mechanical work

Note: In cold environments negative (-) values could be used instead of the (+) that indicates heat gain (especially relevant for R and C). R,C,K and C(rsep) can be in either direction [46].

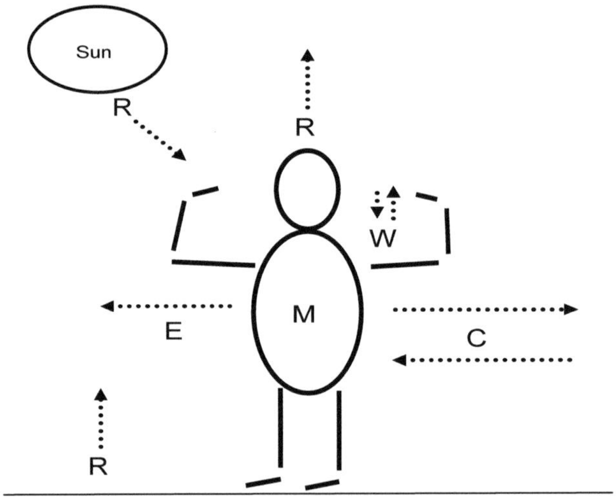

Fig. 1. Schematic representation of heat transfer where R = radiation, M = metabolism, E = evaporation, C = conduction, W = mechanical work

In addition to the heat gained by personnel in these hot environments, high metabolic heat loads associated with heavy working tasks have also been reported [50]. For example, the task of shovelling has been measured to range from between 266 W·m^{-2} and 407 W·m^{-2} [14, 15], while drilling has been found to range from 217 W·m^{-2} to 290 W·m^{-2} [15, 16]. Shovelling at 266 W·m^{-2} for a 75 kg individual without the capacity to cool could increase T_c by ~0.1°C·min^{-1}. According to the International Standards Organization 7243, such work intensities correspond to high and very high metabolic rates [17]. If heavy work intensities are performed during environmental conditions previously described, the onset of a heat-related illness can occur [18], causing symptoms ranging from central and/or peripheral fatigue [19-22], decreased focus/concentration, oedema of the periphery [23], up to a more serious and sometimes fatal heat stroke [23].

International Standards Organization (ISO), World Health Organization (WHO), National Institute for Occupational Safety and Health (NIOSH), and the American Conference of Governmental Industrial Hygienists (ACGIH) are some of the governing bodies that have developed/implemented heat stress guidelines and/or indices to allow for safe repeated bouts of heat exposure by industrial personnel. There are several criteria deemed as a safe upper limit of T_c. These limits which have been developed by industrial governing bodies are: (1) a 1°C increase above resting T_c values [51], (2) a maximum T_c of 38.0°C [51], and (3) a T_c of 38.5°C if workers have been medically screened [51]. Despite these conservative limits, the incidence of heat stress related illnesses remains high, particularly in an Australian mine during the summer months (43/million-man hours on average throughout the year versus 147/million-man hours during February) [18]. Higher cases of heat illness during the summer months (May and September (88%)) were also observed among US marine corps [52]. With higher cases being reported during hotter months, one could suggest that workers and their managers are violating these imposed thermal limits and that improved heat stress interventions are required.

Thus, it seems important for occupational hygienists and managers to be aware of the severe consequences of a hot working environment and the potential risk for heat-related injuries. Some of the currently implemented interventions involve, establishing maximal exposure durations to stressful environments through heat stress indices [53-56], educating workers on hydration [57], and modification of the ambient working environment [50, 58]. By complementing these heat stress strategies with newer approaches, the incidence of heat related injuries in industry may be reduced. Therefore, the purpose of this review is to identify some approaches already taken to reduce heat stress in industry-highlighting some restrictions these interventions may have, and to provide an alternative solution which may compliment currently implemented heat stress interventions.

Environmental conditions in industry, as previously described, can place high and sometimes uncompensatable heat loads on workers. In order to help protect workers from heat stress related illnesses, heat stress indices or measurements have been created. These indices can be classed into three general categories; direct, rational and empirical indices. Direct indices involve the use of standard ambient measuring equipment. The more popular direct index used in industry is the ISO 7243 - WBGT [17]. Rational indices are measurements based more on physiological parameters such as sweating, T_c, heart rate, and metabolic work. Examples of rational indices include but are not limited to: predicted heat strain [59], heat stress index [56], and ISO 7933. Empirically based indices are those measurements which are based on meteorological parameters such as temperature, humidity and wind speed. Examples of empirically based indices are: effective temperature [60], corrected effective temperature and the predicted four hour sweat rate (P_4SR) [54].

Some approaches in addressing the issue of heat stress range from monitoring and manipulation of the ambient working environment (heat stress indices and ventilation practices), altering work practices and work schedules (mechanical equipment and rest to work ratios), primary care (acclimation of workers), implementation of safety equipment (cooling garments), to education of workers (hydration practices). Some challenges in creating a universal heat stress index are the multitude of variables which exist in the working environment. Such variability includes the identification of metabolic demands for tasks between workers, phenotype of workers, health status of the worker, tolerance to heat, heat sources (natural and artificial), mechanisation of occupation, interference of thermolytic mechanisms, level of intermittent work, and the ambient environment. Accounting for each variable in a single heat stress index may not be feasible for industrial applications. As a result, several indices have been developed to assist with protecting the worker and predicting heat loads. Regardless of its type, as summarized by Epstein and Moran [61], an index should: (1) be feasible and accurate through a range of conditions, (2) integrate important variables, (3) represent the workers exposure and (4) reflect increased physiological and psychological safety and health.

Described below are several heat stress indices and other heat stress interventions used in industry with a brief review of their function and in some cases, the variables measured and limitations.

4. Heat stress indices

Thermal Work Limit (TWL) - This index is defined as the limiting or maximal sustainable metabolic rate that a euhydrated, acclimatized individual can maintain in a specific thermal environment within safe limits of both deep body core temperature (38.2°C) and sweat rate (< 1.2 $kg{\cdot}hr^{-1}$) [62]. This index has been reported to be more appropriate and realistic than the WBGT during a field study performed by Miller and Bates [63]. The index incorporates various physiological limits in thermolysis to define its scale. From these physiological limits and environmental variables (WB, DB, barometric pressure and wind speed), a portable electronic device then determines a limit value. This value is compared to a table which then determines a safe sustainable metabolic level. Although this index may provide better accuracy in determining a safe working limit, the use of this index is difficult without the aid of the calculating device.

ISO 7243 - Wet Bulb Glob Temperature (WBGT) - An empirical index which is a compromise between an easy to use measure of ambient conditions and a reduced precision index for industrial environments. It is regarded as an exploratory method [17] to determine heat stress through the calculation of radiative, dry bulb, and wet bulb values.

The WBGT has been generally accepted amongst governing bodies upon which their recommendations and standards are founded [64]. This index allows for a maximal rectal temperature (Tre) of 38.0°C. The WBGT is calculated and then referenced against a table for tolerable exposure times, metabolic intensities and work ratios. Weighting for spatial variation in temperature accounts for the temperature at the head (having a weighting factor of two), abdomen and ankles divided by four. Also, there is a time weighting factor which is based on the work to rest ratio. The measurement is averaged over each work period. The simplicity of this index makes it an easy field assessment tool as it requires minimal equipment and training. In addition to the averaging of body segments and time, this index has two variations; the inclusion of radiative or solar heat loads. Typically they are used indoors or outdoors:

Indoors:

$$WBGT = 0.7\ t_{nw} + 0.3\ t_g \tag{2}$$

Outdoors:

$$WBGT = 0.7\ t_{nw} + 0.2\ t_g + 0.1\ t_a \tag{3}$$

t_{nw} = natural wet bulb

t_g = globe temperature

t_a = air temperature (dry bulb temperature)

In conjunction with WBGT values, estimated metabolic rates are given in five broad categories. This index also provides work/rest ratios adjusting for ambient conditions. The reference values provided are for a normally clothed individual (0.6 Clo), physically fit for the activity being considered and in good health and both acclimated and non-acclimated individuals [17].

While the usability of this index is easy, dry bulb measurements towards the top end of the scale may be over emphasised [30]. Further, the index may not adequately consider air flow during hot and humid conditions, and is insensitive to air flows above 1.5 $m{\cdot}s^{-1}$ [30]. This index is unable to accommodate for differences in metabolic rates; however, concomitantly using another ISO standard can correct for this shortcoming. The insulative component of clothing is not accounted for during the calculation of this index; although, another ISO standard can be used to correct for insulation. Despite the correction factors available from other indices, constantly referring to them may make this index cumbersome to use.

ISO 7933 – Ergonomics of the thermal environment – Analytical determination and interpretation of heat stress using calculation of the predicted heat strain - Predicting sweat rates and T_c are described by ISO 7933. The objectives of ISO 7933 are twofold; (1) to evaluate the working environment where rises in T_c or excessive water loss typically occur, and (2) determine exposure times where physiological strain is acceptable.

As the ISO 7933 index estimates strain in Western populations, this specificity may discriminate against other ethnicities based on phenotype. McNeill and Parsons [65] investigated the accuracy of this heat stress index during a simulated tea leaf picking task in conditions similar to those found in India. They used Western participants in the study and observed differences in the accuracy of measured sweat rates, metabolic rates and insulative properties of clothing. The appropriateness of the index was found to be mainly directed towards Western countries as opposed to those regions where anthropometrically different people habituate. ISO 7933 states within its introduction that it is not applicable to cases where special protective clothing is worn [59], which include reflective clothing, active cooling and ventilation clothing, impermeable clothing and PPE.

ISO 8996 – Ergonomics of the thermal environment – Determination of metabolic rate – Here, the ISO 8996 specifies different methods for determining metabolic rates in assessment of working practices, jobs and activities. These estimates are based on an individual of 30 years of age, weighing 70 kg and standing 1.75 m tall (BSA 1.8 m^2) for men, and weighing 60 kg and standing 1.70 m tall (BSA of 1.6 m^2) for women [51].

The index is divided into four different assessment levels for metabolic estimates with each level having different levels of accuracy. Level 1; screening - this assessment quickly characterizes the mean workload of the occupation, but contains a high risk of error in estimation. Level 2; observation - a time motion analysis is performed for the occupation which includes workload estimates for body segments and postures. The accuracy of this level is ± 20%. Level 3; analysis - the estimation of metabolic rate is determined through heart rate. The accuracy of this level is ± 10%. Lastly, level 4; expertise - indirect calorimetry. Accuracy of this method is ± 5%, however it is limited by the measurement, duration or motion being evaluated.

Observer experience in the interpretation of task intensity, as defined by ISO 8996, plays a key role. Additionally, the grading of an activity can vary with the appraiser's level of fitness, age, experience and training level [66]. It was found that the difference between two groups of appraisers before visual training ranged between 18-60%. After training, the largest difference in a measurement was found to be 24%. These findings highlight the importance of intra-observer experience to accurately assess metabolic demands for heat stress purposes.

ISO 9886 – Ergonomics – Evaluation of thermal strain by physiological measurements – several methods are provided to measure physiological parameters which are to be used in conjunction with other ISO standards. The parameters included in this standard are: body temperature, skin temperature, heart rate and body mass loss. The index provides several methods to measure each parameter with an emphasis on body temperature. ISO 9886 provides limit values for the various physiological parameters.

Using heart rate as an indicator of thermal strain may be subjective as heart rate increases with work and heat. Physiological responses to heat may vary between individuals and setting an upper limit of an increase in HR of 33 bpm may be conservative. Nielsen and Meyer [67] attempted to calculate $\dot{V}O_2$ from measuring HR and observed both over and underestimation in $\dot{V}O_2$ due to differences in temperature, posture, and whether there were static or dynamic movements and non-steady state types of activities performed. Using HR as a factor to limit work may require further investigation.

Predicted 4 hour Sweat Rate (P_4SR) – developed by McArdle and colleagues [54], with the aim to create a simple index or method of assessing the physiological effects of any combination of temperature, humidity, radiation and air movement on personnel wearing different clothing types and working at various intensities. A nomograph encompasses these variables for ease of use. As with all indices, some limits were implemented in its derivation. This includes the dry bulb or globe temperature range, wet bulb, air movement speeds, metabolic rates and an upper sweat rate limit of 4.5 L in a four hour period. Once environmental variables have been obtained, lines are drawn on the nomograph and the required sweat rate can be determined along with the predicted rise in T_{re} at the end of a 4 hour period.

The inherent limitations are described within the index itself, however, the application of this index to acclimated individuals can be challenging since such individuals can easily achieve a sweat rate of 4.5 L in a period of four hours (1.125 $L \cdot hr^{-1}$), and in fact, Wyndham et al. [68] showed acclimated individuals had a P_4SR range between 4.95 and 5.35 L. Therefore, a sweat rate of 4.5 L could be an overly conservative estimate. In as much as the investigators provide a nomograph for calculating sweat rates and rise in T_{re}, deciphering the graph provides a further challenge to the field use of the index. Furthermore, this index accounts for partial clothing to be worn by personnel, and therefore does not consider fully encapsulating garments, which could be problematic.

Physiological Strain Index (PSI) –an 11 point scale (0 to 10) is used to indicate the level of stress which is based on two physiological parameters; heart rate and T_{re} [69]. The PSI is simple to use and it does not discriminate between environmental conditions, nor the clothing worn by individuals; hence the functionality of the index. The evaluation of heat strain can be preformed instantaneously by a supervisor or the workers themselves at any time, which is advantageous; however, the social acceptance of T_{re} monitoring and its invasiveness are questionable.

$$PSI = 5(T_{ret} - T_{re0}) \cdot (39.5 - T_{re0})^{-1} + 5(HR_t - HR_0) \cdot (180 - HR_0)^{-1} \qquad (4)$$

T_{ret} and HR_t are simultaneous measurements of rectal and heart rate

T_{re0} and HR_0 are the initial rectal and heart rate measurements

Conversely, the PSI could be considered a reactive rather than a proactive index. It is reactive in that, the workers would already have been or are currently being exposed to high heat loads. It is only when they stop work that their physiological responses are measured. These measurements could be a misrepresentation as a critical core temperature could have already been reached. It has been previously shown that modifications to work practices begin to occur as ambient conditions increase [11], reducing the effectiveness of this index.

Heart rate – ISO 9886 [51] - includes equations to estimate heat strain in workers based on heart rate. These equations include a limit of heart rate (HR_L) that should not be exceeded:

$$HR_L = 185 - 0.65 \cdot \text{age} \tag{5}$$

or a sustained heart rate;

$$HR_{L,\,\text{sustained}} = 180 - \text{age} \tag{6}$$

It is suggested to set the upper limit for a change in heart rate of 33 bpm which is associated to a thermal strain being experienced by the worker (ΔHR_T). Despite these suggested limits, as with T_c, there are circumstances in which this limit can be exceeded, provided there is medical supervision. During these circumstances, the upper limit for HR would be 60 bpm.

4.1 Limitations to current heat stress interventions

Heat stress interventions typically do not consider individual variability. As such, individuals will respond differently to the same condition. Therefore, the accuracy of the index will vary. The development of a heat stress index is based on the statistical probability that most of the population will be protected and this probability will then either over protect or not protect at all. Those individuals who are considered to be at either one of the tail ends of the probability curve may not be adequately protected. Over the past century, there have been many indices developed that are aimed at protecting workers; however, the one major shortcoming of all indices is that they do not consider the unique characteristics of each individual during its prediction. In addition to the limitation of accuracy, a new index can be difficult to implement or regulate.

Creation of a new heat stress index could take years to accurately develop and trial. Manipulating the working environment can prove to be too costly and implementing cooling PPE would provide benefits when adhered to. As all workers are required to drink at rest breaks or during work, therefore supplying personnel with a specific type of drink could be an effective cooling intervention to implement. Drinking a solution which changes physical states, solid to liquid, has the potential to provide additional cooling to the worker during work.

4.2 Drinking a cold liquid as a heat stress intervention

The consumption of cold liquid water ($H_2O_{(aq)}$) results in an expansion of the body's natural heat sink. As the body warms the cooler consumed $H_2O_{(aq)}$, heat energy is exchanged between the body and the $H_2O_{(aq)}$ until a thermal gradient no longer exists. Therefore, the heat energy that would have been otherwise stored in the body is transferred to the $H_2O_{(aq)}$.

The consumption of cooler quantities of $H_2O_{(aq)}$ will theoretically allow even larger quantities of heat energy to be transferred from the body to the solution. In order to increase the temperature of $H_2O_{(aq)}$ by 1°C, approximately 4210 $J \cdot g^{-1} \cdot K^{-1}$ of heat energy is required to be transferred into the liquid. Thus, the specific heat equation 7 is used to calculate the quantity of heat transferred to 500 g (assuming the density of water is 1.000 ($kg \cdot m^{-3}$)) of 0°C $H_2O_{(aq)}$ consumed by an individual (body temperature of 37°C).

$$Q = m \cdot C_p \cdot \Delta T \tag{7}$$

Q is the quantity of heat gained or lost (kJ)

m is the mass of the substance (kg)

C_p is the specific heat capacity of the substance ($kJ \cdot kg^{-1} \cdot K^{-1}$)

ΔT is the change in temperature (°K)

Using this equation, it can be determined that approximately 77.9 kJ of energy is required to equilibrate the water to body temperature. In other words, by consuming 500 g of 0°C water, 77.9 kJ of cooling capacity is administered to the individual.

An ice slurry (combination of both solid ($H_2O_{(s)}$) and $H_2O_{(aq)}$ water; $H_2O_{(is)}$) results in an even greater thermodynamic potential for heat energy to be exchanged with the body. If left undisturbed, $H_2O_{(aq)}$ begins to change physical states from liquid to solid at a temperature of approximately 0°C. However, if $H_2O_{(aq)}$ is continuously stirred, the liquid forms small ice crystals and changes into an $H_2O_{(is)}$. By maintaining both physical states (solid and liquid), the $H_2O_{(is)}$ drink may provide a subtle, but significant advantage to reducing heat strain in thermally challenging conditions This advantage is due to the phase changing feature of the $H_2O_{(is)}$ when $H_2O_{(s)}$ is converted to $H_2O_{(aq)}$. $H_2O_{(s)}$ has a different specific heat capacity (C_p) (2108 $J \cdot g^{-1} \cdot K^{-1}$) to that of $H_2O_{(aq)}$. Comparing $H_2O_{(aq)}$ and $H_2O_{(is)}$, the $H_2O_{(is)}$ would have a greater C_p as a result of having both phases of water in its solution; this ultimately increases the solution's heat sink capacity. Therefore, if the C_p of $H_2O_{(s)}$ is used as a conservative approximation for $H_2O_{(is)}$ at temperatures below 0°C, and the C_p of $H_2O_{(aq)}$ is used for temperatures above 0°C, $H_2O_{(is)}$ results in a greater heat sink capacity than $H_2O_{(aq)}$ alone.

An additional factor which contributes to the larger $H_2O_{(is)}$ heat sink capacity is the energy required to change the physical state of a solid to a liquid. That is, the energy required to change the physical state of $H_2O_{(s)}$ to $H_2O_{(aq)}$ without a change in temperature. This is termed the latent heat of melting or 'enthalpy of transformation'. For water, the energy required is 334 $kJ \cdot kg^{-1}$. To estimate the cooling capacity of $H_2O_{(is)}$ from equation 7 while incorporating both the enthalpy of transformation and the C_p of $H_2O_{(s)}$, the cooling capacity for 500 g of $H_2O_{(is)}$ at -1°C becomes 245.9 kJ. Again, using equation 7 to determine the change in T_c for a 75 kg individual drinking 500 ml of $H_2O_{(aq)}$ or $H_2O_{(is)}$, a change of 0.299°C and 0.945°C would occur, respectively.

While the thermodynamic effect of $H_2O_{(is)}$ consumption has been investigated in animals. Vanden Hoek et al. [70] infused a 50 ml $\cdot kg^{-1}$ solution of either saline slurry or saline water of equal temperature in 11 swine over a 1 hr period. Brain temperature was reduced by 5.3 ± 0.7°C with saline slurry compared with 3.4 ± 0.4°C using saline water. Another study by Merrick and co-workers [71] showed how phase changing cryotherapy modalities were able to produce colder superficial skin temperatures (ice bag; from 35.6 ± 0.9 to 27.8 ± 3.5°C at 1 cm, 36.3 ± 0.7 to 31.8 ± 2.2°C at 2 cm, wet-ice; from 35.7 ± 0.8 to 27.2 ± 3.4°C at 1 cm, 36.2 ± 0.7 to 30.6 ± 3.0°C, and gel pack; from 35.49 ± 0.8 to 29.5 ± 2.4°C at 1 cm, 36.1 ± 0.9 to 32.1 ± 1.5°C at 2 cm) at a depth of 1 and 2 cm compared with non-phase changing cryotherapies. Kennet and colleagues [72] investigated the cooling efficiency of four different cryotherapeutic agents and showed that crushed ice (19.6 ± 3.8°C) reduced skin temperatures more than a gel pack (13.2 ± 5.1°C), frozen peas (14.6 ± 4.2°C), and ice-water immersion (17.0 ± 2.8°C). Lee et al. [73], demonstrated that cold (4°C) versus warm (37°C) drinks administered prior to and during cycling exercise lowered mean T_{re} during exercise (37.3 ± 0.4°C versus 38.0 ± 0.4°C) and extended time to exhaustion (63.8 ± 4.3 vs. 52.0 ± 4.1 min; cold versus warm drink, respectively). More recently, Siegel et al. [74] showed that consuming 7.5 $ml \cdot kg^{-1}$ ice slurry resulted in a lower pre-exercise T_c, which remained lower for the first 30 min of treadmill running compared with ingesting cool liquid of the same composition. This supports the notion of ice slurry having a greater cooling capacity than cool liquids of equal volumes. Additionally, time to exhaustion was significantly (P = 0.001) increased in the ice slurry (50.2 ± 8.5 min) versus cold liquid (40.7 ± 7.2 min). While a thermodynamic advantage should theoretically be gained through the phase change properties of solid versus liquid water, the physiological effects of consuming such a mixed solution during exercise have only recently been reported [72, 74].

With a greater theoretical cooling capacity of an ice slurry over a liquid, ingesting this as an additional cooling source should aid in regulating heat during work. In addition to the cooling potential of an ice slurry, the capacity to hydrate also increases as the ice slurry provides a source of fluid replacement. Replacing fluids, as described below, with an ice slurry could theoretically better attenuate the rate of rise in body temperature and increase exercise performance compared to water alone.

5. Recent research

Recent heat stress research in the LNG industry by Maté et al. [75] focused on identifying which heat stress indices best attenuated heat stress in on and off shore workers. The authors measured the physiological responses to a typical work day, as deemed by personnel during March. Body temperature, skin temperature, heart rate, hydration status and estimated metabolic work were measured throughout the work day. The interesting findings from the study were, the P_4SR was most accurate for both cohorts, ISO 8996 did not accurate predict workloads and the majority of personnel were dehydrated upon the start and completion of their work shift. These findings question the appropriateness of specific heat stress indices to be used while dehydrated.

A subsequent study by the same authors [76] investigated a practical cooling intervention on an off shore oil platform. They compared the physiological responses to drinking a cold liquid to drinking ice slurry. The same physiological measurements were recorded as in the previous study. Results from the study indicated that complete replacement of fluid during working hours (excluding meal breaks) by ice slurry, although not statistically significant, can attenuate the heat load experienced by personnel. Interestingly, the hydration status of workers was similar between studies as well as ambient working conditions. It could therefore be concluded that the physiological attenuation of heat gain is attributed to the ingestion of ice slurry.

The results from both studies indicate the P_4SR and ingestion of ice slurry will mitigate heat stress in personnel, a *caveat* must be applied to each study. Sample sizes were small and the sample population were from one location and time of year. Although these limitations do exist, the findings hold promise for using ice slurry as a cooling modality. It is easily implementable, cost effective and personnel enjoyed drinking the new beverage. Future focus should be placed on educating the work force on the importance of hydrating. Once adherence to maintaining hydrated has been firmly implemented in the working culture, heat loads experienced by personnel can be accurately determined.

6. Recommendations for further research

Occupational heat stress is one issue which is most likely to remain within industry. In order to attenuate the effects of heat on personnel, a two pronged approach can be proposed. This consists of 1) better prediction of heat loads and 2) identifying those individuals whom are better suited physiologically to work in the hot environment. Irrespective of the approach, the task to effectively minimize heat stress related disorders in industry is monumental.

Predicting heat loads which personnel will experience can be further dissected into environmental and metabolic. Environmental considerations vary according to atmospheric conditions and the immediate working vicinity. Controlling the atmosphere is not probable; however, manipulating the immediate working environment is. This cost can be substantial; which suggests more research into better conditioning techniques and efficiently running and cooling machinery. Engineering examples for environmental modification can include but are not limited to more efficient machinery, better insulated components, and separation of heat producing sources and personnel.

In addition to conditioning of the environment, modification of the physicality of tasks can further attenuate heat loads. For example, rather than manually lifting boxes from point A to point B, have boxes delivered as close as possible to the destination and also at a height which is mechanically and spatially practical. This may be an area where ergonomist could provide better and more detailed evaluations of work space.

Heat stress indices attempt to predict heat loads experienced by personnel which are dependent on the environmental and metabolic loads. The accuracy and precision of the index is also dependent on the accuracy of the values entered into the various equations. Should an estimated temperature be entered into the equation, an estimated predicted heat load will be provided. The calculated value may or may not be a true reflection of the actual heat load experienced. That estimate may in turn over or under protect the worker. In the field, obtaining accurate environmental measurements are relatively easy and simple. Obtaining metabolic measurements of tasks are unfortunately not as simple. A similar type of error may occur as with an inaccurate temperature reading. If a task is assumed to be not as physically demanding than it is in reality, then the worker will be expected to work longer in unsafe conditions. This type of situation can jeopardize the safety and health of the worker. Therefore, investigating the metabolic costs associated with specific occupations or even tasks could increase the protectiveness of current heat stress indices.

Methods to identify physiologically suitable individuals for work are also required. Practically speaking, attainment of a thermal neutral working environment with minimal physical exertion is not likely for those industries where manual labour is the only method of production. Therefore, a closer inspection of those variables which allows one individual to work in a more heat stressful environment than another is warranted.

There may be some specific genotypical predisposition between individuals that determines the quantity of stress which can be tolerated. In addition to genotype, the tolerance developed by acute or chronic exposure to heat may also contribute to this tolerance. Changes in physiology which occur as a result of heat acclimation have been described above. As mentioned previously, this process attenuates heat stress related illnesses but does not eliminate the issue or susceptibility.

The precise physiological modifications which occur from acclimatization are not well understood; however, several hypotheses have been proposed. It is thought that a modification in the cellular functioning is what ultimately defines the capacity of one individual to do work over another. Recently, interest has grown into measuring cellular protein concentration levels as a defence to acute episodes to heat shock. It is this protein, called heat shock protein (HSP), which stabilises other cellular proteins. Further reading can be found at [77-82]. With the HSP safeguarding other protein structures within the cell, destruction as a result of heat exposure is attenuated. There is an abundant quantity of literature on plant and animal testing, however, limited research has been done in humans. Therefore, investigation in the cellular modifications which occur as a result of heat insult is an area of research which is growing and could possibly explain the physiological changes responsible for acclimation.

7. References

[1] McMichael, A., et al. *National Climate Change Adaptation Research Plan Human Health.* 2008; Available from: http://www.nccarf.edu.au/national-adaptation-research-plan-human-healt.

[2] Pengelly, L.D., et al., *Anatomy of heat waves and mortality in Toronto: lessons for public health protection.* Can J Public Health, 2007. 98(5): p. 364-8.

[3] Schulte, P.A. and H. Chun, *Climate change and occupational safety and health: establishing a preliminary framework.* J Occup Environ Hyg, 2009. 6(9): p. 542-54.

[4] Luginbuhl, R.C., et al., *Heat-related deaths among crop workers in the United States, 1992-2006.* Journal of the American Medical Association, 2008. 300(9): p. 1017-8.

[5] Plogg, B.A., *Fundamentals of Industrial Hygiene.* 5th ed, ed. B.A. Plogg and P.J. Quinlan. 2002, Washington: National Safety Council.

[6] Bonauto, D., et al., *Occupational heat illness in Washington State, 1995-2005.* Am J Ind Med, 2007. 50(12): p. 940-50.

[7] Di Corleto, R., G. Coles, and I. Firth. *Heat stress standard & documentation developed for use in the Australian environment.* in *Australian Institute of Occupational Hygienists.* 2003. Melbourne, Australia.

[8] Buono, M.J., J.H. Heaney, and K.M. Canine, *Acclimation to humid heat lowers resting core temperature.* American Journal of Physiology - Regulatory Integrative and Comparative Physiology, 1998. 274(5 43-5).

[9] Ye, Q., *Commodity booms and their impacts on the Western Australian economy: The iron ore case.* Resources Policy, 2008. 33(2): p. 83-101.

[10] Kalkowsky, B. and B. Kampmann, *Physiological strain of miners at hot working places in German coal mines.* Industrial Health, 2006. 44(3): p. 465-473.

[11] Brake, D.J. and G.P. Bates, *Deep body core temperatures in industrial workers under thermal stress.* Journal of Occupational and Environmental Medicine, 2002. 44(2): p. 125-135.
[12] Weller, R., *The environmental hazards encountered in potash mining*. 1981, University of Notthingham.
[13] Marx, W.M., *Providing an acceptable working environment in ultra deep mines.* Journal of the Mine Ventilation Society of South Africa, 1998. 51(2): p. 57-60.
[14] Bethea, N., Bobo, M., Ayoub, MM. *The physiological response to low coal mining.* in *Proceedings of the human factors society 24th annual meeting*. 1980.
[15] Leithead, C., Lind, AR., *Heat Stress and Heat Disorders*. 1964, London: Cassell.
[16] Graves, R.J., et al., *Thermal conditions in mining operations.* 1981, Edinburgh: Institute of Occupational Medicine.
[17] ISO, *ISO 7243,1989, Hot environments - Estimation of heat stress on working man, based on the WBGT-index (wet bulb globe temperature). Geneva: International Standards Organization* 1989.
[18] Donoghue, A.M., M.J. Sinclair, and G.P. Bates, *Heat exhaustion in a deep underground metalliferous mine.* Occupational and Environmental Medicine, 2000. 57(3): p. 165-174.
[19] Nybo, L., *Hyperthermia and fatigue.* J Appl Physiol, 2008. 104(3): p. 871-8.
[20] Nybo, L. and B. Nielsen, *Perceived exertion is associated with an altered brain activity during exercise with progressive hyperthermia.* J Appl Physiol, 2001. 91(5): p. 2017-23.
[21] Saldanha, A., M.M. Nordlund Ekblom, and A. Thorstensson, *Central fatigue affects plantar flexor strength after prolonged running.* Scand J Med Sci Sports, 2007.
[22] Todd, G., et al., *Hyperthermia: a failure of the motor cortex and the muscle.* J Physiol, 2005. 563(Pt 2): p. 621-31.
[23] Coris, E.E., A.M. Ramirez, and D.J. Van Durme, *Heat illness in athletes: the dangerous combination of heat, humidity and exercise.* Sports Med, 2004. 34(1): p. 9-16.
[24] Gramling, R., *Oil in the Gulf: Past Development, Future Prospects*, U.D.o.t.I.M.M. Service, Editor. 1995, Gulf of Mexico OCS Region: New Orleans, LA, USA.
[25] Storey, K., *Fly in fly-out and fly-over: Mining and regional development in Western Australia.* Australian Geographer, 2001. 32(2): p. 133-148.
[26] *Australian Government Bureau of Meteorology (2011)*. Available from: www.bom.gov.au.
[27] Yamazaki, F. and K. Hamasaki, *Heat acclimation increases skin vasodilation and sweating but not cardiac baroreflex responses in heat-stressed humans.* Journal of Applied Physiology, 2003. 95(4): p. 1567-1574.
[28] Senay, L.C., D. Mitchell, and C.H. Wyndham, *Acclimatization in a hot, humid environment: body fluid adjustments.* J Appl Physiol, 1976. 40(5): p. 786-96.
[29] Shvartz, E., A. Magazanik, and Z. Glick, *Thermal responses during training in a temperate climate.* Journal of Applied Physiology, 1974. 36(5): p. 572-576.
[30] Taylor, N.A., *Challenges to temperature regulation when working in hot environments.* Ind Health, 2006. 44(3): p. 331-44.
[31] Nadel, E.R., et al., *Mechanisms of thermal acclimation to exercise and heat.* J Appl Physiol, 1974. 37(4): p. 515-20.
[32] Garden, J.W., I.D. Wilson, and P.J. Rasch, *Acclimatization of healthy young adult males to a hot-wet environment.* J Appl Physiol, 1966. 21(2): p. 665-9.
[33] Yousef, M.K., S. Sagawa, and K. Shiraki, *Heat stress: a threat to health and safety.* J Uoeh, 1986. 8(3): p. 355-64.
[34] Shvartz, E., et al., *A comparison of three methods of acclimatization to dry heat.* J Appl Physiol, 1973. 34(2): p. 214-9.
[35] Nag, P.K., et al., *Human work capacity under combined stress of work and heat.* J Hum Ergol (Tokyo), 1996. 25(2): p. 105-13.

[36] Wyndham, C.H., et al., *Tolerance times of high wet bulb temperatures by acclimatised and unacclimatised men.* Environ Res, 1970. 3(4): p. 339-52.
[37] Wyndham, C.H. and G.E. Jacobs, *Loss of acclimatization after six days of work in cool conditions on the surface of a mine.* J Appl Physiol, 1957. 11(2): p. 197-8.
[38] Gopinathan, P.M., G. Pichan, and V.M. Sharma, *Role of dehydration in heat stress-induced variations in mental performance.* Arch Environ Health, 1988. 43(1): p. 15-7.
[39] Sharma, V.M., et al., *Influence of heat-stress induced dehydration on mental functions.* Ergonomics, 1986. 29(6): p. 791-9.
[40] Saboisky, J., et al., *Exercise heat stress does not reduce central activation to non-exercised human skeletal muscle.* Exp Physiol, 2003. 88(6): p. 783-90.
[41] Thomas, M.M., et al., *Voluntary muscle activation is impaired by core temperature rather than local muscle temperature.* J Appl Physiol, 2006. 100(4): p. 1361-9.
[42] Martin, P.G., et al., *Reduced voluntary activation of human skeletal muscle during shortening and lengthening contractions in whole body hyperthermia.* Exp Physiol, 2005. 90(2): p. 225-36.
[43] Hohnsbein, J., et al., *Effects of heat on visual acuity.* Ergonomics, 1984. 27(12): p. 1239-46.
[44] Ramsey, J.D., *Task performance in heat: a review.* Ergonomics, 1995. 38(1): p. 154-65.
[45] Nielsen, B., et al., *Brain activity and fatigue during prolonged exercise in the heat.* Pflugers Arch, 2001. 442(1): p. 41-8.
[46] Plogg B., A. and P. Quinlan, J. , *Fundamentals of Industrial Hygiene (5th ed); NSC.* 2002.
[47] Di Corleto, R., G. Coles, and I. Firth, *Heat stress standard & documentation developed for use in the Australian environment.* 2003, Australian Institute of Occupational Hygienists, Tullamarine, Vic.
[48] Mekjavic, I.B., C.J. Sundberg, and D. Linnarsson, *Core temperature 'null zone'.* Journal of Applied Physiology, 1991. 71(4): p. 1289-1295.
[49] Buskirk, E.R., *Temperature regulation with exercise.* Exercise and Sport Sciences Reviews, 1977. 5: p. 45-88.
[50] Mate, J., Hardcastle, S.G., Beaulieu, F.D., Kenny, G., Reardon, F.D., *Exposure Limits for Work Performed In Canada's Deep Mechanised Metal Mines©*, in *Challenges in Deep and High Stress Mining*, J.H. Y. Potvin, T.R. Stacey, Editor. 2007, Australian Centre for Geomechanics: Perth. p. 527-536.
[51] ISO, *ISO 9886, 2004, Ergonomics - Evaluation of thermal strain by physiological measurements, Geneva: International Standards Organization.* 2004.
[52] Kark, J.A., et al., *Exertional heat illness in Marine Corps recruit training.* Aviat Space Environ Med, 1996. 67(4): p. 354-60.
[53] ACGIH, *Threshold limit values for chemical and physical agents and biological exposure indices, American Conference of Governmental Industrial Hygienists, Cincinnati.* ISBN 1-882417-58-5, 2005.
[54] McArdle, B., et al., *The Prediction of the Physiological Effects of Warm and Hot Environment.* Medical Research Council, 1947. 47: p. 391.
[55] Yaglou, C.P., and Minard, D., *Control of Heat Casualties at Military Training Centers.* American Medical Association Archives of Industrial Health, 1957. 16: p. 302 - 316.
[56] Belding, H.S., and Hatch, T.F., *Index for Evaluating Heat stress in Terms of Resulting Physiological Strains.* Heating and Piping Air Conditioning, 1955. 27: p. 129-136.
[57] Brake, D.J. and G.P. Bates, *Fluid losses and hydration status of industrial workers under thermal stress working extended shifts.* Occupational and Environmental Medicine, 2003. 60(2): p. 90-96.
[58] Hardcastle, S.G. and C.K. Kocsis, *The ventilation challenge.* CIM Bulletin, 2004. 97(1080): p. 51-57.

[59] ISO, *ISO 7933, 2004, Ergonomics of the thermal environment - Analytical determination and interpretation of heat stress using calculation of the predicted heat strain. Geneva: International Standards Organization.* 2004.
[60] Houghton, F.C., and Yaglou, C.P., Trans American Society of Heating and Ventilation Engineering, 1923. 28: p. 163 - 176 and 361 - 384.
[61] Epstein, Y. and D.S. Moran, *Thermal comfort and the heat stress indices.* Ind Health, 2006. 44(3): p. 388-98.
[62] Brake, D.J. and G.P. Bates, *Limiting Metabolic Rate (Thermal Work Limit) as an Index of Thermal Stress.* Applied Occupational and Environmental Hygiene, 2002. 17(3): p. 176-186.
[63] Miller, V.S. and G.P. Bates, *The Thermal Work Limit Is a Simple Reliable Heat Index for the Protection of Workers in Thermally Stressful Environments.* Ann Occup Hyg, 2007. 51(6): p. 553-561.
[64] Parsons, K.C., *International heat stress standards: a review.* Ergonomics, 1995. 38(1): p. 6-22.
[65] McNeill, M.B. and K.C. Parsons, *Appropriateness of international heat stress standards for use in tropical agricultural environments.* Ergonomics, 1999. 42(6): p. 779-797.
[66] Kahkonen, E., et al., *The effect of appraisers in estimating metabolic rate with the Edholm scale.* Appl Ergon, 1992. 23(3): p. 186-90.
[67] Nielsen, R. and J.P. Meyer, *Evaluation of metabolism from heart rate in industrial work.* Ergonomics, 1987. 30(3): p. 563-72.
[68] Wyndham, C.H., et al., *Limiting rates of work for acclimatization at high wet bulb temperatures.* J Appl Physiol, 1973. 35(4): p. 454-458.
[69] Moran, D.S., A. Shitzer, and K.B. Pandolf, *A physiological strain index to evaluate heat stress.* Am J Physiol, 1998. 275(1 Pt 2): p. R129-34.
[70] Vanden Hoek, T.L., et al., *Induced hypothermia by central venous infusion: saline ice slurry versus chilled saline.* Crit Care Med, 2004. 32(9 Suppl): p. S425-31.
[71] Merrick, M.A., L.S. Jutte, and M.E. Smith, *Cold Modalities With Different Thermodynamic Properties Produce Different Surface and Intramuscular Temperatures.* J Athl Train, 2003. 38(1): p. 28-33.
[72] Kennet, J., et al., *Cooling efficiency of 4 common cryotherapeutic agents.* J Athl Train, 2007. 42(3): p. 343-8.
[73] Lee, J.K., S.M. Shirreffs, and R.J. Maughan, *Cold Drink Ingestion Improves Exercise Endurance Capacity in the Heat.* Med Sci Sports Exerc, 2008. 40(9): p. 1637-44.
[74] Siegel, R., et al., *Ice Slurry Ingestion Increases Core Temperature Capacity and Running Time in the Heat.* Med Sci Sports Exerc, 2010. 42(4): p. 717-725.
[75] Maté, J., J. Oosthuizen, and G. Watson, *Appropriateness of heat stress indices used in the on and offshore liquefied natural gas industry.* (Submitted), 2011.
[76] Maté, J., J. Oosthuizen, and G. Watson, *Field investigation of a laboratory tested heat stress intervention using an ice slurry drink.* (Submitted), 2011.
[77] Sandstrom, M.E., et al., *The effect of 15 consecutive days of heat-exercise acclimation on heat shock protein 70.* Cell Stress Chaperones, 2008. 13(2): p. 169-75.
[78] Lindquist, S. and E.A. Craig, *The heat-shock proteins.* Annu Rev Genet, 1988. 22: p. 631-77.
[79] Kregel, K.C., *Heat shock proteins: modifying factors in physiological stress responses and acquired thermotolerance.* J Appl Physiol, 2002. 92(5): p. 2177-86.
[80] Moseley, P.L., *Heat shock proteins and heat adaptation of the whole organism.* J Appl Physiol, 1997. 83(5): p. 1413-7.
[81] Asea, A., *Mechanisms of HSP72 release.* J Biosci, 2007. 32(3): p. 579-84.
[82] Marshall, A., et al., *Human physiological and heat shock protein 72 adaptations during the initial phase of humid-heat acclimation.* Journal of Thermal Biology, 2007. 32: p. 341 - 348.

Part 6

Environmental Justice

14

Educating Latina Mothers About U.S. Environmental Health Hazards

Andrea Crivelli-Kovach, Heidi Worley and Tiana Wilson
Arcadia University, USA

1. Introduction

Environmental justice emphasizes health equality among all groups and cultures, so that no one group suffers disproportionately from environmental conditions over another group. The Environmental Protection Agency (EPA) defines environmental justice as "the fair treatment and meaningful involvement of all people regardless of race, color, national origin, or income with respect to the development, implementation, and enforcement of environmental laws, regulations, and policies" (EPA, 2011).

Environmental justice entitles everyone to healthy housing and protection from indoor environmental hazards. Yet there remain low-income families in urban areas of the United States whose living conditions adversely affect their health. Specific health issues include inadequate housing, indoor environmental health hazards, lack of health insurance, and barriers to health care (Sharfstein, Sandel, Kahn, & Bauchner, 2001).

2. Health disparities for minorities in the United States

Minority groups are disproportionately affected by the large number of health consequences from indoor environmental hazards. Latinos, compared to Caucasians, experience increased exposure to asthma triggers, lead poisoning, second-hand smoke, pest problems, dust mites, dangerous cleaning chemicals and pesticides, as a result of environmental inequity (Miller, Pollack, & Williams, 2011).

Progress has been made to curb some exposures, but disturbing disparities remain, especially among children. Blood lead levels decreased from 8.6% during 1988-1991 in US children ages one to five to 1.4% from 1999-2004 (Jones, Homa, Meyer et al., 2009). Despite this decrease, roughly 250,000 American children between one and five have blood lead levels of 10 µg/dL or greater, a level known to adversely affect a child's well-being (ATSDR, 2007; CDC, 2011a). Moreover, the Natural Resources Defense Council (2004) found that Latino children are twice as likely as Caucasian children to have blood lead levels that exceed 10 µg/dL. Elevated blood lead levels in children have been linked to decreased IQ levels as well as behavioral problems. A major source of lead exposure in homes is lead paint dust found in homes built before 1978 which can be ingested by babies and young children (Gilbert & Weiss, 2006; Jones, Homa, Meyer et al., 2009; Pearce, 2007).

Asthma is a common disease afflicting more than 23 million Americans in the United States (Bloom, Cohen, & Freeman, 2009; Pleis, Lucas, & Ward, 2009). Nearly 9.5 million (13%) of these individuals are children under the age of eighteen (Bloom, Cohen, & Freeman, 2009). Asthma attacks may occur in children when there is exposure to indoor asthma triggers (i.e., mold, dust mites, second-hand smoke, pest problems, and dangerous cleaning chemicals), and several studies emphasize the need to decrease or eliminate these triggers (Akinabi, Moorman, Garbe, and Sondik, 2009; Chipps, 2004; Lwebuga-Mukasa, Wojcik, Dunn-Georgiou, & Johnson, 2002).

Nationally, 14% of children from birth to eighteen years had ever been diagnosed with asthma in 2009 and Latino children were 60% more likely to have asthma than their Caucasian counterparts (National Center for Health Statistics, 2010; U.S. Department of Health and Human Services, 2009). While Latinos overall had the lowest prevalence of asthma nationally (6%), Puerto Ricans had the highest prevalence (14%) followed by African Americans (10%) and Caucasians (7%) (CDC, 2010b).

From 2007-2008, approximately 88 million Americans were exposed to second-hand smoke. This figure includes nearly 22 million (53.6%) children between the ages of 3 and 11 years (CDC, 2010a). The potential negative health effects of second-hand smoke include SIDS, respiratory and ear infections, and severe asthma (Melen, Wickman, Nordvall, van Hage-Hamsten, & Lindfors, 2001; U.S Department of Health and Human Services, 2006). Exposure to second-hand smoke in the unborn child can result in growth retardation, preterm labor, and low birth weight (Khader, Al-Akour, Alzubi, & Lataifeh, 2011; Law, Stroud, LaGasse et al., 2003).

Pests such as mice and cockroaches have taken a toll on the health of low-income Latino children, through the development of asthma or allergies from pest allergen sensitization (Stelmach, 2002). To eliminate pests and the negative health consequences associated with them, those who are suffering from infestation in their homes generally use pesticides and dangerous cleaning chemicals. However, these chemicals have been associated with miscarriages, birth defects, brain damage, and cancer (National Center for Healthy Housing, 2008; March of Dimes, 2011). A disease can lay dormant for several years only to manifest years after the initial exposure. Even exposure to low levels of dust mite allergen is related to asthma morbidity, suggesting that there is no safe level of exposure to dust mites (Jalaludin, Xuan, Mahmic et al, 1998; Kuehr, Frischer, Meinert et al., 1994). Additionally, dust mite exposure is associated with a decrease in lung function as well as asthma severity (Carter, Peterson, Ownby et al., 2003; Suppli & Backer, 1999).

3. Pennsylvania Latinos

The Latino population in Pennsylvania has been steadily increasing. A significant influx of Latinos moved to Pennsylvania between 2000 and 2009, bringing with it a 64% increase (394,088 to 646,524) in Latinos over the course of the decade (Pennsylvania Department of Health, 2011a). Meanwhile, the African American population grew by 11.4% (1,224,612 to 1,364,549) and the Caucasian population grew just 2.8% (10,484,203 to 10,773,983) in the same time period. This trend is striking considering these rates do not include the number of undocumented pregnant or newly parenting Latina women who migrate to the United States every year.

Latino children are particularly at risk of living in poverty. In 2008, almost one third (31%) of Latino children eighteen years or younger nationwide lived below the poverty level and half of Latino children in Philadelphia lived at the poverty level (Pew Hispanic Center, 2008). Babies and children of low-income minority parents are at a higher risk for indoor environmental health issues. In 2008, 5% of the Pennsylvania population was Latino, and Latina women between the ages of 15 and 44 accounted for 8% (12,000) of all live births in Pennsylvania (Pew Hispanic Center, 2008).

Even with the national decrease of the fertility rate among Latinas from 3.4 in 1990 to 2.6 children per woman in 2003 (Navarro, 2004), the number of pregnant Latina women ages 15-44 years in Pennsylvania reached 10,513 (6% of the total pregnant population) in 2002 (Pennsylvania Department of Health, 2002). From 2005-2008 Latinos had an 14% increase in live births in Pennsylvania (12,145 to 13,883) compared with Caucasians who experienced a 1% decrease in live births (108,795 to 107,623) (Pennsylvania Department of Health, 2010).

In Pennsylvania, asthma prevalence for children under 18 was 10% (285,000) and children ages 0-4 had the highest asthma hospitalization admission rate (48.5 per 10,000) among age groups. In 2009, Philadelphia had an asthma hospitalization rate nearly 3 times that of the whole state at 54.1 admissions for every 10,000 residents (Pennsylvania Department of Health, 2011b). Latinos also had the highest number of age-adjusted hospital admissions at 35.3 per 10,000 verses Caucasians at a rate of 11.8 per 10,000 residents.

In 2007, 2,246 Philadelphia children had lead poisoning - half the number of children that were affected in 2001 (Public Citizens for Children and Youth, 2008). This figure has decreased significantly in large part because organizations have been making homes lead safe, but there are still many homes with lead paint that have yet to be remedied since eighty percent of Pennsylvania homes were built before 1980 when lead paint was phased out (U. S. Census Bureau, 2000).

4. Needs assessments of environmental health disparities in the Latino community

Pennsylvania can draw on experiences from other programs. The Seattle Healthy Homes Program found that using community health workers to educate minority groups most at risk for environmental health hazards was an effective intervention for reducing the exposure to environmental health hazards in the home (Krieger, Takaro, Song, Beaudet, & Edwards, 2009). The Centers for Disease Control's Childhood Lead Poisoning Prevention Branch developed a web-based Healthy Housing and Lead Poisoning Surveillance System which tracks lead and non-lead housing risk factors and identifies groups that require assistance (CDC, 2009).

The Finance Project, a non-profit firm in Washington D.C., helps to improve linguistic and cultural barriers in health care (Lind, 2004). It offers strategies such as tailoring services to the community, providing oral and written translation when needed, and holding health education campaigns in many languages in order to reach a greater number of people.

5. Maternity Care Coalition: "Healthy at Home" program in Philadelphia

Maternity Care Coalition (MCC) is a private non-profit community-based organization in Philadelphia that works with individuals, families, health. Care providers, and the community to improve maternal and child health MCC's signature program, the MOMobile®, utilizes community health Advocates to identify and support pregnant and newly parenting women and their families in Philadelphia. MCC's Advocates live within the community where they work to implement the MOMobile® program. The Advocates' effectiveness lies in their ability to relate to and understand the culture and lifestyle of their clients.

"Healthy at Home" was a MOMobile® educational intervention developed to address indoor environmental health hazards including lead poisoning, pests, second-hand smoke, asthma, and noxious cleaning products. This program was aimed at pregnant Latina women and new parents living within the city of Philadelphia, to address the high rates of asthma and lead poisoning.

A "Healthy at Home" assessment was conducted to evaluate the knowledge gained by Latina women who participated in the program and to evaluate its effect on their behavior regarding the proper management of environmental hazards in their homes.

The majority of women received high scores in all environmental content (knowledge gained) areas. There were significant behavioral changes concerning environmental pests, the use of cold water to reduce lead exposure, and effective cleaning techniques. There were also significant knowledge increases related to lead poisoning and asthma (Wilson, Crivelli-Kovach, & Worley, 2010).

5.1 Case study: Environmental justice interviews with Latina mothers

5.1.1 Participants

Once the "Healthy at Homes" program was completed, Latino women were invited to participate in a follow-up study exploring their views of environmental justice and how it related to their homes and community.

In October 2004, MOMobile® Advocates from MCC recruited ten pregnant and/or newly parenting Latina women to participate in an interview discussing environmental justice. Inclusion criteria were:

- pregnant or newly parenting Latina women who participated in the first year of the "Healthy at Home" project implemented at the Latina MOMobile® site in Philadelphia, PA, and
- current clients of MCC.

Women were included whether they spoke English or Spanish. Questionnaires were developed in both languages and the interviews conducted in the language of choice of the interviewee.

5.1.2 Methodology

Design

Data were collected for this study using face-to-face interviews in the participants' homes to investigate the impact of the "Healthy at Home" intervention on the beliefs of Latina women about environmental justice issues and to explore the degree to which Latina women become socially active as a result of increased awareness of environmental hazards.

Instrument

The questionnaire was developed based on the literature and was provided to the women in both English and Spanish depending on the woman's language of choice. A panel of experts including Advocates from the Latina MOMobile® (Maria, Jenny, and Carmen) reviewed the questionnaire for content validity.

Data Collection

MCC Advocates recruited interview participants via telephone, inviting Latina women who had completed the "Healthy at Home" program to participate in the interviews. Advocates scheduled home visits with each participant so that the researcher could interview them in their home. The researcher was accompanied by one of the Advocates. The interviews took approximately twenty minutes to half an hour to complete. The interview also incorporated the collection of basic descriptive data including age, number of children, type of housing, and income.

Data Analysis

SPSS was used to analyze demographic data in the environmental justice interviews. N-VIVO was used to identify and analyze content themes in the qualitative data obtained from the interviews.

5.1.3 Results

Demographics

All of the Latina women who participated in the environmental justice interview were Puerto Rican between the ages of twenty and twenty-nine with a mean age of 24. Each woman had between 2 and 7 children but the largest number of women (4, 40%) had two children.

The number of individuals who lived in a house verses an apartment was nearly half (6, 60% vs. 4, 40% respectively) and 8 (80%) of the women rented their homes. Four (40%) lived where they currently did due to family and 2 (20%) reported that cost of living was a factor.

Eight women (80%) were not currently employed and all of the women (100%) had an educational level of high school equivalency or below. The average number of years of education among the women was 10.2 years.

Eight of the women (80%) were the sole primary caregivers for their children. Seven (70%) did not have a live-in partner or a partner who worked or contributed money to benefit their child(ren).

Several themes emerged from the environmental justice interviews. Three of these themes – (a) health behavior change leading to health promotion, (b) government's role in society, and (c) trust and distrust -- were linked qualitatively with the results of the "Healthy at Home" survey pre- and post- tests (Wilson, Crivelli-Kovach, & Worley, 2010).

Theme 1: Health behavior change leading to health promotion

Out of the ten women, 8 (80%) made some type of change within their home after the "Healthy at Home" program. Four women (40%) started dusting and washing their homes with baking soda and vinegar. Two (20%) individuals, including one who dusted, also mentioned that they had pest problems and attempted to fix that as well; one through pest control and the other on their own.

Every health behavior change that the women made in the home promoted better health for the parents and the children. Two (20%) of the women said they had specifically changed their cleaning habits to benefit their children. Three out of the 5 (60%) families who had one or more family members with asthma began smoking outside, rather than in the home. Half of the women who were interviewed reported that the education made it easier to make changes in the home, whereas only 2 (20%) found that "trying to do everything" and having to watch the kids made it more difficult.

Theme 2: Government's role in society

Though none of the women became more involved in their community by rallying for environmental equity, 5 (50%) voted in the most recent presidential election and 5 (50%) shared environmental health education with others.

The Latina women had mixed feelings about the government's responsibility for environmental issues in the home. While half of the women indicated that it was their sole responsibility to protect their children from environmental hazards in the home, three (30%) expressed that it was the responsibility of both parents and all levels of government to protect their children.

Half of the women said they believed the government was able to make important laws and policies based on environmental concerns.

Theme 3: Trust and distrust

Trust and distrust were prominent themes throughout the interviews, on many levels. Overall, issues of trust were revealed through questions that explored the government-U.S. citizen relationship, the Advocate-client relationship in the "Healthy at Home" program, and the interviewer-interviewee relationship. As previously mentioned, half (50%) of the clients trusted the government to take care of environmental laws and policies.

Given that the Advocates came from the same community as the Latina women and were bilingual, the women who participated in the interviews embraced the Advocates, trusted them to help the mothers with health issues and deliver the environmental health information (i.e., pamphlets discussing lead poisoning and asthma) that the mother's needed.

However, a few of the women still seemed cautious of the interviewer and skeptical about the interview. Additionally, the women were given a choice between conducting the interviews in English or Spanish, and 3 (30%) chose English even though their primary language was Spanish. The same women spoke English as well, and there was only one (10%) individual who asked for the questions to be verbally stated in both English and Spanish so they could fully comprehend it.

Finally, the community-individual trust relationship was revealed in one question, which asked the women if they had shared information about the consequences of asthma and lead poisoning with others they knew. Over half (60%) of the women provided family or friends with environmental hazard information, while the remaining women (4 or 40%) did not inform anyone at all.

5.1.4 Discussion

Latinos generally have more children and are younger than the general population when they first become pregnant (McDonald, Suellentrop, Paulozzi, & Morrow, 2008; Taylor, Ko, & Pan, 1999; Wingo, Smith, Tevendale, & Ferré, 2011). Some researchers attribute early age of pregnancy to the cultural background and norms of the Latino community.

Latinos overall complete fewer years of formal education than the general population (McDonald, Suellentrop, Paulozzi & Morrow, 2008). The level of educational attainment found in the interviews is similar to a study performed by Giachello (1994). According to Giachello, while 85 percent of Caucasian mothers and 70 percent of African American mothers had 12+ years of education, only 46 percent of Latina mothers achieved the same level of education.

Theme 1: Health behavior change leading to health promotion

The health behavior changes that the women made in the home promoted better health for the parents and the children. One woman stated, "I do it for my children."

The women's changes were comparable to those made by the parents of inner-city African American and Latino youth by the NIAID and NIEHS, whose actions produced a decrease in passive smoking, pest problems, dust mites, animal dander, and mold within the home (Morgan, Crain, Gruchalla et al., 2004). This decrease eventually led to a greater than 30% decrease in hospitalizations due to asthma.

The percentage of families who had one or more family members with asthma smoke outside is somewhat similar to that of another study (Krieger, Takaro, Allen et al., 2002) where 20% of those who received smoking education and patches quit smoking.

Theme 2: Government's role in society

Voting in the presidential election marked the first step to environmental justice by getting Latinos involved in the political system. The women may have felt that voting was their social action, since it focused on a national level as opposed to a community event.

One mother reported that she was not politically involved now but "I want to because it will help my children." Another wanted to be more involved in her community and politics. However, due to unarticulated reasons, she had some difficulty accomplishing it. She declared, "I wanna rally for a lot of things but it's not like it's gonna happen." When asked why, she responded with a shrug.

One individual stated that it was the responsibility of "me and my husband but the government needs to keep the houses fixed up and safe and secure. There's already a crack in our house and it's not even been a year."

One woman voiced her opinion regarding the government role in implementing important laws and policies saying that "they gotta do what they gotta do." Even with laws and policies put into effect by the government, inequities still occur among minority groups, as seen in the case of the Warren County incident of 1982 (Ringquist, 2000), where PCB-contaminated soil was dumped in a landfill in a primarily African American neighborhood.

Importantly, women who were open about the way they felt toward the government and politics before the tape recorder started to record were less open during the interview itself.

The fact that many of the parents responded that they should be responsible for their homes yet trusted the government to make appropriate laws and policies to change indoor environmental health issues gives the impression that what goes on inside the home is the family's business and the government's focus is on the entire Latino community's health rather than that of individual families.

Theme 3: Trust and distrust

The finding that half of the clients trusted the government to take care of environmental laws and policies is slightly less than the national average where over sixty percent of Latinos trust that every level of government can solve various issues (National Public Radio, 2000). Another study, The Pew National Hispanic Survey (Pew Hispanic Center, 2002), found that over 15% of Latinos trusted the government completely verses 13% of Caucasians and 9% of African Americans.

The Advocates provided a safe atmosphere for pregnant and newly parenting women who were trying to support themselves. One of the interviewees became so attached and grateful to one of the Advocates that she started to have her kids call the Advocate "grandma" in Spanish.

The women's skepticism regarding the interviewer and the interview itself could be related to their fears that the interview might not be anonymous or the government might hear what they were saying. However, all of the women were reassured before the interviews that there would be no identifying information linking them to their responses.

One of the four women who did not inform anyone about environmental health hazards reported, "I don't have friends to explain it to." Still, some of the women who took part in the environmental justice interviews did not portray that sense of community where they lived; in reality, certain women faced social isolation. They moved from one neighborhood to the next every few years and did not have the time or the energy to make bonds with people in their communities. Many had most if not all of their relatives still in Puerto Rico. Some of the women were just struggling to survive and take care of their children. They may have been more focused on the basic needs of their children rather than making the extra effort to correct indoor environmental health dangers and telling other people about the environmental problems.

Putnam (2000) emphasized the importance of social capital among communities. He found that there has been a gradual increase over the years of people looking out for themselves rather than the community as a whole. Contrary to this belief, the Social Capital Community Benchmark Survey of 2000 (Roper Center for Public Opinion Research, 2000) found that social capital was high among the Latino community. In fact, 83% of Latino population in America said they had old or new friends who gave them a sense of community.

6. Program and policy implications

The knowledge and insight of the environmental justice interview led to several recommendations for future program development. It became apparent that a number of issues needed to be addressed in the "Healthy at Home" program. Either there should be an increase in overall indoor environmental household changes through stronger education or the concentration should be on just one or two indoor environmental health issues, in order to achieve a greater rate of behavior change. The language used in the environmental justice questionnaire could be designed more in layman's terms.

Policy recommendations highlight the need for leadership and participation. With such a large number of women who rent their homes, landlords need to become involved to improve indoor environmental health. Leaders who facilitate addressing public health concerns are best supplied by their respective local communities. These leaders need to work with public health officials and the government to improve the community's overall health. Finally, steps need to be taken to increase the Latina women's trust.

6.1 Housing policies

Eight (80%) of the women rented homes. The government and health professionals need to work with landlords to try to decrease housing concerns. Even with laws in place, many are not enforced to protect the rights of minorities. But some strides are being made.

For example, in order to protect people from housing discrimination the government passed the Fair Housing Act in 1986 which was later amended in 1974 and again in 1988. Race or color, national origin and familial status (i.e., someone with children or pregnant) are all included under the Act (U.S. Department of Housing and Urban Development, 2004). By law, no one can refuse to rent or sell housing or have different rules or conditions for the rental or sale of housing based on an individual's background, color of their skin, national origin or whether or not they have children. These stipulations include Latinos and other minority groups who continue to be discriminated against and have had to deal with residential segregation where they have less access to jobs and transportation as well as a higher concentration of lead poisoning and asthma (National Low Income Housing Coalition, 2008).

In spite of all the available literature about the consequences of lead poisoning, lead screening has not been universally mandatory. Nevertheless, a couple of states have created statewide policy requiring children to be screened for it. Massachusetts passed 105 CMR 460,050 in 1990. This law enforces yearly screening in all children throughout Massachusetts, between the ages of nine months and four years (Sargent, Brown, Freeman et al., 1995). Sargent et al. evaluated this lead screening and found that a child is seven to ten times more likely to have lead poisoning based on whether they were living in poverty, whether or not the child lived in a home from before the 1950's, and whether or not the parents owned the home. Connecticut started universal blood lead level screenings in 2009 due to Public Act 07-2 (Connecticut Department of Public Health, 2009). Universal screening is important because if there is no screening, there would be no way of knowing if those most at risk need treatment for it. By screening everyone, and especially, those most at risk, one can insure that treatment brings the lead poisoning levels down and hopefully decreases incidence rates.

In 2004 the Washington Post listed Philadelphia as one of several cities around the country that either discarded the city's water test if it showed high lead levels or refused to test homes that are at high risk for lead problems (Leonnig, 2004). Leonnig reported that Senate members are trying to increase laws to reduce lead in water and make the general public aware of any exposure to lead poisoning. Various government officials are investigating whether the EPA is doing its job at protecting high-risk populations.

California put the Pesticide Prevention Act and the Healthy Schools Act into effect in 2000 so that schools must tell parents when they use pesticides, keep records of the pesticides they use, and develop a safer pest management program (California Department of Pesticide Regulation, 2001).

Thirty states are currently working to pass the Safer Alternatives Bill which calls for the use of safer alternatives to dangerous chemicals in everyday cleaning products (The Alliance for a Healthy Tomorrow, 2011). They are also working to change the Toxics Substances Control Act of 1976 which continues to allow dangerous and untested chemicals to be used in everyday products.

Governor McGreevey from New Jersey authorized an environmental justice executive order to improve quality of life and reduce the disproportionate amount of exposure to environmental health hazards that affect low-income and minority groups (State of New Jersey, 2004). The Department of Environmental Protection plays a significant role in this law because it must correct health information to meet the needs of minorities who speak English as a second language, and examine currently available health research to improve industrial and commercial sites located in low-income and minority neighborhoods to reduce undue exposure to environmental health hazards. The environmental justice executive order includes the need for increased community involvement in environmental health policy through the help of government agencies. By addressing all of these issues successfully, environmental justice may become part of a political discourse and action plan in other states.

In both minority and low-income families, children bear a great extent of the burden of negative health outcomes from indoor environmental hazards (Powell & Stewart, 2001). As children are not yet capable of protecting themselves, they become fully dependent upon their parents to guard them from exposure to indoor health hazards. Parents may accomplish this through personal indoor environmental health change, their appeal for environmental health programs and through new environmental laws and policies.

6.2 Distrust of government

Half (50%) the women interviewed trusted the government. The level of trust in the government will most likely increase when the community sees that the government is serious in following through on environmental laws and policies that will decrease the environmental health problems in Latino homes. Several studies including Krieger et al. (2009) and Perez et al. (2006) have found community leaders to be effective in changing health behavior because individuals related to and trusted them. Additionally, by getting policy leaders involved with a particular community, as seen in the case of the Kaiser Permanente Community Health Initiative (Kramer, Schwartz, & Cheadle et al., 2010), it may help to facilitate the policy process. It can make the transition easier for individuals within the community to speak out and become more involved in the legalities and policies of environmental health.

It is important to establish community leaders in the Philadelphia Latino community. Intuitively it is best for leaders to come from within the community than to be brought from outside. LeBlanc et al (1989) performed a study that found that community leaders were effective in changing the attitudes the community had towards cancer because the community trusted them.

Half the women trusted the government but there should be an even higher level of trust between government and the Latino community. The Latino mother needs to have someone to depend on such as the government and community leaders. Once community leaders have been established, they need to represent the rest of their community and have constant interaction with public officials and health professionals who can improve the community's health situation.

Finally, many of the women were reluctant to talk in general, and more specifically, about certain issues like the government. As mentioned previously, this may be connected with the women's fear of someone hearing what they have to say and the fact that they wanted their statements to be anonymous. For example, if the women said something bad against the government, they might fear that their welfare or insurance benefits would be negatively affected. It is important to find out how to elicit more information from women, whether it is to handwrite interviews, have several meetings with the women beforehand, or have the Advocates conduct interviews.

7. Future directions

Although each of the covered topics are equally important, the focus of the "Healthy at Home" program may need to change in order to cover just one or two topics rather than emphasize several at one time. It is important to note that fewer than 50% of individuals diagnosed with asthma have been taught how to avoid asthma triggers and of those that did receive education, 52% percent followed most of the recommendations (CDC, 2011b). MCC may also want to perform a needs assessment within the Latino community to see which topics are most important to the members of the community. For example, individuals might want to know more about lead poisoning than the other given topics. Once the majority of the community has reached a decision about what it feels it needs, program planning and implementation can go from there.

Half (5, 50%) of the women shared information about environmental hazards with family or friends. With respect to social action, many women felt that voting was their social action, demonstrating a perspective more national than local. Future studies will prove beneficial in finding ways to improve self empowerment for the Latino individual, social interaction within the Latino community itself as well as increase trust toward the government in order to promote environmental health change.

8. References

Akinbami, L.J., Moorman, J.E., Garbe, P.L., Sondik, E.J. (2009). Status of childhood asthma in the United States, 1980-2007. *Pediatrics,* 123(suppl 3):S131–S145.

Agency for Toxic Substances and Disease Registry. (2007). Toxicological profile for lead. Retrieved March 28, 2011 from http://www.atsdr.cdc.gov/PHS/PHS. asp?id=92&tid=22.

The Alliance for a Healthy Tomorrow. (January 2011). Mass. and 29 other states announce chemical reform legislation. Retrieved July 24, 2011, from http://www. healthytomorrow.org/2011/01/legislation-announcement.html.

Bloom, B., Cohen, R.A., Freeman, G. (2009). Summary health statistics for US children: National Health Interview Survey, 2008. National Center for Health Statistics. *Vital Health Statistics, 10*(244):1-81.

California Department of Pesticide Regulation. (2001). Overview of the California School IPM Program. Retrieved October 26, 2004, from http://www.cdpr.ca.gov/cfdocs/apps/schoolipm/overview/main.cfm?crumbs_list=1,3.

Carter, P.M., Peterson, E.L., Ownby, D.R., Zoratti, E.M., & Johnson C.C. (2003). Relationship of house-dust mite allergen exposure in children's bedrooms in infancy to bronchial hyperresponsiveness and asthma diagnosis by age 6 to 7. *Annals of Allergy Asthma and Immunology, 90*: 41–44.

Centers for Disease Control and Prevention (CDC). (2011b). Asthma in the U.S.: Growing Every Year. Retrieved July 20, 2011, from http://www.cdc.gov/VitalSigns/ Asthma/index.html.

Centers for Disease Control and Prevention (CDC). (2009). Childhood Lead Poisoning Data, Statistics, and Surveillance. Retrieved March 26, 2011, from http://www.cdc.gov. nceh/lead/data/index.htm.

Centers for Disease Control and Prevention (CDC). (2011a). Lead. Retrieved July 20, 2011, from http://www.cdc.gov/nceh/lead/.

Centers for Disease Control and Prevention. (2010b). 2007 National Health Interview Survey Data. Table 4-1 Current Asthma Prevalence Percents by Age, United States: National Health Interview Survey, 2007. Atlanta, GA: U.S. Department of Health and Human Services, CDC.

Centers for Disease Control and Prevention (2010a). Vital Signs: Nonsmokers' Exposure to Secondhand Smoke—United States, 1999–2008. *Morbidity and Mortality Weekly Report, 59*(35):1141–6. Retrieved July 19, 2011, from http://www.cdc.gov/mmwr/preview/mmwrhtml/mm5935a4.htm?s_cid=mm5935a4_w.

Chipps, B.E. (October 2004). Determinants of asthma and its clinical course. *Annals of Allergy, Asthma, and Immunology, 93*(4): 309-15.

Connecticut Department of Public Health. (January 2009). Mandatory Universal Blood Lead Screening begins in Connecticut. Retrieved July 24, 2011, from http://www.ct.gov/ dph/cwp/view.asp?A=3659&Q=434526.

Giachello, A.L. (1994). Maternal/Perinatal Health. In CW Molina & M Aguirre-Molina (Eds.), *Latino Health in the US: A Growing Challenge*. Washington, DC: American Public Health Association.

Gilbert, S.G., & Weiss, B. (2006). "A rationale for lowering the blood lead action level from 10 to 2 microg/dL.". *Neurotoxicology*, 27 (5): 693–701.

Jalaludin, B., Xuan, W., Mahmic, A., Peat, J., Tovey, E., & Leeder, S. (1998). Association between *Der p*1 concentration and peak expiratory flow rate in children with wheeze: a longitudinal analysis. *Journal of Allergy and Clinical Immunology, 102*: 382-386.

Jones, R. L., Homa, D. M., Meyer, P. A., Brody, D. J., Caldwell, K. L, Pirkle, J. L., et al. (2009). Trends in blood lead levels and blood lead testing among US children aged 1 to 5 years, 1988-2004. *Pediatrics, 123*(3): e376-e385.

Khader, Y.S., Al-Akour, N., Alzubi, I.M., & Lataifeh, I. (2011). The Association Between Second Hand Smoke and Low Birth Weight and Preterm Delivery. *Maternal and Child Health Journal, 15*(4): 453-459.

Kramer, L., Schwartz, P., Cheadle, A. Borton, J.E., Wright, M., Chase, C. & Lindley, C. (2010). Promoting policy and environmental change using photovoice in the Kaiser Permanente community health initiative. *Health Promotion Practice, 11*(3):332-339.

Krieger, J., Takaro, T.K., Song, L., Beaudet, N, & Edwards, K. (2009). The Seattle-King County Healthy Homes II Project: A Randomized Controlled Trial of Asthma Self-management Support Comparing Clinic-Based Nurses and In-Home Community Health Workers. *Archives of Pediatrics and Adolescent Medicine, 163*(2):141-149.

Krieger, J.K., Takaro, T.K., Allen, C., Song, L., Weaver, M., Chai, S., et al. (2002).The Seattle-King County healthy homes project: implementation of a comprehensive approach to improving indoor environmental quality for low-income children with asthma. *Environmental Health Perspectives, 110* (Suppl 2), 311-322.

Kuehr, J., Frischer, T., Meinert, R., Barth, R., Forster, J., Schraub, S. et al. (1994). Mite allergen exposure is a risk for the incidence of specific sensitization. *Journal of Allergy and Clinical Immunology, 94*, 44-52.

Law, K.L., Stroud, L.R., LaGasse, L., Niaura, R., Liu, J., & Lester, B.M. (2003). Smoking during pregnancy and newborn neurobehavior. *Pediatrics, 111*(suppl):1318.

LeBlanc, D., Lusero, G., Joyce, E., Hannigan, E., & Tucker, E. (1989) Cervical Cancer, A Major Killer of Hispanic Women: Implications for Health Education. *Health Education Quarterly*, 23-28.

Leonnig, C.D. (2004). Senators Urge Probe of EPA on Lead in Water. Retrieved October 27, 2004, from http://www.washingtonpost.com/wp-dyn/articles/A95502004Oct5.html.

Lind, C. (2004). Addressing Linguistic and Cultural Barriers to Access for Welfare Services. Retrieved July 24, 2011, from http://www.financeprojectinfo.org/publications/ addressinglinguisticRN.pdf.

Lwebuga-Mukasa, J.S., Wojcik, R., Dunn-Georgiou, E., Johnson, C.: Home environmental factors associated with asthma prevalence in two Buffalo inner-city neighborhoods. *Journal of Health Care for the Poor and Under-Served, 13*(2):214-228.

March of Dimes. (2011). Environmental Risks and Pregnancy. Retrieved July 19, 2011, from http://www.marchofdimes.com/stayingsafe_indepth.html.

McDonald, J.A., Suellentrop, K., Paulozzi, L.J., & Morrow, B. (2008). Reproductive health of the rapidly growing Hispanic population: data from the Pregnancy Risk Assessment Monitoring System, 2002. *Maternal and Child Health Journal, 12*:342-356.

Melen, E., Wickman, M., Nordvall, S.L., van Hage-Hamsten, M., & Lindfors, A. (2001). Influence of early and current environmental exposure factors on sensitization and outcome of asthma in pre-school children. *Allergy, 56*:646-652.

Miller, W.D., Pollack, C.E., Williams, D.R. (January 2011). Healthy Homes and Communities: Putting the Pieces Together. *American Journal of Preventive Medicine, 40* (1) (suppl 1):S48-S57.

Morgan, W.J., Crain, E.F., Gruchalla, R.S., O'Connor, G.T., Kattan, M., Evans, R., III et al. (2004). Results of a home based environmental intervention in urban children with asthma--The Inner City Asthma Study. *The New England Journal of Medicine 351(*11):1068-1080.

National Center for Healthy Housing. (2008). Pesticides. Retrieved July 19, 2011, from http://www.nchh.org/What-We-Do/Health-Hazards--Prevention--and-Solutions /Pesticides.aspx.

National Low Income Housing Coalition (NLIHC). (2008). The National Low Income Housing Coalition 2008 Advocates' Guide to Housing and Community Development Policy. Retrieved July 8, 2011, from http://www.nlihc.org/doc/ AdvocacyGuide2008-web.pdf.

National Center for Health Statistics. (2010). Summary health statistics for U.S. children:

National Health Interview Survey, 2009. Vital *Health Stat., 10*(247). Retrieved July 24, 2011, from http://www.cdc.gov/nchs/data/series/sr_10/sr10_247.pdf.

National Public Radio. (2000). Americans Distrust Government, but Want It to Do More. Retrieved March 29, 2005, from http://www.npr.org/programs/specials/ poll/govt/summary.html.

Natural Resources Defense Council. (2004). Hidden Danger: Environmental Health Threats in the Latino Community- Executive Summary. Retrieved December 27, 2004, from http://www.nrdc.org/health/effects/latino/english/execsum.asp.

Navarro, M. (December 5, 2004). For Younger Latinos, a Shift to Smaller Families. *New York Times*, p.35.

Pearce, J.M. (2007). Burton's line in lead poisoning. *European Neurology, 57* (2): 118–119.

Pennsylvania Department of Health. (2011a). Minority Health Disparities in Pennsylvania: Population (1990-2009)-Data Highlights. Retrieved July 20, 2011, from http://www.portal.state.pa.us/portal/server.pt?open=18&objID=1059252&mode=2.

Pennsylvania Department of Health. (2011b). Pennsylvania Asthma Fact Sheet. Retrieved July 20, 2011, from http://www.portal.state.pa.us/portal/server.pt/document/1038364/january__2011_asthma_fact_sheet_pdf.

Pennsylvania Department of Health. (2010). 2010 Pennsylvania Title V Needs and Capacity Assessment. Retrieved July 20, 2011, from https://perfdata.hrsa.gov/MCHB/TVISReports/Documents/NeedsAssessments/ 2011/PA-NeedsAssessment.pdf.

Pennsylvania Department of Health. (2002). Reported Pregnancy Data Tables. Retrieved September 21, 2004, from http://www.dsf.health.state.pa.us/health/lib/health/ 2002_preg.pdf.

Perez, M., Findley, S.E., Mejia, M., & Martinez, J. (2006). The impact of community health worker training and programs in NYC. *Journal of Health Care for the Poor and Underserved, 17*(1) (suppl): 26-43.

Pew Hispanic Center. (2008). Demographic Profile of Hispanics in Pennsylvania, 2008. Retrieved March 28, 2011, from

http://pewhispanic.org/states/?stateid=PA.
Pew Hispanic Center. (2002). The Pew Hispanic Center and the Kaiser Family Foundation 2002 National Survey of Latinos. Retrieved March 28, 2011, from http://pewhispanic.org/files/reports/15.pdf.
Pleis, J.R., Lucas J.W., Ward, B.W. (2009). Summary health statistics for U. S. adults: National Health Interview Survey, 2008 *Vital and Health Statistics. Series, 10*(242). Washington, D C: Government Printing Office.
Powell, D.L., & Stewart, V. (2001). Children. The unwitting target of environmental injustices. *Pediatric Clinics of North America, 48*(5), 1291-1305.
Public Citizens for Children and Youth (PCCY). (2008). The Lead Court and Healthier Children: The Philadelphia Story- 2008. Retrieved July 20, 2011, from http://www.pccy.org/userfiles/file/ChildHealthWatch/Courting%20Healtier%20Lead%20Report.pdf.
Putnam, R. (2000). Bowling Alone: The Collapse and Revival of American Community. New York: Simon & Schuster.
Ringquist, E.J. (2000). Environmental Justice: Normative Concerns and Empirical Evidence. In: Vig, N and Kraft, M (eds.), Environmental Policy in the 1990s, 4th edition. Washington, DC: Congressional Quarterly.
Roper Center for Public Opinion Research. (2000). Social Capital Community Benchmark Survey. Retrieved July 8, 2011, from http://www.ropercenter.uconn.edu/data_access/data/datasets/social_capital_community_survey.html.
Sargent, J.D., Brown, M.J., Freeman, J.L., Bailey, A., Goodman, D., & Freeman, D.H., Jr. (1995). Childhood Lead Poisoning in Massachusetts Communities: Its Association with Sociodemographic and Housing Characteristics. *American Journal of Public Health, 85*, 528-534.
Sharfstein, J., Sandel, M., Kahn, R., & Bauchner, H. (August 2001). Is Child Health at Risk While Families Wait for Housing Vouchers? *American Journal of Public Health, 91*(8): 1191–1192.
State of New Jersey. (2004). Governor Pledges to Build a Better New Jersey Through Commitment to Environmental Justice. Retrieved October 25, 2004, from http://www.state.nj.us/cgibin/governor/njnewsline/view_article.pl?id=1760.
Stelmach, I., Jerzynska, J., Stelmach, W., Majak P, Chew G, & Kuna P. (2002). The prevalence of mouse allergen in inner-city homes. *Pediatric Allergy and Immunology, 13*(4):299-302.
Suppli, U.C., & Backer, V. (1999). Markers of Impaired Growth of Pulmonary Function in Children and Adolescents. *American Journal of Respiratory and Critical Care Medicine,* 160 (1), 40-44.
Taylor, F.M., Ko, R., Pan, M. (1999). Prenatal and Reproductive Health Care. In EJ Kramer, SL Ivey, & Y-W Ying (Eds.), *Immigrant Women's Health: Problems and Solutions*. San Francisco, CA: Jossey-Bass, Inc.
U.S. Department of Health and Human Services. (2006). The Health Consequences of Involuntary Exposure to Tobacco Smoke: A Report of the Surgeon General. Atlanta, GA: U.S. Department of Health and Human Services, Centers for Disease Control and Prevention, Coordinating Center for Health Promotion, National Center for Chronic Disease Prevention and Health Promotion, Office on Smoking and Health.

U.S. Department of Health and Human Services: Office of Minority Health. (2009). Retrieved July 24, 2011, from http://minorityhealth.hhs.gov/templates/content.aspx?lvl=3&lvlID=532&ID=6173

U.S. Department of Housing and Urban Development (HUD). (2004). Fair housing: Equal opportunity for all. Retrieved January 24, 2005, from http://www.hud.gov/ offices/fheo/FHLaws/yourrights.cfm.

U. S. Census Bureau. (2000). 2000 Census Summary File 3, Matrices H36, H37, H38, and H39. Retrieved July 20, 2011, from http://factfinder.census.gov/servlet/QTTable?_bm=y&-geo_id=04000US42&-qr_name=DEC_2000_SF3_U_QTH7&-ds_name=DEC_2000_SF3_U.

U. S. Environmental Protection Agency (EPA). (2011). Environmental Justice. Retrieved July 19, 2011, from http://www.epa.gov/environmentaljustice/.

Wilson, T., Crivelli-Kovach, A., Worley, H. (2010). Healthy at Home: Latina Mothers Knowledge and Behavior Regarding Indoor Environmental Health Hazards. *Environmental Justice, 3*(3): 103-109.

Wingo, P.A., Smith, R.A., Tevendale, H.D., & Ferré, C. (2011). Recent Changes in the Trends of Teen Birth Rates, 1981-2006. *Journal of Adolescent Health, 48*(3): 281-288.